COUNSELING IN
GENETICS

COUNSELING IN GENETICS

Editors

Y. Edward Hsia

Departments of Genetics and Pediatrics
John A. Burns School of Medicine
University of Hawaii at Manoa

Kurt Hirschhorn

Division of Medical Genetics
Department of Pediatrics
Mt. Sinai School of Medicine
New York, New York

Ruth L. Silverberg

Department of Pediatrics
Yale University School of Medicine
and
Genetics Clinic
Yale University
New Haven, Connecticut

Lynn Godmilow

Division of Medical Genetics
Department of Pediatrics
Mt. Sinai School of Medicine
New York, New York

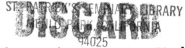
Alan R. Liss, Inc., New York

Address all Inquiries to the Publisher
Alan R. Liss, Inc., 150 Fifth Avenue, New York, NY 10011

Copyright © 1979 Alan R. Liss, Inc.

Printed in the United States of America

Library of Congress Cataloging in Publication Data

Main entry under title:

Counseling in genetics.

Includes bibliographical references and index.
1. Genetic counseling. I. Hsia, Yujen Edward,
1931—
RB155.C68   613.9   79-3038
ISBN 0-8451-0205-2

DEDICATION

This book is dedicated to the families who have taught us all that
we know about genetic counseling.

Contents

Contributors

Robin J. Caldwell, Department of Human Genetics, Medical College of Virginia, Virginia Commonwealth University, Richmond, Virginia (Presently at Department of Medicine, Division of Medical Genetics, University of North Carolina at Chapel Hill, 27514) **[121]**

Barton Childs, Department of Pediatrics, The Johns Hopkins Hospital, Baltimore, Maryland 21205 **[xvii]**

Lynn Godmilow, Division of Medical Genetics, Department of Pediatrics, Mount Sinai School of Medicine, New York, New York 10029 **[281]**

Marjorie Guthrie, Committee To Combat Huntington's Disease, Inc., New York, New York 10019 **[329]**

Kurt Hirschhorn, Division of Medical Genetics, Department of Pediatrics, Mount Sinai School of Medicine, New York, New York 10029 **[1, 261]**

Paula E. Hollerbach, Center for Policy Studies, The Population Council, New York, New York 10017 **[155, 189]**

Y. Edward Hsia, Medical Genetic Services, Departments of Genetics and Pediatrics, John A. Burns School of Medicine, University of Hawaii 96826 **[1, 261]**

Marc Lappé, Department of Health, Office of Health, Law, and Values, Sacramento, California 95814 **[295]**

Audrey T. McCollum, Department of Pediatrics, Child Study Center at Yale University School of Medicine, New Haven, Connecticut (Presently in private practice) **[239]**

Barbara R. Migeon, Department of Pediatrics, Johns Hopkins University, Baltimore, Maryland 21205 **[111]**

Orlando J. Miller, Departments of Human Genetics and Obstetrics and Gynecology, College of Physicians and Surgeons, Columbia University, New York, New York 10032 **[81]**

Walter E. Nance, Department of Human Genetics, Medical College of Virginia, Virginia Commonwealth University, Richmond, Virginia 23298 **[121]**

John Pearn, University of Queensland, Department of Child Health, Royal Children's Hospital, Brisbane, Queensland, Australia 4029 **[223]**

Marian L. Rivas, Neurological Sciences Institute of Good Samaritan Hospital and Medical Center, Portland, Oregon **[43]**

Philip Reilly, Yale Law School, Yale University, New Haven, Connecticut 06511 **[311]**

I.M. Rosenstock, Department of Health Behavior and Health Education, The University of Michigan, Ann Arbor, Michigan 48104 **[139]**

Joy Ruth Cohen, Yale-New Haven Hospital, New Haven, Connecticut 06504 **[31]**

Marlene B. Rudnick, Department of Social Services, Westchester County, New Rochelle, New York 10801 **[31]**

Ruth L. Silverberg, Department of Pediatrics, Yale University School of Medicine, and Genetics Clinic, Yale University, New Haven, Connecticut 06511 (Presently in private practice) **[239, 281]**

The number in brackets following each contributor's name is the opening page number of that author's chapter.

Foreword

If the life of a witch doctor is politically precarious, it is at least uncomplicated by question of his authority; his practice is autocratic, and a universal acceptance of his prescriptions is expected. But the modern doctor is being challenged by an increasingly skeptical public, some members of which are knowledgeable enough to put probing questions; others are simply no longer willing to accept pronouncements ex cathedra, as it were. Physicians have begun to recognize that this less-than-reverential attitude can result in private, occasionally irrational decisions based on distortion, misunderstanding, or neglect of their instructions; investigations of this "noncompliance," as it is called, have revealed its alarming extent. In consequence, it has become necessary to examine the processes of communication between doctor and patient; indeed, between an increasingly massive and diverse medical establishment and the recipient of its benefits, the public.

And it turns out to be much more complicated than anyone expected. It appears that context is everything; that what we can learn in a session with a doctor or other counselor depends on what we bring to it: our knowledge, past experiences, and willingness and ability to learn. Without a receptive, expectant attitude, we may hear nothing; without knowledge, we may be able to grasp little; and without experience of life, it may be difficult to translate new information into sensible action.

Until recently, physicians, like witch doctors, were constrained mainly by the rules of their own profession — rules that were mainly of their own devising. But today's physician, possessing weapons of great power both to heal and to hurt, must observe new social and legal obligations designed to maximize the healing and minimize the hurt. What all this means is that medicine is being woven more intimately into the fabric of society than ever before, and at a rate that taxes the capacity of many physicians to adapt.

One of the latest and most rapidly proliferating disciplines that doctors must reckon with is medical genetics. Until about a generation ago, genetics was perceived to be the business of botanists, zoologists, and agricultural husbandmen, but now nearly all medical schools and teaching hospitals have divisions of medical genetics, and state and city health departments have developed screening and other services for the prevention and treatment of genetic illnesses.

Among these services is genetic counseling: the information, advice, and other support that enables patients and their relatives to understand a disorder, to adapt to it, and to make plans for the future, including reproduction. At first, genetic counseling was practiced by nonmedical geneticists who, recognizing the vacuum created by the ignorance of physicians, attempted to fill it. Accordingly, initial published reports of experience with this service dealt only with modes of inheritance and reproductive odds, and with few lessons in genetics for patients whose knowledge of genetics was limited to the observation that diseases sometimes "run in families," or whose high school biology, if any, left them unprepared to grasp either the fact of genetic disease or that such diseases might recur with predictable regularity. Also, because the patients who presented themselves for counseling were those who saw their need and who could be expected, therefore, to grasp its meaning and to use the experience to profit, little attention was given to evaluation of the process or, indeed, to define what a successful outcome might be. But later, as medially trained people entered the field of genetics and as medicine itself became more socially integrated, the educational, psychological, sociological, ethical, and legal aspects of genetic counseling were revealed and the process of critical evaluation was begun. Nowadays genetic counseling is an essential element of the management of patients referred to genetic clinics and a necessary part of screening services of any kind.

This book is an outcome of much study, experience, and discussion of genetic counseling, processes which the book itself shows not yet to be exhausted. Its authors are physicians, social workers, nurses, sociologists, psychologists, lawyers, ethicists, and consumer advocates, and some are more than one of these. In inviting these people to present their experience and wisdom, the editors have presented the reader a comprehensive view of genetic counseling and, because each author sees this transaction from a different, though sometimes overlapping, position, the manifold complexity of what once seemed to be a simple transaction is revealed. The book also shows, and not just coincidentally, how rapidly medicine is being secularized. Shamanism is no longer fashionable; the public wants to collaborate in the maintenance of its health.

Barton Childs, MD
The Johns Hopkins Hospital
Baltimore, Maryland

Preface

Genetic counseling is not telling families what they should do; rather it is telling families what they can do [1]. This book is about this process: how to tell families and how they respond. It is written for those interested in broad multidisciplinary discussions of genetic counseling. It includes practical contributions from experienced physicians, geneticists, social workers, and nurses about the process of genetic counseling. It also includes overviews from behavioral scientists, demographers, an ethicist, a lawyer, and a consumer about their perspectives of genetic counseling. Some of these professions regard counselees as patients and others as clients, but the emphasis throughout is on counselees as individual persons. The attitudes, needs, and responses of those receiving genetic counseling are the recurring themes unifying all the chapters. This book is not meant to be a text on medical genetic disorders. There are many excellent monographs on the recognition, classification, and analysis of these disorders [2–10, 35]. It is not meant to be a practical primer [11–14] because we believe the process of genetic counseling cannot be condensed into an inflexible routine without loss of the sensitivity required to respond to the personal needs of individual counselees. It is certainly not intended to be an encyclopedia of genetic counseling, because the number of disorders is too vast [1, 7, 10]. Our current knowledge of individual responses to genetic information is too uncertain and the various approaches to delivery of genetic information are too diverse to be contained in a single volume [15–18].

Despite the intense interest in genetic counseling by professionals, students, and the general public [19, 20] there are still many naive misconceptions about how genetic counseling is delivered and inordinately high expectations about what geneticists can and cannot do [11, 15, 21]. There is a rapidly growing demand for genetic counseling and gradually increasing financial support for expanding genetic counseling services throughout the world [23–26]. Much has been written about medical genetics, but little about the process of counseling in genetics.

Medical training is expected to give physicians the competence and experience to recognize genetic problems [27–30] and to help their patients understand how to cope with these problems. In large medical centers, special multidisciplinary teams have been assembled to deliver medical genetic services [21, 24, 25, 31]. Genetic training programs are developing new types of health professionals to meet the anticipated manpower needs. Regional and community screening projects are being conducted to find people with genetic susceptibilities or risks [23]. The number of fetal diagnostic tests is rapidly expanding [32]. All of these diverse activities converge on the common function of genetic counseling, yet there is no unanimity about this function [1, 15, 17].

Recent rapid expansion of technical expertise and scientific knowledge in the fields of genetics has dramatically increased the analytical precision [33, 34] and laboratory sophistication of what can be done for families with genetic problems. The very substantial advances in some areas of genetics contrast starkly with large remaining gaps in our knowledge of other areas. Keeping abreast of advances is a continual challenge for all health professionals, especially those in medical genetics. In this book we aim to provide a theoretical and practical foundation for counseling in genetics, without claiming to have current data on recent advances, because these can be found only in the latest periodicals. While striving for scientific accuracy, we have stressed the importance of maintaining a balance between factual knowledge, the need for effective communication, and the duty to provide humane service. Professional duties and moral responsibilities imply legal liabilities. In genetic counseling, the truth can hurt, and errors can certainly be harmful. Whoever offers genetic information or advice, therefore, should be wary of the possible repercussions from mistaken, misunderstood, or misused information [15, 26].

The editors have shared many years of experience in genetic counseling. We have found it challenging, sometimes frustrating, often rewarding, but always absorbing. We are still learning about the complexities of genetic problems and the rich diversity of human nature evinced by people trying to cope with these deeply personal problems. We trust that practitioners and students of genetic counseling will find the distillation of our own experiences and the contributions of our colleagues in this book interesting and useful.

This book would not have been possible without the devoted thoughtful assistance of many colleagues and friends. Particular tribute must be paid to Mrs. Leatrice Herold, Mr. Sidney K. Silverberg, Mrs. Anita Waters, and Ms. Juliet Y.M. Yuen, who all know how vital their contributions have been. Responsibility for any misrepresentations or errors, however, while wholly unintentional, must lie with the authors and editors.

The Editors
June 1979

ACKNOWLEDGEMENTS

We are grateful to our colleagues who shared their experiences with us and helped to shape our ideas in discussions and debate. The work on which our contributions are based was supported in part by National Foundation–March of Dimes Medical Service grants C-41, C-155, and C-297.

REFERENCES

1. Fraser FC: Genetic Counseling. Am J Hum Genet 26:636–659, 1974.
   A formal definition of genetic counseling by a committee of the American Society of Human Genetics.
2. DeGrouchy J, Turleau C: "The Clinical Atlas of Human Chromosomes." New York, Wiley, 1977.
   A useful brief catalogue of known chromosome abnormalities in man.
3. Bondy PK, Rosenberg LE: "Duncan's Diseases of Metabolism," Ed. 7. Philadelphia: W.B. Saunders, 1974.
   Detailed scholarly reviews of many areas of human metabolism, including many genetic disorders (two volumes).
4. Gardner LI (ed): "Endocrine and Genetic Diseases of Childhood and Adolescence," Ed 2. Philadelphia: W.B. Saunders, 1975.
   A good text with discussion of most genetic disorders.
5. Goodman RM, Gorlin RJ: "Atlas of the Face in Genetic Disorders." St. Louis: CV Mosby, 1977.
   A helpful illustrated reference for facial malformations.
6. Holmes LB, Mack C, Moser HW, Pant SS, Halldórsson S, Matzilevich B: "Mental Retardation: An Atlas of Diseases with Associated Physical Abnormalities." New York: Macmillan, 1972.
   An outstanding atlas with succinct descriptions of each disorder.
7. McKusick VA: "Mendelian Inheritance in Man. Catalogues of autosomal dominant, autosomal recessive, and X-linked phenotypes." Baltimore: Johns Hopkins University Press, 1978, p 837.
   An essentail reference with brief computerized summaries and key bibliography for virtually all known and suspected single gene disorders.
8. Smith, DW: "Recognizable Patterns of Human Malformation: Genetic, Embryologic and Clinical Aspects," Ed 2. Philadelphia: W.B. Saunders, 1976.
   An outstanding, richly illustrated atlas with helpful brief discussions which give perspective to this entire field.
9. Stanbury JB, Wyngaarden JB, Fredrickson DS (eds): "The Metabolic Basis of Inherited Diseases," Ed 4. New York: McGraw-Hill, 1978.
   Detailed chapters on inherited disorders in many selected areas of metabolism.
10. Warkany J: "Congenital Malformations: Notes and Comments." Chicago: Year Book, 1971.
    A unique monograph with detailed discussions of the causes and clinical features of congenital malformations.
11. Kelly PT: "Dealing with Dilemma: A Manual for Genetic Counselors." New York Springer-Verlag, 1977.
    A sensitive practical discussion of counseling techniques and relationships by an experienced counselor.

12. Lynch HT: "Dynamic Genetic Counseling for Clinicians." Springfield, Illinois: CC Thomas, 1969.
    A treatise on genetic counseling for various types of disorders by one of the first medical geneticists.
13. Reed SC: "Counseling in Medical Genetics." Ed 2. Philadelphia: WB Saunders, 1963.
    A highly readable account of experiences in genetic counseling by the geneticists who first coined this term.
14. Stevenson AC, Davison BCC, Oakes MW: "Genetic Counseling," ed 2. Philadelphia: JB Lippincott, 1976.
    Contains listings of many genetic disorders.
15. Capron AM, Lappé M, Murray RF, Powledge TM, Twiss SB (eds): "Genetic Counseling: Facts, Values and Norms." New York: Alan R. Liss, for The National Foundation—March of Dimes. BD:OAS 15(2): 1979.
    Ethical discussions about approaches to genetic counseling.
16. Hilton B, Callahan D, Harris M, Condliffe P, Berkley B (eds): "Ethical Issues in Human Genetics." New York: Plenum, 1973.
    A symposium on genetic research, illness, treatment and counseling.
17. Lubs HA, de la Cruz F (eds): "Genetic Counseling." New York: Raven, 1977.
    Proceedings of a conference on studies of genetic counseling.
18. Motulski AG: "Genetic Counseling – Collected Works." New York: MSS Information, 1973.
    Papers on genetic counseling by many leading medical geneticists.
19. Milunsky A: "Know Your Genes." New York: Avon, 1977.
    A simple readable text for the lay public.
20. Riccardi VM: "The Genetic Approach to Human Disease." New York: Oxford University Press, 1977.
    A simple readable text for all health professionals.
21. Hook EB, Porter IH (eds): "Service and Education in Medical Genetics." New York: Academic (in press).
    Proceedings of a symposium.
22. Milunsky A (ed): "The Prevention of Genetic Disease and Mental Retardation." Philadelphia: WB Saunders, 1975.
    Many useful chapters.
23. Childs B, Simopoulos AP (eds): "Genetic Screening." Washington, DC: National Academy of Sciences—National Research Council, 1975.
    A special symposium on the many issues involved in genetic screening programs.
24. Cohen BH, Lilienfeld AM, Huang PC (eds): "Genetic Issues in Public Health and Medicine." Springfield, Illinois: CC Thomas, 1978.
25. Lynch HT, Guirgis H, Bergsma D, Paul NW: "International Directory of Genetic Services." Ed 5. White Plains, New York: The National Foundation—March of Dimes, 1977.
    A directory of all medical centers in the world claiming to provide genetic services.
26. Reilly PR: "Genetics, Law, and Social Policy." Cambridge, Massachusetts: Harvard University Press, 1977, 275pp.
    A review of recent legislation and background issues, focusing mainly on genetic screening projects.
27. Fraser G, Mayo O (eds): "Textbook of Human Genetics." Oxford: Blackwell Scientific, Glossary and Indices pp 524, 1975.
    A textbook suitable for medical students.
28. Nora JJ, Fraser FC: "Medical Genetics: Principles and Practices." Philadelphia: Lea & Febiger, 1974.
    A textbook for medical students.

29. Roberts JAF, Pembrey ME: "An Introduction to Medical Genetics," Ed 7. London: Oxford University Press, 1978.
    A textbook for medical students.
30. Thompson JS, Thompson MW: "Genetics in Medicine," Ed 3. Philadelphia: WB Saunders, 1979.
    A textbook for medical students.
31. Bergsma D, Hecht F, Prescott GH, Marks JH (eds): "Trends and Teaching in Clinical Genetics." New York: Alan R. Liss, for The National Foundation—March of Dimes. BD:OAS 13(6): 1977.
32. Milunsky A (ed): "Hereditary Disorders and the Fetus." New York: Plenum (in press).
33. Emery AEH: "Methodology in Medical Genetics: An Introduction to Statistical Methods." Edinburgh: Churchill Livingstone, 1976.
34. Murphy EA, Chase GA: "Principles of Genetic Counseling." Chicago, Year Book, 1975.
    An exhaustive lucid exposition of the logical and mathematic principles underlying risk calculations in genetics.
35. Bergsma, Daniel (ed): "Birth Defects Compendium, Second Edition." New York: Alan R. Liss for The National Foundation – March of Dimes, 1979.

1

What is Genetic Counseling?

Y. E. Hsia, BM, MRCP, DCH, and K. Hirschhorn, MD

"WILL OUR NEXT CHILD BE NORMAL?"

When this question is asked because of specific concern about a real or imagined genetic problem the questioner deserves an accurate, helpful answer. Since an honest answer can never be "yes" and is rarely "no," genetic counseling is the art of helping the questioner understand the scientific basis behind a qualified "maybe."

The fascination of genetic counseling lies in the challenge of combining the science of genetics with the art of counseling. This attractive fascination can be dangerous, however, for genetic counseling can have dire consequences if it is mistaken, misunderstood, or misguided. Therefore the task of answering genetic questions should not be taken lightly or handled casually, because of its importance.

DEFINITION

The term "genetic counseling" was coined by Sheldon Reed [1] to describe how he conscientiously gave careful answers to genetic questions asked by anxious parents. Recently, in reviewing the history of genetic counseling, Reed has expressed regret [2] about how the term has become a catch-phrase, meaning different things to different users. The function of genetic counseling is undertaken consciously or unconsciously by general physicians, other health professionals, medical geneticists, trained genetic associates, and also informally by well-intentioned lay advisors. People in each of these groups use the term to define very different activities and responsibilities. What these definitions all share is the answering of a genetic inquiry. A unifying definition, therefore, is proposed that views genetic counseling from the perspective of the recipient.

Genetic counseling is the process whereby an individual or family obtains information about a real or possible genetic problem.

This definition should prove to be generally applicable. Analysis of genetic counseling and the purposes it serves, from this viewpoint, will show what genetic counseling means to the recipient and how this general definition should be qualified in order for genetic counseling to be accurate, accepted, and beneficial.

The Recipient's Viewpoint

Once aware of a problem, an inquirer wants to be informed about the nature and gravity of the problem, may need emotional support and reassurance, often desires guidance in decision-making, and may require access to relevant resources— eg, fetal diagnostic testing. Thus, from the inquirer's viewpoint, desire for genetic knowledge is fulfilled by receiving relevant information. Genetic counseling also has to be psychologically supportive and needs to be backed up by practical health services. (Whether guidance in decision-making should be directive or nondirective is debatable, and is discussed in Chapter 13 [2a].) The motivated inquirer wants to understand, wants to make wise decisions, wants to be able to carry out these decisions, and wants moral support.

The expected answer. All the inquirer asks for is a simple, direct answer to his or her genetic question. The answer is never altogether simple, however, and every inquirer perceives information in an individual way, because he or she has different backgrounds, strengths, and vulnerabilities. Whoever offers answers to genetic questions should keep in mind how the answer appears to an inquirer and should prepare and present the answer accordingly.

Accepting the answer. The information to be given, if it is to be beneficial, must be desired, understood, remembered, believed, and accepted as having personal relevance. The constructive purposes for which this information could then be used include the making of informed decisions, the implementation of these decisions, and adjustment to the realities of a genetic problem (see Chapter 12).

Genetic Counseling Is Educational

Insofar as the acquisition of information is a learning process, genetic counseling is educational [3].

Any educational function is a multi-stage process, with input from many sources. In the same way, learning answers to genetic questions builds upon prior knowledge (or misconceptions). In addition to whatever genetic knowledge is retained from formal schooling, an inquirer may be alerted to a genetic problem from mass media, obtain considerable information by a library search, and glean partial answers to a genetic question from several successive physicians or geneticists. In a broad sense, all of these sources have contributed to genetic counseling.

Preparation for Genetic Counseling

An adequate response to a genetic question demands thorough preparation, careful, personalized presentation, and responsible follow-up. All these are essential for the information to be used constructively by a counselee, unhampered by barriers to rational decisions, actions, or attitudes.

Two very different kinds of preparation are required, related to objective genetic facts and subjective personality characteristics. The first, genetic preparation, has to include confirmation that the genetic diagnosis is correct (Chapters 4–6), ascertaining how the genetic trait has been distributed in the family, predicting the probabilities of its affecting family members (Chapter 3), and checking on the options available for dealing with the genetic problem. The second, personality assessment, is to discover a prospective counselee's educational status, cultural beliefs, health behavior patterns, concept of odds, attitudes toward reproduction, and any personality foibles or intrafamilial stresses that could impede the transfer of genetic information or its utilization (Chapters 8–11, 13). Without adequate genetic preparation, the answer presented may be erroneous, so this preparation is critical; without careful personality assessment, presentation of the answer may be ineffective, so this assessment is necessary to enhance the acceptance and utilization of the genetic information by the inquirer.

Erroneous Definitions

According to our definition, it would be wrong to use the term "genetic counseling" as though it meant "genetic advice," equivalent to psychotherapeutic help or marriage guidance; "genetic comforting," equivalent to religious comforting or grief comforting; or just "genetic instruction," equivalent to diet instruction or exercise instruction. It should not be directive "advice," because its purpose is to inform rather than to recommend; it should not be mere "comforting," because a discomfortingly honest answer may be needed to forewarn the inquirer of unpleasant truths [4]; it is much more than "instruction," because its purpose is not to give directions for following a prescribed regimen, but rather to give understanding for informed decision-making.

Neither is genetic counseling just "diagnostic counseling," "disease counseling," "treatment counseling," "risk counseling," or "decision counseling." Explanations of diagnostic findings, the nature of a disease, or its treatment may all be requested, but these requests should be answered in the same manner regardless of whether a disease is genetic or nongenetic, so response to these requests is not unique to genetics. For a particular person or situation, these explanations may have to precede genetic counseling or be a part of genetic counseling. Genetic counseling does not have to include explanations about a medical condition, but must always include explanations about risks of the condition to family members, with encouragement to decide rationally among the choices available. The responsibilities of genetic counseling, however, include more than just risk prediction and help in decision-making, because a correct diagnosis should be determined beforehand and follow-up support should be provided afterwards.

To consider that genetic counseling refers to a "genetic consultation," genetic interview," or "genetic discussion" falsely confines the process of genetic information transfer to a single episode or context. Many events prior to a formal genetic interview could have helped to lay the groundwork for this information, and many experiences subsequent to formal genetic counseling may reinforce — or undermine — the information.

Hitherto, the term genetic counseling has been generally used to describe a function, but recently it has been used also to define a profession. To consider genetic counseling as being restricted to trained professionals would be unfortunate, since many more people ask genetic questions and would benefit from genetic answers than could be efficiently or economically served by the present small band of trained medical geneticists and their associates. It would be unrealistic to ignore the fact that many health professionals are giving genetic information to their patients and clients and impractical to channel all genetic inquiries to formally trained genetic counselors.

Definition of the Genetic Counselor

From the viewpoint of the inquirer, the genetic counselor is the health professional who provides a genetic answer. In this sense, when genetic counseling is regarded broadly as a function and not as a specialty, many health professionals participate in this function, hopefully collaboratively and constructively.

It would be wrong either to assume that any person who knows the objective facts is always suited to give genetic counseling or to insist that genetic counseling can only be given by professional "counselors." When the problem has been recognized, the question has been heard, and the answer is known, the answer should sometimes be presented by the one who knows the inquirer best, and sometimes by the one who knows the answer best, but often the questioner will benefit from receiving the answer coordinately from both sources.

Responsibilities of genetic counseling. The traditional responsibilities of a physician are to diagnose, to intervene, and to advise about an illness affecting an individual patient. These diverge somewhat from the responsibilities in genetic counseling to recognize, to predict, and to inform about risks of an illness for present and future relatives in a family. Some physicians are unfamiliar with the recognition of specific genetic disorders, uncertain of the predictive risks, or uncomfortable with the interactive tasks of helping people understand both health-related and probability-related topics. He or she may wish to consult a medical geneticist or to call for the help of a specialist experienced in genetic counseling [5].

Whoever provides genetic counseling has a further responsibility of following through to ensure that information has not been misunderstood, rejected, or forgotten; that the information has not aggravated existing problems, or created new ones; that assistance is available to implement decisions that have been made, and that the counselee is making satisfactory adjustments to the problem. In this way, the person giving genetic counseling can learn from his or her mistakes, gain encouragement from successes, and improve genetic counseling skills with experience. As in all other activities, careful preparation, conscientious execution, and prior experience enhance the effectiveness of genetic counseling.

Training. The perfect genetic counselor would be a trained geneticist, experienced clinical subspecialist, skilled psychologist, sensitive social worker, effective teacher, supportive advocate, and efficient coordinator of health resources. It would also help if the person had strong ethnic, cultural, and religious identity with each family who seeks genetic counseling, could devote unlimited time and mobilize boundless resources for each family.

Some of these attributes are innate personality traits which cannot be acquired by training; others are so demanding that they cannot all be learned within a lifetime. And so, this paragon of genetic counseling does not exist.

Short of this ideal model, practical compromises are the provision of genetic counseling by primary physicians, by a trained medical genetic team, or by a peripheral team, composed of a trained genetic associate working with a primary physician.

The primary physician. Training in medical genetics and genetic counseling for the primary physician or nongenetic specialist is necessarily limited by all the other demands on his or her skill and time. Since very few physicians have had comprehensive formal genetic education during their training [6], much of their genetic learning has to be by postgraduate courses, conferences, consultations, or personal reading [7]. An interested committed physician can learn enough from these sources to give effective genetic information to a patient, provided this is done with careful attention to accuracy of objective information and presented with sensitive awareness of the subjective state of the patient. The long-term association of the primary physician with the patient means that the patient's personal characteristics and family background are already well known to the physician and that continuity of care is assured. These two major advantages often make the primary physician ideally situated to give genetic counseling.

The medical genetic team. A team can either be greater or less than the sum of its parts (see Chapter 13). An effective medical genetic team should include expertise in medical diagnosis and genetic analysis; skills in objective and subjective data collection; experience in information presentation and family support. How these various functions are shared among various members should be determined by the individual strengths and talents available in each team. Someone on the team should have strong abilities in medical diagnosis; it is usually best for a genetically trained clinician to supervise the team. Other functions can be assigned according to demands on the time and skills of each team member.

A quantitative geneticist can provide sophistication in genetic analysis at a higher level than most medical geneticists can attain; a social worker can serve as a psychosocial evaluator and patient advocate (see Chapter 11); a nurse or genetic associate can collect family information, coordinate all team activities, and provide follow-up support. Research and teaching activities are often additional functions, which mean that students and observers are added to the team. When including students and observers, it is poor practice to sacrifice any quality of service for the sake of training. This means that a trainee should not be allowed to intrude on the privacy of an individual receiving genetic counseling, except with the knowledge and consent of that individual, and with reasonable precautions to prevent the trainee's presence from being distracting.

Formal training of genetic associates at the Master's degree level has been offered by several universities, some with emphasis more on technical aspects of genetic tests, and some with emphasis more on psychological aspects of genetic explanations. The actual job potentials of these trained genetic associates are not yet clear. Many have become integral team members in medical genetic units, but often with functions and roles quite different from those for which they were trained. It is expected that with increasing support and demand for genetic services, the role of the genetic associate will become better defined, and more career opportunities will open up for people with this type of training.

The peripheral team. If a physician has insufficient genetic expertise, this cannot be fully provided by a trained genetic associate, and so this combination would be unacceptable unless there were strong back-up support. When there is a medical genetic service at a large medical center, its outreach could be either via satellite visiting clinics staffed by their own team members [8] or via close liaison with a trained genetic associate, stationed peripherally in association with a group of local physicians. This peripheral team concept has not yet been tested, but it might become a useful economic means to fulfill the genetic counseling needs of scattered populations.

PREREQUISITES FOR GENETIC ENQUIRY

Awareness: Who Needs Genetic Counseling?

The existence of a genetic problem may not be recognized by either a patient's family or physician; conversely, an imagined problem, with no basis in fact, may seriously trouble a family. Even when a problem is imaginary, the *concern* is real and should be allayed if at all possible. Convincing reassurance that concerns have no factual basis can be highly beneficial to an anxious inquirer, whereas a casual dismissal of imagined concerns, if unconvincing, could well divert an inquirer to unorthodox health systems. Time, money, and hope are often squandered in seeking comforting promises based on unproved fancy rather than scientific fact [9]. Too often, patients seek these remedies because they perceive their own physicians as preferring to dispense tranquilizers than to listen, discuss, and explain [10].

The responsibilities of the primary health professional are to recognize the presence of a genetic disorder and to judge whether the genetic component of the disorder has aroused or should arouse concern in the affected patient and the patient's relatives. Having made this judgment, the best response to these concerns can then be planned.

Who has a genetic disorder? *Recognition.* Recognition of a condition as being genetic may be simple for some of the more common genetic disorders, but it is often overlooked. For example, when preoccupied with the urgent medical needs of a middle-aged man with myocardial infarction, the physician may neglect to ask whether the man had underlying autosomal dominant type II hyperlipoproteinemia, with a 50–50 risk of the same genetic susceptibility to coronary occlusion affecting his brothers, sisters, and children. Genetic recognition may be very difficult for rarer disorders, and when the genetic basis of a problem is not recognized by either the patient or the physician, recognition sometimes comes from unexpected sources.

Mr. and Mrs. A had a three-year-old boy with chronic ear infections, a protuberant abdomen, and delayed speech. His speech therapist remarked that his features resembled a photograph in her textbook of a patient with mucopolysaccharidosis. The parents indignantly reported this unsolicited slur on their son's appearance to his physician, who consulted a medical geneticist. The boy was confirmed to have the typical features of mucopolysaccharidosis.

Recognition can often be facilitated or confirmed by a suggestive family history.

Mrs. A had a brother who died at age three during anesthesia for tonsillectomy. His physician had written to the parents, explaining that a thorough autopsy had been uninformative "except for unexplained enlargement of the liver and spleen." Undoubtedly, Mrs. A's brother, too, had mucopolysaccharidosis, which is associated with increased anesthetic hazards from airway obstruction. This suggested the X-linked recessive inheritance pattern of the Hunter syndrome, type II mucopolysaccharidosis. Eliciting this history and examining Mrs. A's son left little room for doubt about the diagnosis, which was clinched by testing for the specific enzyme deficiency.

A physician's responsibility for his or her patient is rarely considered to extend beyond that patient, unless the patient's condition threatens the health of others.

This concept of responsibility for threat to others applies to relatives-at-risk for genetic disorders. Familial disease may be of vital concern to relatives both for preventive treatment and for warning of risks to future children. Recognition of a genetic disorder in one family-member may lead to its recognition also in relatives previously unaware of the existence of any disorder.

> Mrs. B had enlarged cystic kidneys and renal failure. She was thought to have autosomal dominant polycystic kidney disease. Not until she developed cancer of the kidneys did her doctors realize that several of her relatives had von Hippel Lindau disease, which does cause kidney cysts, but also kidney cancer, and tumors of the eye or brain. A cousin had been diagnosed and presented at a medical conference 15 years earlier, but no information about the condition and its chance of affecting relatives had been given to the family. When informed about this disease, many members of the family were eager to cooperate in a genetic study, which detected over 15 additional affected relatives, including some with treatable brain tumors and others with treatable kidney cancer [11].

This extension of a physician's responsibilities to relatives has even succeeded in breaking through the protective anonymity of adoption agencies.

> Diagnosis of autosomal dominant precancerous colonic polyps in Miss C, who was adopted, led her physician to seek out her biological relatives. This resulted eventually in the discovery of several affected relatives, who benefited from early preventive treatment and genetic counseling [12].

Search. Some genetic disorders that threaten progeny can be identified before a family has had an affected member. Prevention of these undesirable and often incurable afflictions before they occur can be achieved if prospective parents who are at risk can be identified. This is possible by the process of parental screening, which is discussed in Chapters 14 and 15.

Particularly where families have not had prior experience with a genetic problem, there often are very ill-defined motives for wanting genetic information, and ill-informed notions about genetic risks and options. Thus, the educational aspect of genetic counseling is of utmost importance. Candidates for any parental genetic screening program, including pregnant mothers having maternal blood alpha-fetoprotein [13] or amniocentesis measurements for maternal age (Chapter 4) should be given a clear understanding of the odds, stakes, and consequences involved when invited to participate in any screening tests [14, 15]. When subjects for genetic testing are being solicited for entry into a screening program, relevant explanations should aim to ensure that informed decisions are made *prior* to participation in the program. Naturally, concern about the consequences of testing will dissipate when the results are negative and will intensify when the results are abnormal. Participants with negative results may be lulled into a false feeling of security, and participants having abnormal results may develop aggravated concerns requiring additional counseling. Education in a screening program, therefore, has to include explanations of the limits and accuracy of negative as well as of abnormal results. Inadequate prior preparation can lead to emotional inability to accept the meaning of test results [16, 17].

Who wants genetic information? When a person has genetic concerns, voicing them and having them heard in a busy physician's office may be difficult. The enterprising, persistent, or garrulous patients will make their concerns known, but the hesitant, diffident, or passive patients may find no suitable opportunity to ask genetic questions (see Chapter 2). This is where a physician's experience and judgment may help to draw out the question, and where a physician's lack of appreciation for these concerns may inhibit a sensitive patient from asking. Sometimes the concern is expressed to other health professionals who may appear to be more receptive. When this occurs, patients should be encouraged to speak to their primary physicians, who can then judge whether their concerns are readily answerable or need referral to a specialist. This judgment is not easy. The tendency to judge that the truth — or too much of the truth — would be too burdensome for families is becoming less generally accepted.

> Mr. and Mrs. A, having been informed of the incurable nature and anesthetic risks of their son's type II mucopolysaccharidosis, became inordinately anxious about a scheduled ear operation, and equally anxious about a move to a distant city. They did understand the genetic risk that future sons might be similarly affected and that the option of fetal diagnosis was available for this condition.

It could be argued that Mr. and Mrs. A would have been better left in a state of ignorant bliss, but the unpleasant consequences — risk of anesthetic death, certainty of progressive mental and physical decline, and threat to future children — would have caught up with them eventually, and so alerting them to the truth was a justified unpleasant necessity. Equally necessary was continued support to help them adjust to the realities of their situation. With expert anesthesia, the operation was successful; with introduction to specialists near their new home, the move was uneventful.

> When parents of children with congenital heart malformations were polled at an informal meeting about whether the 1 in 20 or 1 in 30 recurrence risk of heart malformations for future children was information they wanted, the unanimous response was that this information was important to them and that it should be offered to all parents with similar problems [18].

It would seem that families' opinions about what they wished to know differed markedly from physicians' frequently facile assumption that it is kinder not to worry them with hypothetical risks. Other polls have shown that parents prefer to be informed early about genetic disorders in their infants [19, 20], and are more often dissatisfied with incomplete information than with being overinformed [21]. They generally prefer knowing the worst to being kept in ignorance.

Dilemmas of overreaction and indifference. Two dilemmas caused by excessive concern or indifference confound attempts at deciding whether to alert someone to genetic risks. Both are due to the unpredictability of human nature.

Mention of a relatively trivial genetic risk to a person may arouse anxieties totally out of proportion to the size or gravity of the risk, so that excessive time and resources are needed to put to rest concerns that might better have been left unawakened. Judgment in this area is often colored by a physician's reluctance to cause undue alarm or to stir up protracted inquiries.

The first dilemma, that once a genetic topic is opened an irreversible step has been taken that could have tiresome, if not unpleasant, consequences is illustrated by the experience of Mr. D.

> Mr. and Mrs. D were invited to participate in a research project for presymptomatic detection of autosomal dominant polycystic renal disease, which had affected Mrs. D's father. Even after several efforts to inform them via written material, family conferences, and appointments for personal interviews, Mr. D refused to involve himself but agreed to his wife and 18-month-old daughter participating. When ultrasound testing diagnosed kidney cysts in both mother and daughter, the couple refused to come for a personal interview and insisted on learning the results by telephone. Although Mr. D assured us he had read the written explanations that presence of cysts would cause no threat to his daughter for decades and that no treatment was available, he telephoned back in a panic that evening, alarmed and indignant that his daughter's pediatrician would not see her until the next day [22].

Clearly, Mr. D became unduly alarmed and had totally misconstrued the meaning of the test results. Part of the problem arose because of pressures from relatives to participate in the project, and part was from a misconception that early treatment was available and effective for this condition. In this instance there can be little room for doubt that the information had caused far more immediate harm than good, despite the best of intentions and attempts to forestall any misapprehensions.

The specter of genetic information causing marital break-up is often raised. This is certainly a very sensitive area, which needs discrete, sympathetic handling, but prudence should dictate caution, not silence. Obviously, an unstable family is liable to fall apart under stress, but close family relationships are often strengthened by adversity. To blame a genetic problem or genetic disclosure for family dissension ignores the probable existence of fundamental pre-existing instabilities from personality conflicts and incompatibilities. Families who are forewarned would be in a stronger position to withstand recriminations and to face genetic realities together. In the current climate of physician—patient relationships, legal accountability also makes it more prudent to inform than to withhold information (see Chapter 15).

The second dilemma, indifference or noncompliance, can be very serious when a health professional can see a definite genetic problem and an appropriate course of action, but the patient is resistant to offers of genetic information. Mr. D's early resistance was an extreme example of such a case. Here the health professional's judgment may be based on correct facts and accurate prediction of consequences, but the patient will not or cannot agree. This situation should still be considered from the viewpoint of the subject, who refuses to seek counseling, and not of the health professional, who thinks he or she knows best. Awareness of a genetic need may be resisted because of educational, socio-familial, or psychological attitudes. When these barriers can be identified, they can often be bypassed by starting the process of genetic counseling from the position of the subject, and slowly introducing the educational elements needed to promote motivation, understanding, and acceptance [23].

> Mr. E had a four-year-old son with the typical characteristics of type II mucopolysaccharidosis, but he refused to believe his physicians, choosing instead to rely on his faith. "In the eyes of God my son is complete. He stands only to lose from your tests." Mr. E changed physicians and refused genetic counseling until his son was eight years old, when the realities of the need for special schooling finally drove him to return for help.

This was a sad example where it took four years for Mr. E's position to shift from vigorous denial to earnest inquiry. Having a person accept genetic information involves the same challenges as having a person comply with medical instructions. It is not what is told that matters, but when and how it is told, whether it is accepted, believed, remembered, and used.

Distracting concerns. Often an inquirer's genetic question is overwhelmed by other more urgent questions that require satisfactory answers before the genetic question can be heard or even voiced. When there already are affected individuals in the family, the nature of their medical problem, its treatment possibilities, and future prospects, all demand explanations in the same way that a patient needs to understand any disease process. Satisfactory explanations and disease counseling should be given by the appropriate physicians or health professionals caring for the affected patient. When a problem is genetic, it threatens the self-image of the family and its members by undermining self-concepts of normalcy from within and cannot be regarded with the same kind of hostile aversion as an external threat, such as an infectious agent. This undoubtedly accounted for much of Mr. E's recalcitrance. Also, by their genetic nature, inherited disorders implicate other family members in a way that acquired diseases do not. Explanations about a genetic disorder include disturbing revelations that parents and other relatives are inherently imperfect, which threatens these people's self-images. Until members of a family have understood explanations of a disease process and accepted its genetic basis, they will not be able to focus on genetic risks or make practical decisions for coping with these risks.

Asking the Genetic Question: Its Components

A second prerequisite for genetic counseling, awareness having been aroused, is motivation (because some families with genetic problems have no need or desire to ask any genetic questions).

> Mrs. F was born with a mild form of short-limbed dwarfism, hypochondroplasia. She suffered no medical complications from this condition, apparently had a satisfactory childhood and a happy marriage. After she had borne three children, two of whom had the same short-limbed dwarfism, she was referred to a geneticist for counseling. It turned out, however, that she had no interest or concern about the genetic aspects of her condition. She was confident that she could give her affected children just as fulfilling an upbringing as she had herself, and so the condition seemed not at all serious to her. The 50–50 probability of a child being affected made no difference in her plans for having children.

Whatever might be the opinion of Mrs. F's physician or others, she and her husband had no place for genetic information in their rational decisions about family size. They perceived no handicap, and so had no genetic questions to ask.

When someone is concerned about a genetic problem and does have genetic questions, these can only be answered within a logical framework: Is the problem genetic? Who is at risk? What are its consequences? How certain is the answer? What are the options? Integrated answers to these component questions will then provide the best available answer to the inquirer.

Availability: Is There an Answer?

Diagnosis is often restricted by current limits to scientific knowledge and by lack of key information about possibly affected relatives. Biological variations and statistical uncertainties both impair predictions about manifestations of a genetic disorder in a family. Despite these shortcomings, answers to genetic questions may have immense practical importance to a family. Also, an answer that is of no use to one family is valued by another. An obvious example is the rejection of fetal diagnosis by one family as absolutely unacceptable emotionally or ethically, but eager acceptance of this option by another family as the practical solution to their plight. Since the acceptability and utility of a genetic answer depends so much on subjective factors, paradoxically, even the proved absence of an answer can be helpful to an inquirer. Many times a family with serious concerns about a possible genetic problem has been thoroughly investigated with entirely negative results, but their concerns have been relieved by the knowledge that all reasonable steps had been taken to try to answer their questions and that serious genetic possibilities have been excluded. Therefore, even "no" and "we do not know" are answers that are of use to some families, although these answers can lead to dissatisfaction with the counseling experience [23a].

Access: Who Has the Answer?

Genetic problems are so protean and so complex that no single person or medical center can possibly have the right answers to all inquiries. A prudent prerequisite for answering any genetic question is that the responder have sufficient expertise to be confident of the diagnosis and to be aware of possible medical and genetic exceptions to a presumptive diagnosis.

> Dr. and Mrs. G's second and fourth children both died at birth of severe multiple malformations. Each time, their obstetrician, a family friend, told them neither he nor his colleagues had ever seen that pattern of malformation before and authoritatively assured them that there could be no risk of recurrence. Their fifth child was similarly affected. It turned out that the condition was an autosomal recessive disorder [24].

To give false assurances beyond one's knowledge may be done out of kindness and could work out well with luck, but statistically one cannot always be lucky. Dr. and Mrs. G's obstetrician friend caused them unnecessary grief and suffering by claiming what he could not know.

With improved data processing and communication, answers to genetic questions are being provided from a network of specialist centers to health professionals and to patients with ever-improving sophistication and precision, virtually regardless of geographic isolation. In the future, therefore, knowledge should become more accessible, and errors in diagnosis or interpretation will be less defensible.

PREPARATION FOR GENETIC COUNSELING

Anyone providing genetic information should prepare accurate, objective information about the inquiry and perceptive subjective information about the inquirer. The section that follows discusses the collection and relevance of objective and subjective family information for genetic counseling.

Objective Information

Objective information is needed to answer each component of the genetic question. This requires medical, genetic, and probabilistic assessment with as much confirmation of facts as is reasonably indicated.

Diagnosis. A correct medical diagnosis often must precede a genetic diagnosis, but is not necessarily equivalent to it (see Chapters 3–6). A thorough medical evaluation of the affected individual is mandatory, whenever possible (this includes autopsy data, when available). Sometimes medical evaluation of other relatives is also indicated. When objective clinical information has already been collected by others, scrutinizing the medical records of relevant family members is a necessary part of the preparation; additional investigations may have to be undertaken as well in preparation for genetic counseling.

For certain conditions it is simple to confirm or exclude a genetic diagnosis, such as when a chromosomal cause is being considered, by appropriate tests. Many disorders caused by a single gene of major effect, especially inherited abnormalities of enzymes and other proteins, can be confirmed by tests of specific protein function or antigenicity. Many other single gene disorders that mimic nongenetic phenocopies (genetic or nongenetic conditions that appear similar), such as congenital heart malformations, or that have variant genocopies, such as the short-limbed dwarfing syndromes, are not easily diagnosed and require many tests. Genocopies (genetic conditions that appear similar) are important when they vary in severity or response to therapy, but they are particularly significant in the genetic counseling context when different patterns of inheritance are involved. For example, the common form of pseudohypertrophic (Duchenne) muscular dystrophy in young boys is inherited via an X-linked gene, but there is a less common, virtually indistinguishable form of muscular dystrophy that is autosomal recessive in inheritance. This means that a young girl with muscular dystrophy probably has the autosomal form, with a one in four risk to future brothers and sisters regardless of sex, and that a young boy with muscular dystrophy is more likely to have the X-linked form, with a one in two risk to future brothers if the mother is a carrier (see Chapter 3). Up to 10% of boys with muscular dystrophy, however, may have the autosomal type, which cannot be differentiated unequivocally until more precise tests can be developed.

Most disorders with a genetic basis are influenced by many genetic factors, each of small effect, which cumulatively may act unfavorably to cause a genetic disorder or weakness. These cases may be arbitrarily classified as either genetic or nongenetic, but from the viewpoint of a prospective parent, the critical question is whether or not a problem will affect future children. A moderately low risk of 1 in 20 to 1 in 50 is considered to be very serious by some families [18, 25]. Many congenital malformations fall into this category (see Chapter 5).

Diagnostic dilemmas are presented by phenocopies, eg, congenital malformations, because some of them can be caused by nongenetic factors, perhaps noxious disturbances during pregnancy (see Chapter 4). If a problem can be associated with a proven external factor during pregnancy, such as a viral infection, then its risk of recurrence can be averted by avoidance of that factor during future pregnancies, and the inquirer can be assured that it is nongenetic. Unfortunately, irretrievable information is sometimes lost by omission of critical tests until too late, such as chromosome testing in a lethally malformed infant, or antibody testing for intrauterine infection in a young infant, or a careful autopsy examination of someone with a possible genetic disease.

Inferential deductions can sometimes be made about the genetic basis of a problem if several relatives are affected, but the coincidence of a disorder among relatives could be from a shared environmental cause, or it might arise by chance alone. The following family illustrates how a genetic diagnosis can be made in the absence of a medical diagnosis.

> Miss H was concerned about a form of dementia, starting in mid-adult life, that had affected her mother, her mother's brother, her paternal grandfather, and his sister. No autopsy information was available on the relatives who had died, and Miss H's older brother, the mother's legal custodian, refused to release any medical information about their mother.

Although no microscopic confirmation of a specific type of presenile dementia could be made [25a], there was sufficient family information to infer that a form of autosomal dominant presenile dementia had affected family members, with a 50–50 risk to the inquirer [25b].

Risk. Construction of an accurate detailed family history is essential for evaluating genetic risk (see Chapter 3). Even when the condition is well-delineated and no one else close to the nuclear family appears affected, brief checking of relatives is important not just for the genetic problem presented, but to ensure that there are no additional unsuspected genetic problems in the family.

Present risk. Among relatives of the inquirer there may be others affected with the genetic problem in question. Some of these may already have symptoms that have not yet been diagnosed, and others may be threatened with serious complications unless timely intervention can be offered. All of them may benefit from genetic information, both for the sake of their own health and for alerting them about risks to future children.

> Miss J was a graduate student who volunteered that she had "Turner syndrome." Upon further inquiry, it was learned that she had had some bony lumps on the head, and the diagnosis was her vague recollection of a physician's off-hand remark. Her mother had had similar lumps, and had a colectomy for cancer of the colon. Investigations revealed Miss J also had colonic polyps, which together with the bony skull tumors established the diagnosis of autosomal dominant Gardner syndrome in this family. Because of the threat of cancerous degeneration of the polyps, she chose to have her colon excised. Her family was given genetic counseling about risks.

In considering a genetic diagnosis, it clearly is unacceptable to assume that a given diagnosis is correct without confirmation. When a genetic diagnosis is under consideration, characteristic inheritance patterns will predict which relatives are most likely to be at risk; often the finding of affected relatives serves to clinch a tentative genetic diagnosis.

Future risk. Accurate prediction of the genetic status of future children is the central focus of genetic counseling. Without this, the rest of genetic counseling would not differ uniquely from disease counseling. This prediction consists of three parts: the nature of the condition, the odds of its occurring, and whether detection or treatment is possible.

Knowing that a condition is genetic does not necessarily provide sufficient information about risks for future children. These risks depend on identifying the genetic makeup of parents-at-risk. With regard to Down syndrome, for the 3–5% of patients who have a translocated chromosome 21 the recurrence risk is quite different, depending on whether both parents have normal chromosomes or whether the mother or the father happens to be the carrier of the translocated chromosome [26, 27].

Occasionally the identification of who is a parent-at-risk for a given genetic problem can be excruciatingly complicated [28]. This pertains particularly to diseases of adult onset (see Chapter 6) and for X-linked recessive conditions where female heterozygotes might transmit an undetected genetic disorder for several generations without a male being affected (see Chapter 3). Correct assignment of the heterozygous state to prospective mothers in such a kindred can be of critical importance to their plans for having children.

Possible consequences. Understanding the consequences of a known risk is a neglected facet of genetic counseling, because a precise numerical risk gives a terribly inadequate one-dimensional prediction about the consequent manifestations and complications of a genetic condition. Again, Down syndrome is a useful example. Every person with Down syndrome has moderately severe mental limitations and some degree of growth failure [26]; severe heart malformations afflict almost 50%; intestinal abnormalities afflict 7%; the risk of leukemia is about 2% [27]. Both morbidity and mortality are obviously very much dependent on the presence or absence of these major complications. Genetically it is possible to derive a numerical risk of Down syndrome for a prospective parent, and to offer intrauterine diagnosis (see Chapter 4), but the medical consequences for an individual with Down syndrome are unpredictably variable. This variability of expression applies to every genetic diagnosis, and objective data on variability are quite sparse for many genetic disorders.

Understanding the consequences of a genetic disorder is very much distorted by one's subjective experience. A person who has lived through the devastation of chronic illness afflicting a close relative needs no description of that condition, but may yet possess a false perspective if the condition is quite variable, perhaps frequently milder, or if improved treatment can be offered. Someone who has had no personal contact with a particular problem, on the other hand, may have great difficulty in appreciating its consequences without very patient descriptions by health professionals or by members of affected families.

Prognostication is just as uncertain for genetic disorders as it is for chronic or grave illnesses. The task of the counselor is to give a balanced prediction of severity that is neither too optimistic nor too gloomy [29], based on realistic expectations.

No one can anticipate with confidence how well or how poorly an individual or a nuclear family might respond to the challenges of a genetically handicapping condition, but in answer to genetic inquiries, the questioner should be given an appreciation both of the odds of a genetic risk and of the stakes involved in being affected with the genetic condition.

A consequence of childbearing that should be fully explained to anyone seeking genetic counseling is the general risk of any child having a serious handicap. In several studies of pregnancy outcome, the incidence of a major handicap has been from 2% to 4% [30] of live births, not counting complications arising from prematurity and birth injury, or learning and behavioral disabilities of later onset (or additional complicating hazards from social factors and standards of health care). Whenever an inquirer is trying to weigh the odds and stakes of a specific genetic risk, this background general risk should be considered; whenever fetal diagnosis is being contemplated, the inability to eliminate this natural background risk should be pointed out.

Certainty of risk. In genetic prediction, certainty is always a multi-faceted factor. In preparing genetic information, estimated certainties are needed of the medical diagnosis, its genetic basis, who in a kindred might be at risk, recurrence probabilities, test reliabilities, and variable severity of the condition. Rarely can every one of these be determined with high precision, and yet errors or unpredictabilities in any one could seriously erode the overall certainty of a genetic prediction.

> Mr. and Mrs. K had two children apparently affected with Tay-Sachs disease who died of their affliction. When Mrs. K again became pregnant, her obstetrician tested the fetus for Tay-Sachs disease. The test result was normal. After the birth of an unaffected child, however, neither parent was found to be a carrier for Tay-Sachs; thus, the fetal testing had been for the wrong disease.

Options. *Unrelated to reproduction.* Helping a family adjust to the realities of a genetic disorder affecting a family member is really disease counseling and not genetic counseling, although it happens to involve a genetic disease. Nonetheless, if a genetic inquirer has overriding concerns in this area, accurate, full information must be offered about the condition, its prospects, treatment possibilities, and available support services, such as training and education. Without satisfying these concerns, genetic information is unlikely to gain the attention or respect of the inquirer. Also, these disease explanations would be equally applicable to future affected offspring, and so should be an integral part of discussion about the consequences of a genetic disorder. All of this information will contribute to the data base an inquirer can use to make informed decisions about genetic problems.

Nonreproductive decisions about genetic problems entail adjustments to the realities of a problem and dealing with the ramifications of that problem. This is the process of coping [31–33]. Learning to cope is a family's capacity to pass through the natural stages of shock, anxiety, guilt, and depression toward adaptation [32]. The responsibility of a genetic counselor is not only to recognize the stage which a family has reached and to help the family gain insight, but also to encourage all family members to find the best possible adjustments to their problem. This may involve, for example, advocating the interests of unaffected brothers and sisters of a seriously handicapped child, since they may be sadly neglected by parents concentrating on the affected child and often feel guilty for being normal. This frequently unwitting rejection of the unaffected children can sometimes be reversed by offering information about how unaffected brothers and sisters might view a genetic problem and be influenced by it.

Related to reproduction. The numerous options open to a person with a genetic problem range from sterilization to procreation, but often include the options of artificial insemination with donor sperm and fetal diagnosis. In giving genetic counseling, information should be given to an inquirer about how each option may or may not be applicable to the particular genetic problem in question. For example, a couple may need information about contraception or about the reversibility of sterilization operations, or about what is involved both physically and emotionally in artificial insemination with donor sperm [34]. Adoption, although not reproductive, can fulfill the parenting drive. Other ways to fulfill this drive include teaching, volunteer activities, and other community leadership responsibilities.

Fetal diagnosis is, at present, a major option for genetic disorders, despite the fact that it can be offered only for a limited number of these problems (see Chapter 4). It often is the only feasible option for a family wanting to have another child and unwilling to accept the risk that the child might be affected. Objective information must therefore be prepared, with medical literature review or consultation with a center active in fetal diagnosis, about applicability of fetal diagnosis for the genetic problem in question. This information has to be carefully evaluated, because technical advances have been so rapid in this field that what recently was impossible has become possible. Caution must be exercised about whether what is possible is actually practical, however, as some procedures such as fetoscopy are being reliably conducted at very few centers, and counselee may not appreciate being referred to a local optimistic experimenter who wants to dabble in an unfamiliar field. The same caution applies to reliance on laboratories with limited experience or expertise.

> Dr. L telephoned to ask for interpretation of a maternal serum alpha-fetoprotein result that had finally been reported one month after it was obtained from a pregnant patient and sent to a commercial laboratory. Dr. L had obtained the specimen because his patient had a previous child with a major brain malformation. The report said the test result was "compatible with hepatocellular carcinoma." Unfortunately, without knowing that laboratory's range of normal concentrations for maternal blood samples at the week of pregnancy when Dr. L obtained the blood, it was impossible to interpret the report.

Subjective Information

Having obtained the most comprehensive objective data possible, the next task of genetic counseling is to make it comprehensible to the inquirer. Fulfillment of this task requires insight about the intellectual, emotional, and personality status of each inquirer (see Chapter 11). Much of this may already be known if the counselor is also the primary physician, and some of it can be obtained in the course of a simple interview. A careful appraisal of an inquirer's subjective strengths, weaknesses, and attitudes can facilitate effective transfer of all health-related information. For genetic information, the task is complicated by special stresses imposed by the implied stigmatization associated with a genetic defect and the vagaries of statistical predictions about children not yet born.

Sensibility. The measurement of emotional attitudes and cognitive strengths are topics of major controversy among behavior scientists. Although precise measurements in these areas are unattainable, anyone offering genetic information as a health professional has a duty to assess the psychological characteristics of the counselee, so that counseling is subjectively acceptable. This requires a deliberate avoidance by the counselor of any personal biases and a conscious effort to view the entire problem from the perspective of the subject (see Chapter 11).

The attribute of sensibility or common sense is not even definable but can be appraised empirically by someone experienced in interpersonal relationships. Dangers arise when erroneous assumptions or snap judgments are made. These can cause irreparable alienation when there is overoptimistic blundering through defensive barriers or, equally, overpessimistic abandonment of attempts to change a person's attitudes.

Astute assessment of a subject's motivation, cognition, affect, self-image, and defenses are discussed in Chapter 11. These should all be considered in planning the level of discussions (and in dispelling any imagined fears).

Demographic factors should be known not only to help in the predicting of genetic risks but also for background about the attitudes of inquirers, which inevitably will be very much colored by cultural and family experience [35–37].

Attitudes. The attitudes of a person or family toward life in general, toward aspects of health behavior [38] (see Chapter 7), toward reproduction (see Chapters 8 and 9), and toward gambling with odds (see Chapter 10) can all exert strong influences on how genetic information is received. Consideration of these attitudes may help to determine how this information is best given.

Personality. All the above factors contribute to personality, which is notoriously complicated. Nonetheless, whether the overall personality is extroverted or introverted, optimistic or pessimistic, brimming with confidence or taut with anxiety, aggressive or passive, amicable or hostile will strongly color the counselee's attitudes and ability to cope.

Strengths and resources. *Family.* The strength of the family fabric is the single most important resource behind a person's ability to cope with a genetic problem. Interpersonal clashes and stresses would aggravate the impact of such a problem, whereas close ties and positive support among relatives can minimize a person's need for help from health and social agencies.

Financial strengths or weaknesses often dictate the flexibility of a family's options; one family could have great hardship traveling to a nearby medical center, but another family would demand access to the best possible expert even halfway around the world. Hence, for genetic counseling about rare disorders, financial status involves more than routine checking about health insurance and third-party coverage of medical costs.

Community. Social, spiritual, and material resources in the community, while not subjective, will supply the options and support available to a person living in that community. For some, the size of this community may be confined to their local church group; for others, it will encompass major state health facilities or the nearest major medical center.

PRESENTING GENETIC INFORMATION

What To Present

Content of genetic information should include both answers to what has been asked and to what should have been asked, with sufficient background information for making reasoned decisions related to the genetic problem. Presentation of excessively detailed or technical explanations of genetic principles would only alienate and confuse a lay inquirer. With planned preparation, the presentation can contain explanations of relevant genetic principles at a level appropriate to the sophistication of the counselee.

With rare exceptions, presentation of genetic information should include all five basic components of the genetic question: whether a condition is genetic, its risks, its consequences, its certainty, and its options. Since the purpose of presenting genetic information is educational, the presentation should be flexible, allowing opportunities for an inquirer to clarify points, explore alternative options, and ask about additional matters arising from the genetic explanations. It should also include reinforcement and repetition, and be open-ended because the goal is imparting knowledge, however long it may take.

How To Present It

Mode. The way in which genetic information is presented can be as varied as the presenter or inquirer desires. The traditional concept is of an interview or formal discussion conducted by a geneticist with a person or a couple. Occasionally a face-to-face interview has to be replaced by a telephone conversation or letter of explanation for inquirers from distant places. When there are several people with re-lated problems, whether they are in the same kindred or not, a larger group discus-sion may be a useful, effective, and efficient way to explore common questions and concerns [39, 40]. The communication process is often more effective if divided into a series of sessions. These sessions could have very highly organized agendas, or sometimes are best left unstructured to allow certain topics to be ex-plored more fully as required [40a].

Medium. Techniques are being developed to provide health-related information via brochures, taped telephone responses, video-tape cassettes, and interactive com-puter programs. For the more common genetic problems, such as those related to congenital heart disease or to fetal diagnosis of spina bifida or maternal age-related chromosome abnormalities, these modalities may prove very useful. For instance, these could provide information to expectant mothers in an obstetrician's waiting room.

With or without input from experienced genetic counselors, writers for the mass media are catering to increasing public demand for genetic information. These writers reach vast audiences and could have powerful influences on the genetic sophistication of the general public. Whenever possible, these writers should be helped by health professionals to ensure that what they write is ac-curate, unbiased, and free of misleading or harmful information.

Use of audiovisual aids and other noninteractive modes can be combined with interactive modes. A multi-media approach is invariably more successful than any of its parts in conveying information. It has become standard practice in many ge-netic services to combine patient interviews with corroborative follow-up letters and to recruit the collaboration of primary physicians in reinforcing explanations about genetic facts and options. A tape-recording of a counseling interview session can also be offered to interviewees, but retrieval of information from a tape is more cumbersome than retrieval from written material.

Manner. There can be no rigid protocols for the manner in which genetic coun-seling should be offered, for it must be a manner which is comfortable for the pre-senter as well as suitable for the recipient. For any one presenter, the manner should be adapted to the subjective needs and receptiveness of each counselee. The presenter should not pretend to be more or less than he or she is, in terms of knowl-edge, culture, or faith. This means that efforts to identify with the inquirer's position should be with respect, free of sham. Equally important, any questions should be considered seriously, regardless of how silly they may appear to be. The only ex-ceptions are questions about another professional's competence. It never is advisable to be drawn into criticisms of previous standards of care given to a patient by others, except in offering expressions of sympathy for unhappy experiences and pointing out that most professionals act in good faith, for the welfare of their patients or clients.

Language. Terms used have to be carefully chosen to be both clear and un-biased. Whenever possible, simple words are better than flowery phrases or techni-cal jargon [41, 42]. The vocabulary and examples used should be drawn from ex-periences familiar to the recipient.

Emotionally charged words (or gestures) can be inadvertently introduced unless the counselor remains alert to this danger. To one person "abortion" is a topic that can be discussed dispassionately, to another it is a battle cry; many figures of speech about "seeing," "hearing," "standing," or "living" can be agonizingly pain-ful to someone who has suffered a loss related to life, limb, or a sense organ.

It is obvious that the counselor and counselee who do not share a common language must use an interpreter, but the quality of interpretation has to include conveying of facts, concepts, and impressions. Ineffectual repetitions of basic points with louder and louder emphasis may appear comical to a bystander, but can lead to tragic misunderstandings. Patients with congenital deafness are a particularly difficult challenge, because lip-reading is always ambiguous, and sign-language is cumbersome for conveying abstract ideas or subtle nuances, since many deaf people live in a silent world bereft of all but the most simple concepts (but with eloquent nonverbal body language).

Nonverbal communication is an integral part of establishing relationships with others [43, 44]. This includes the ambience of the surroundings. When a couple who has lost a child is seen for genetic counseling in a pediatric clinic, sitting in a waiting room among children can be terribly upsetting; similarly, a family con-templating fetal diagnosis can be frightened by seeing a number of multiply handi-capped children in the waiting room. Obviously many stresses are unavoidable, but frustrating tensions caused by difficult-to-find offices or unfeeling receptionists are disruptive and can be avoided with anticipatory planning.

Decor, furnishings, and the presence or absence of telephone interruptions all may affect how readily an inquirer can concentrate on genetic explanations, so choice of locale and time of day should be considered in making appointments for genetic counseling.

Dress and manners can be of utmost importance. Some people would feel much more comfortable if the counselor wore a white coat and pocketed a stethoscope, others would far prefer a less clinical image. Political slogans on lapel buttons can win instant friends, but could also create instant enemies. Therefore, for most situations a moderately neutral outward appearance would allow in-quirers to focus more on the content of what is said rather than on the speaker.

Stance and mannerisms can also help or hinder the communication process. Traditional bedside manner conjures up the image of an erect authority-figure towering over a recumbent patient. Clearly, for free reciprocal information inter-change a more egalitarian arrangement would be more effective.

The dress, mannerisms, and posture of the interviewees can also promote or in-hibit the counseling process and give continuing signals about the attitudes and moods of the subjects. These are especially revealing when a couple is interviewed together; the way the partners sit and whether they touch or exchange glances are powerful clues to their attitudes and to how they share decisions [45] (see Chapter 10). If a counselor is to communicate effectively with *both* partners, their interactions and relationships have to be appreciated. Inadvertent favoritism may alienate one partner or stir conflict between them (see Chapter 11).

Culture. Cultural barriers are particularly difficult. In dealing with someone of a different culture, it can be helpful to invite a representative of that culture to act as an advocate (see Chapter 11) during collection of subjective information and presentation of genetic explanations. Often this representative can be a relative who is more assimilated into the mainstream culture. Other suitable candidates to represent an unfamiliar culture include clergy, community leaders, or health professionals from that culture.

Two possible drawbacks, prejudice and breach of confidentiality, apply to any of these representatives. The person should be chosen prudently, with prior approval by the counselee, and with preparative discussion of that person's expected role and contribution with the representative. This is important if that person is also to interpret the genetic information into a language foreign to the counselor.

The cultural representative can make major contributions in several ways. Explanations and interpretations of cultural norms to the counselor will facilitate the conduct of interviews, helping the counselor to understand cultural orientations and to avoid unintentional gaffs. The mere presence of the representative will be reassuring to the inquirer, because potential misunderstandings can be allayed, and because this presence confers the implied endorsement of genetic counseling by members of that culture.

The most important contribution of a cultural representative is for follow-up and support. However well a genetic explanation is given to recipients, what ultimately happens to their use of the information is determined in very large part by their cultural as well as personal orientations. Since the genetic information will be weighed and used within a cultural framework, introducing this information within the appropriate cultural context from the outset will make it much more likely that the information be used to the best advantage. When the genetic counselor has recruited a representative of that culture as an ally, that person can be a valuable resource to an inquirer for support and reinforcement of decisions made. Cultural and religious beliefs may isolate inquirers from rational science and medicine, when Western medicine is regarded merely as a competing philosophy with no more than equal claims on credibility or faith. It is never wise to belittle any belief, as this will only antagonize, without serving any constructive purpose. This applies to all mystic faiths, ranging from one of the major religions of the world to the unorthodox neighborhood faddism.

Mood. Formality or informality of the relationship between a genetic counselor and an inquirer is of little importance, provided that both feel at ease. Cordiality should be shown, while both frivolous levity and funereal sobriety are inappropriate. If the atmosphere becomes too tense, a brief interlude or distraction may help, but interruptions may often break a train of thought or shatter a communicative mood.

Emotional expressions of grief, anger, and even hostility may be entirely appropriate for a counselee who is under stress, and who has pent-up feelings with few opportunities to find suitable outlets [32, 33]. It is unrealistic to expect someone to be able to discuss very upsetting personal fears and anxieties dispassionately. The counselor has to accept emotional outbursts as perfectly natural reactions, and neither discourage them by word or manner nor become so emotionally involved as to lose professional objectivity. An emotional outburst that is permitted sympathetic expression can clear the atmosphere for improved communication, but if recovery of emotional control is not possible, further discussion may best be deferred.

This does not mean that a person's innermost feelings should be probed and exposed mercilessly by someone unskilled in the professional handling of psychological disturbances. Often a person under severe stress can function only behind irrational psychological defenses. Breaching these defenses can cause irreparable harm unless the person can be helped to replace them with coping mechanisms [33]. Any person who is thought to have psychiatric instabilities or who appears to have a fragile psyche should be given genetic information only in a very supportive situation, preferably with psychiatric assistance.

Who Participates in Genetic Counseling?

Recipients. Genetic counseling is usually given to a couple or to a nuclear family. This can be a most comfortable situation when family members are mutually harmonious. In fact, unless impossible or contraindicated, genetic counseling should be offered to husband and wife together. In certain families other relatives can and should be included; at other times an inquisitive grandmother, an intrusive in-law, or a distracting child should be discouraged from joining a genetic counseling session. If there are no time constraints, a combination of individual interviews and joint sessions may work well. The optimal arrangement for each family can be discussed as part of the contractual process of planning genetic counseling (see Chapter 13). Drawbacks to seeing husband and wife together exist when one has private genetic information too embarrassing to share with the spouse, or when there are open or hidden conflicts between them.

Counselors. Genetic counseling is often given by a single physician, but in other situations it may best be given by a group of physicians, each with a specific role; for example, the primary doctor with a subspecialist, geneticist or advocate (see Chapter 11). It can be intimidating, however, for several professionals to participate. When each has an important role in the intake process of gathering information or conducting tests, each may be familiar enough to the patient to be accepted if they are all present at an explanatory session, but even so it is generally best to limit the number of professionals at any one session so that they do not overwhelm the inquirers. If the session is reasonably informal, several professionals can offer information preferably with a minimum of quibbling or disagreement; if the session is very formal and one person assumes the lion's share of the talking, there is little reason to have colleagues present.

An advocate for the inquirer (see Chapter 11) can be instrumental in helping a person or family feel comfortable with the genetic counseling situation. This is particularly so for people who regard a physician as an authority figure to be held in awe and not to be questioned. Of course, the advocate's responsibility in this situation is to encourage a dialogue and not to disturb the process by acting only as an ego-deflator for the counselor (see Chapter 13).

Supportive tasks, especially in follow-up, can often be fulfilled satisfactorily by sensitive, experienced allied health professionals such as social workers or genetic associates. These personnel should work in close conjunction with the family physician and be supervised by a medical geneticist.

Observers. Any observer can be intrusive and distracting. For the sake of learning, trainees of various disciplines have to attend counseling situations to gain first-hand exposure, and other observers may on occasion have valid reasons to be present at counseling sessions. For some patients this can be perfectly acceptable or even welcome, whereas for others extraneous observers would be disturbing or even humiliating. Whenever a trainee is to be exposed to a counseling session, assignment of contributory tasks to the trainee, such as collection of family information, can facilitate acceptance by patients.

When To Give Information

Readiness. Learning answers to genetic questions takes time; it cannot start until a genetic problem has been recognized. But after recognition, a person or family may still not be ready to face genetic implications of the problem [46].

Readiness is a psychological state that cannot be forced upon an individual, yet sensitive intervention may help a person resolve inner defenses and conflicts. This means that timing of each phase of the genetic counseling process can be a critical factor in determining whether genetic information will be accepted or rejected.

When there is acute shock or grief at the initial revelation of the existence of a genetic problem, the single item of information that should be conveyed is whether genetic information is available. Resolution of grief and fulfillment of mourning take time, but can be facilitated with appropriate sympathetic handling [47]. A person in an acute emotional state will not be able to concentrate on complex explanations, but could be comforted by assurance that important information will be discussed at a more propitious time. Persons in a chronic state of depression also need to accept more enlightened self-awareness before they will have any desire for genetic information.

For immature family members at risk for a genetic problem the same principle applies – that they be made aware of the availability of important information so that when they are ready they can ask for it. In such families the parents are the natural agents for conferring this initial awareness, but they may need expert help later in conveying genetic information.

Giving genetic information too soon may not only be ineffective, but could have a negative effect, for instance by alienating the intended recipients of the information. Giving information too late also has very obvious and sometimes tragic consequences.

> Miss M had two brothers with a rare form of muscular deformity and a cousin with epilepsy. Under the mistaken assumption that she could not have normal children, she shunned social contact with male peers until she was in her mid-thirties, when her psychiatrist referred her for genetic counseling.

Repetition. The process of learning genetic information has many facets, and repeated exposure to relevant background information through formal schooling, mass media, and multiple exposures via various health professionals all contribute to the foundation upon which specific medical genetic information is to be based.

Timing of genetic counseling should therefore be planned according to the state of readiness of an individual and the complexity of the information to be conveyed. Time should be allowed for any questions to be thoroughly discussed, and often multiple sessions are preferred in order that information be assimilated and reinforced. It is less wasteful to spend time reinforcing information than to have it misunderstood or forgotten because the presentation was rushed.

SUMMARY AND CONCLUSIONS

Genetic counseling is the educational process whereby an individual or a family obtains relevant information about a real or possible genetic problem affecting or threatening living or future generations. This process is preceded by recognition of individuals who want to ask genetic questions. It requires that the genetic basis of a problem be identifiable, that its chances of affecting present or future relatives is predictable, and that there are feasible options for dealing with the problem. For effective communication of the genetic information, presentation should be geared to the individual questioner's subjective needs and personality characteristics. The better these are understood and addressed by the provider of genetic information, the less the danger that the information will be misunderstood or rejected.

To be complete, genetic counseling should include explanations of probable causes, risks, options, and consequences, and the degrees of certainty about each of these.

Comprehension of genetic information is a learning process that takes time and will be facilitated by careful preparation, enhanced by lucid presentation, and reinforced by repetition, perhaps with the collaboration of a health professional team.

To be helpful, the information has to be used in the shaping of attitudes and the making of decisions.

Use of genetic knowledge cannot be predetermined by the counselor. Wise use of the information can only be in the context of personal concerns and desires that are very private. Every health professional has a responsibility to recognize valid genetic questions that a patient might have. This involves recognizing the genetic components of medical disorders, and genetic concerns about the disorders.

Whoever is answering genetic questions should be responsible for ensuring that the answers are factually correct and sympathetically presented, lest they cause harm to the recipients. The provider of genetic answers should either offer follow-up support or direct an inquirer to where support can be obtained.

When genetic counseling is properly conducted, the information can be of great benefit to recipients, and the task can be very rewarding to the provider.

ACKNOWLEDGMENTS

We are grateful to our colleagues who shared their experiences with us and helped to shape our ideas in discussions and debate.

The work on which our contributions are based was supported in part by National Foundation March of Dimes Medical Service grants C-41 and C-297.

ANNOTATED REFERENCES

1. Reed SC: "Counseling in Medical Genetics," Ed 2. Philadelphia: W B Saunders, 1963, p 278.
2. Reed SC: A short history of genetic counseling. Soc Biol 21:332–339, 1975.
   A fascinating historical review by a founder of genetic counseling.
2a. Capron AM, Lappé M, Murray RF, Powledge TM, Twiss SB (eds): "Genetic Counseling: Facts, Values, and Norms." BD:OAS, Vol 15(2). New York: Alan R. Liss for The National Foundation-March of Dimes.
3. Fraser FC: Genetic counseling. Am J Hum Genet 26:636–659, 1974.
   Formal committee report to the American Society of Human Genetics.
4. Bok S: "Lying: Moral Choice in Public Life." Westminister, Maryland: Pantheon, 1978.
5. Kushnick T: When to refer to the geneticist. JAMA 235:623–625, 1976.
6. Childs B: A place for genetics in health education, and vice versa. Am J Hum Genet 26: 120–135, 1974.

7. Hsia YE, Bucholz KK, Austein CF: Genetic knowledge of Connecticut pediatricians and obstetricians: Implications for continuing education. In Hook EB, Porter IH (eds): "Service and Education in Medical Genetics." New York: Academic Press (in press).
    A questionnaire survey of genetic knowledge and learning preferences.
8. Riccardi VM: Health care and disease prevention through genetic counseling: A regional approach. Am J Public Health 66:268–272, 1976.
9. Ingelfinger FJ: Quenchless quest for questionable cure. N Engl J Med 295:838–839, 1976.
10. Firman GJ, Goldstein MS: The future of chiropractic: A psychosocial view. N Engl J Med 293:639–642, 1975.
    An argument that chiropractors are needed because physicians have no time to listen.
11. Lamiell JM, Salazar FG, Polk NO, Hsia YE: Pre-symptomatic surveillance for von Hippel Lindau disease in a large kindred. Am J Hum Genet 30:57a, 1978.
12. Crane RJ: The case of the illegitimate gene. Postgrad Med J 51:637–642, 1975.
13. Dunelm J: Ethical problems of screening for neural tube defects. Lancet 2:148, 1978.
14. Reilly P: "Genetics, Law and Social Policy." Cambridge, Massachusetts: Harvard University Press, 1977, p 275.
    Review of policies, statutes and litigation related to genetic screening projects and genetic counseling.
15. Childs B, Simopoulos AP (eds): "Genetic Screening." Washington DC: National Academy of Sciences – National Research Council, 1975.
16. Stamatoyannopoulos G: Problems of screening and counseling in the hemoglobino-pathies. In Motulsky AG, Ebling FJG (eds): "Birth Defects: Proceedings of Fourth International Conference." Amsterdam: Excerpta Medica, 1974, pp 268–176.
    How information about carriers had harmful social effects in some communities.
17. Grover R, Wethers D, Shahidi S, Grossi M, Goldberg D, Davidow B: Evaluation of the expanded newborn screening program in New York City. Pediatrics 61:740–749, 1978.
    An important discussion of pitfalls and problems met in screening programs.
18. Halloran KH, Hsia YE, Rosenberg LE: Effect of genetic counseling for congenital heart disease in a pediatric cardiac clinic. J Pediatr 88:1054–1056, 1976.
19. Gayton WF, Walker L: Down syndrome: Informing the parents. A study of parental preferences. Am J Dis Child 127:510–512, 1974.
20. Pueschel SM, Murphy A: Assessment of counseling practices at the birth of a child with Down's syndrome. Am J Ment Defic 81:325–330, 1976.
21. Anon: Having a congenitally deformed baby. Lancet 1:1499–1501, 1973.
22. Wolf B, Rosenfield AT, Taylor KJW, Rosenfield N, Gottlieb S, Hsia YE: Presymptomatic diagnosis of adult onset polycystic kidney disease by ultrasonography. Clin Genet 14:1–7, 1978.
23. Lasagna L (ed): "Patient Compliance." Mount Kisco, New York: Futura Publishing, 1976.
23a. Aodmilou L, Hirschhorn K: Evaluation of genetic counseling. In Lubs HA, de la Cruz F (eds): "Genetic Counseling." New York: Raven Press, 1977, pp 121–130.
24. Hsia YE, Bratu M, Herbordt A: Genetics of the Meckel syndrome. Pediatrics 48:237–247, 1971.
25. Hsia YE, Leung F, Carter LL: Attitudes toward amniocentesis: Surveys of families with spina bifida children. 1974, 1977. In Hook EB, Porter IH (eds): "Service and Education in Medical Genetics." New York: Academic Press (in press).
25a. Poser CM: The presenile dementias. JAMA 233:81–84, 1975.
25b. Tsuang WT: Genetic counseling for psychiatric patients and their families. Am J Psychiatr 135:1465–1475, 1978.
26. Smith DW, Wilson AA: The child with Down's syndrome (Mongolism): Causes, characteristics and acceptance. Philadelphia: W.B. Saunders, 1973, p 106.
    An excellent monograph for parents and health professionals.

27. Breg WR: Down's syndrome. In Gardner LI (ed): "Endocrine and Genetic Diseases of Childhood and Adolescence," Ed 2. Philadelphia: W B Saunders, 1975, pp 730–762.
28. Murphy EA, Chase GA: "Principles of Genetic Counseling." Chicago: Year Book Medical Publishers, 1975, p 391.
     Quantitative principles underlying risk prediction are explained thoroughly in this book.
29. Siegler M: Pascal's wager and the hanging of crepe. N Engl J Med 293:853–857, 1975.
30. Holmes LB: Prospective counseling for hereditary malformations in newborns. In Lubs HA, de la Cruz F (eds): "Genetic Counseling." New York: Raven Press, 1977, pp 241–252.
31. McCollum AT: Coping with prolonged health impairment in your child. Boston: Little Brown, 1975.
32. Falek A: Use of the coping process to achieve psychological homeostasis in genetic counseling. In Lubs HA, de la Cruz F (eds): "Genetic Counseling." New York: Raven Press, 1977, pp 179–191.
33. Rainer JD: Psychiatric considerations in genetic counseling. In Hook EB, Porter IH (eds): "Service and Education in Medical Genetics." New York: Academic Press (in press).
     An excellent examination of this important topic.
34. Strickler RC, Keller DW, Warren JC: Artificial insemination with fresh donor semen. N Engl J Med 293:848–853, 1975.
35. Tips RL, Lynch HT: The impact of genetic counseling upon the family milieu. JAMA 184:117–120, 1963.
36. Sultz HA, Schlesinger ER, Feldman J: An epidemiologic justification for genetic counseling in family planning. Am J Public Health 62:1489–1492, 1972.
37. Leonard CO, Chase GA, Childs B: Genetic counseling: A consumer's view. N Engl J Med 287:433–439, 1972.
38. Simons RC, Pardes H (eds): "Understanding Human Behavior in Health and Illness." Baltimore: Williams & Wilkins, 1977, p 718.
     Contains discussion of the three models of the doctor–patient relationship (pp 397–404), Activity–Passivity, Guidance–Cooperation and Mutual Participation.
39. Headings VE: Alternative models for genetic counseling. Soc Biol 22:297–303, 1975.
40. Bracken MB, Grossman G, Hachamovitch M, Sussman D, Schrier D: Abortion counseling: An experimental study of three techniques. Am J Obstet Gynecol 117:10–20, 1973.
40a. Kelly PT: "Dealing with Dilemma: A Manual for Genetic Counselors." New York: Springer-Verlag, 1977.
41. Freemon B, Negrete VF, Davis M, Korsh BM: Gaps in doctor-patient communication: Doctor-patient interaction analysis. Pediatr Res 5:298–311, 1971.
42. Raimbault G, Cachin O, Limal JM, Eliacheff C: Aspects of communication between patients and doctors: An analysis of the discourse. Pediatrics 55:401–405, 1975.
     Disturbing examples of patient misunderstandings in the Turner syndrome.
43. Fast J: "Body Language." New York: M Evans, (JB Lippincott, Philadelphia), 1970, p 192.
44. Leventhal H, Fischer K: What reinforces in a social reinforcement situation — words or expressions? J Pers Soc Psychol 14:83–94, 1970.
45. Slovic P, Fischhoff B, Lichtenstein S: Behavioral decision theory. Ann Rev Psychol 28:1–39, 1977.
46. Zola LK: Studying the decision to see a doctor: Review, critique, corrective. Adv Psychosom Med 8:216–236, 1972.
47. Lewis E: The management of stillbirth: Coping with an unreality. Lancet 2:619–620, 1976. An eloquent plea to help parents grieve realistically.

2

Who Should Have Genetic Counseling: Case Finding

Joy Ruth Cohen, RN, MSN, CNM, and Marlene B. Rudnick, BA

This chapter focuses on people. on what they want, and how they express their need for genetic counseling. The case studies offered here will demonstrate the relevance of genetic assessment and counsel.

OVERVIEW

Most people, even some physicians, are not aware that a medical specialty, genetic counseling, exists. In addition, people may not know where to get such counseling, how to use it, or how to make it available to persons who do need it. Perhaps to some, genetic counseling is suggestive of the same stigma formerly attributed to the necessity for psychiatric care. To others, perhaps it is a suggestion of self or family fraility, a diminution of the ego, and a shadow on the future.

The quality of future generations depends upon the fertilization of undamaged ova by genetically sound sperm. If a genetically defective zygote survives, the infant born can cause disastrous financial burdens, intense anguish, and years of unresolved guilt for the families so afflicted. To these people, genetic counseling can become an integrated and essential component of family planning. They seek ways to avoid inflicting upon their progeny, hazards inherent in their own genetic structure, when it is established that such hazards exist. Some couples clearly desire that reproduction stop with them, because of the potential clinical devastation for a child born of their union.

Often, major genetic risks are taken by couples because there is such a paucity of accurate and comprehensible information. Advice about genetic problems is dangerous if it is inaccurate, but it is equally dangerous for advice to be given in such a way that it is not understood or if it antagonizes the recipients. Decisions based on sound genetic counsel can offer various options for a couple. For example, they may choose to go ahead with procreation and seek prenatal diagnostic testing at the time of pregnancy, or they may decide on complete contraception and adopt children. Not all genetic risk is indication for contraception, or if contraception fails, for abortion. There are cases in which the problem can be corrected surgically or medically. This, too, has implications for genetic counseling which will be discussed below.

31

At times, couples present carefully compiled clinical manuscripts. This broad base of data may include pedigrees, statements of cost from care facilities, psychiatric and obstetrical recommendations, hormonal studies, and even photographs. In some cases, a family member whose physical appearance vividly demonstrates the nature and extent of the problem is brought to the counselor. Conversely, there are those who are much less articulate. They grope for answers, guidance, and justification for their existence and their desire to procreate. Some of these people seek confirmation and reinforcement for prior decisions while others seek guidance from a knowledgeable counselor who will listen, will piece together the relevant parts of the puzzle, and who will explain empathetically those parts of the picture that are applicable to that couple's life plan.

There are many ways by which people come to the realization that they need genetic counseling. Unexpected information may be found through routine diagnostic tests or special genetic screening tests. This may occur during an otherwise normal pregnancy. There are others who are stunned by a genetically determined abnormality at the birth of a long-awaited, already loved infant. At that time, the parents are shocked by a less than perfect, less than healthy infant, who may enjoy a less than fulfilling life. Often, a genetic problem becomes apparent only after successive family members develop an illness, such as Huntington's disease, which could have been predicted had adequate knowledge and counseling been available earlier.

No matter what precipitates the need for genetic counseling, many of the people who seek it come with a combination of hopefulness and hopelessness, with the fear of being too hopeful and the plague of feeling hopeless. People also protect themselves from further hurt by presenting their own defensive facades. Some assume an open and smiling attitude and eagerly anticipate positive words of assurance and hope. Others openly plead for any scrap of information which might reverse the negative direction in which they see their lives moving. Some verbalize or behaviorally demonstrate their feelings of fear, anxiety, and frustration. Some wring their hands; still others cry; and some stoically parrot medical terms without any understanding of the "why" and "how." Others adamantly deny the existence of any problem, and may refuse to seek help, or may refuse to listen to any counsel. While it is easy to say these things, it is ironic that pitifully few persons who might benefit from genetic counseling are aware that it exists, and is obtainable.

Each person involved in health care delivery systems should be sensitive to, and ever mindful of, the individual's right to information about himself or herself, as an individual, as a family member, and as a procreative member of society. In the eyes of the public, genetic counseling is viewed as new, and possibly threatening, because many of its negative applications have been publicized widely. Certainly then, we need to stress the positive aspects of genetic counseling as a tool by which to enhance the quality of one's own life, as well as the life of one's progeny. Therefore, it becomes clear that genetic counseling is a special and essential type of preventive medicine.

APPLICATIONS

Despite the fact that the potential benefits of genetic counseling have been demonstrated, one should not assume that these concepts have been or will be fully implemented. If we assume, however, that genetic counseling is freely available, we can go on to discuss when it is needed most: those years during which a woman is fertile.

At present, couples appear to investigate and then consider the options available to them more carefully than ever before. Whether it is conventional or not, the number of couples who live together during a premarital period to develop and "try out" a relationship has increased markedly. More and more, these couples seek information, guidance, and specific methods of contraception. Thus, family planning facilities are increasingly well utilized. It is through these facilities that genetic counseling should be available and publicized. Family planning, whether contraception or conception, enjoys a reciprocity with genetics. Therefore, health care services for young women, men, and couples should include an investigation of their pedigrees as an integral part of total care. First, questions concerning the genetic background of a couple should be asked in the initial interview, then written into the primary health status assessment, and finally, incorporated into the individual and family history. All this information could be labeled collectively as the "genetic data bank." Furthermore, the couple must be viewed, not only as a unit, but as two separate individuals; as such, they are descendants of two specific families. For example, families belonging to certain ethnic groups are more susceptible to particular genetic disorders, such as Tay-Sachs disease and sickle cell and Cooley anemia. What should be applied in each individual case history is a checklist of group related genetic problems. After the problems on this checklist are eliminated, more specific information as to individual family related problems then can be investigated. If any familial problems do exist, it then must be determined if they are truly genetic in origin. If either the man or the woman has a family history of possible genetic disorder, it must be determined if this is a dominant, recessive, or polygenic trait. In any case, since potential danger does exist, to a greater or lesser extent, this information should be included as part of the "genetic data bank." In other words, the ideal is to have an effective method designed to assess ancestral health consistently and to measure its influence on present and future generations.

In addition, there is a need to listen — not only to the heart beat, the lung sounds, and the description of symptoms — but to the incidental remark, the casual question, the subtle hint that a cause for further questioning or examination might exist. Indeed, there is a need to listen more purposefully. This differs fundamentally from the need to ask random questions in a conversational way, in order to put the individual or couple at ease during the examination. Direct, honest, pointed dialogue with the patient is necessary to extract the broadest base of factual background possible, so that high quality, safe, and effective care can be provided consistently.

Next, action is required. That action must be knowledgeable, effective, and efficient, and must take into consideration the total family. It should not be directed toward just one person. This action may take a variety of forms, but it must reflect the purpose of the service offered within the context of total health care, of which genetic counseling is one part. Those families who have experienced genetic problems should be counseled before they plan to have another child. However, it seems that the majority of family planning agencies, as well as physicians, direct their efforts toward contraception with little or no thought to advising the couple about having children.

Finally, it is important that the action taken, that is, referral to a genetic counselor, be validated. In other words, there must be feedback from the geneticist as to the propriety of the referral, the interpretation of the genetic information, and the content of the counsel given. A list of options for the couple must be formulated, presented, and reinforced by various members of the health care team. These options are subject to the couple's approval, implementation, or amendment.

One of the options for a couple to consider may be therapeutic abortion. Although few people would have problems accepting the inevitability of spontaneous abortions, therapeutic abortions present problems of a different nature. This type of abortion is performed electively; often it is performed because the fetus is not normal, or because the prospective mother's health is jeopardized. When the medical indications are obvious, it may not be too difficult for a couple to handle the situation emotionally. On the other hand, the emotional impact may be greater than appreciated, despite the fact that the abortion was indicated medically.

Most spontaneous abortions occur because the fetus was not viable, or because the intrauterine environment was not conducive to its development. Often, a genetic problem is responsible, and referral to a genetic counselor is indicated, particularly when there are recurrent miscarriages. However, nutritional, psychological, and pastoral counseling also might be indicated.

If an abortus presents with an anomaly that may be evidence of a genetic problem, too often it is either ignored or overlooked by the attendant physicians and nursing personnel. Conversely, the anomaly may have a nongenetic cause. For example, defects may occur when a drug (ie, thalidomide) is given which changes the intrauterine environment, particularly during the first trimester of pregnancy.

Elective abortions, those induced for nonmedical reasons, (ie, the preference of one or both of the parents) may present more emotional overtones for the couple. Despite a desire not to have a child at a specific time, the couple may feel very uncomfortable because of various moral, religious, and societal pressures. (The decision to have an abortion is unacceptable to a substantial number of people in our society.) On the other hand, when an elective abortion terminates a pregnancy which would have produced an anomalous infant, there is less emotional upheaval because the abortion is defensible. The parents are able to rationalize and justify the action; therefore, guilt is mitigated. In this type of situation, genetic counseling is strongly indicated and more readily accepted than in situations where the baby was really wanted, and where the loss is felt in greater depth.

The following case studies are illustrative of situations in which genetic counseling would have application. The histories are about real people; no case has been fabricated.

Case 1

Donald and Marilyn A. were married four months after they met. Eleven months after marriage, Marilyn was delivered of a 6 pound, 3 ounce boy following a long and difficult labor. The infant's Apgar* score was 3 at 1 minute and 5 at 5 minutes following birth. Despite intensive care and consultation with skilled neonatologists, the infant died 5 hours later. Autopsy revealed that the infant's lungs were so underdeveloped that they were unable to support life. When told of the probable cause of death, Marilyn shook her head and disclaimed any knowledge of a problem such as this in her family. Meanwhile, Donald paled visibly. He remembered a younger brother who had died shortly after birth of "bad lungs." Upon subsequent enquiry, Donald was told by his family that this respiratory weakness was a part of the family history and had manifested itself over several generations. No member of his family had spoken of it since they believed that it would "serve no useful purpose."

Even if a precise prediction might not have been possible (no specific genetic diagnosis is possible here without more information), this is a clear illustration of how genetic counsel could have been of benefit. If a full family history had been known before they had children, Donald and Marilyn could have been forewarned about the possibility of a lung disorder. Therefore, the trauma of this experience would have been mitigated, although not necessarily eliminated. Further, the problem might have been predictable by recently developed diagnostic techniques.

Cases 2 and 3

James B. and Pamela C. planned to be married. Each went to a private physician to obtain the traditional clean bill of health and the standard blood tests.

During the examination, Pam's physician asked routine questions to elicit her personal and family history. Almost as an afterthought, he asked about her mother's

*The Apgar score is a measure of vital functions. At birth it is normally above 7, and is usually 9 or 10.

obstetrical history. Pam related that her mother had been pregnant four times, although only two children, both girls, had been carried to term. These pregnancies had been successful only after Pam's mother had been given a special hormone (diethylstilbestrol). She said, "The medicine had an odd and very long name." She added, "My Mom used to call us her 'D-E-S-perate babies!'" Pam laughed. Her physician smiled at the "D-E-S-perate babies" remark, but made plans to screen Pamela's vaginal and cervical mucosa, because this hormone may cause vaginal cancer in females exposed during fetal life. He told Pamela that he was concerned that her mother's medication of 18 years before might cause her (Pam) serious health problems. She accepted his explanation of the risk of vaginal cancer and hoped that proper care would eliminate the problem. Another of her concerns, however, was whether, like her mother, she would be unable to carry a pregnancy to term.

Meanwhile , James had also had his premarital examination and was given a clean bill of health. When advised of the results of Pam's examination, he was shocked. Together, they suffered through discussions filled with piercing questions and brutal honesty. James wanted very much to be the father of a large family. Pam, too, had anticipated parenthood, although she had wanted to have only one or two children. James could not accept the fact that Pamela was what he considered to be an "unhealthy female." He looked at her in a different, less caring way, seeing her as an impediment to his deep desire to father his own children. The two of them were advised to seek further medical and genetic counsel. Although they did so, James barely participated in the counseling sessions. They agreed not to marry.

Pamela pursued genetic counseling as a source of information and guidance. She brought her sister and her mother into the discussions and played a responsible role in securing medical care for them. Three years later, Pamela married another man. She and her husband decided to adopt children rather than run the risk of repeated spontaneous abortions.

In this case history we see that an option to discontinue a relationship was made possible by appropriate counsel. This couple's decision was not made haphazardly, but was based on sound reasoning, for them. Obviously, this was only one of several options available to Pamela and James. In spite of the fact that a reconciliation was not possible for this couple, genetic counseling allowed an intelligent decision to be made by them.

Couples who experience the devastation brought on by the appearance of chromosomal anomalies at the birth of a child are another group of people who unexpectedly need genetic counseling. They require effective counseling quickly. Although a couple may not be able to understand and utilize all that the geneticist has to offer until after the initial shock and acute grief have passed, they need to be made aware of the existence of genetic counseling and what it offers. They should be given clarification about the cause of their baby's problem, a projection for the baby's future, specific information about the risks of recurrence with future children, and appropriate counsel about reproductive options. To withhold this kind of direction from such a couple under the guise of kindness, as is so often the practice, is a medical *unkindness* which must not be allowed to continue. It is erroneous to assume that individuals involved in personal grief cannot accept and respond to therapeutic help.

Nancy and Jack D. had an obstetrical experience that certainly warranted such help. Consider the birth of their third child.

Case 4

Nancy's obstetrical history, including this pregnancy, was essentially normal. Together, the couple had participated actively in the birth of each of their children. They had shared the excitment of each pregnancy with formal preparation and happy anticipation. This excitement had culminated with the birth of each baby. There had been no reason to expect that the birth of their third child would be any different. Then came the shock. At the time of delivery, they saw a gray, limp baby with un unusually large, rather translucent head. The rest of the infant's body seemed puny by comparison. Although Jack and Nancy wanted to look at the baby, the little that they could see, frightened them.

Nancy related her emotional turmoil as a series of disconnected thoughts. She said that she felt as though she were shouting.

Please help me, I'm frightened!

Why don't I hear the baby?

Why are there so many people suddenly coming into the room?

What's wrong?

What was that shot they just gave me?

Is it a boy or a girl?

Is it alive?

Please, let me hold the baby.

I feel so tired.

What's wrong?

I want to look at the baby.

I'm frightened!

"Somehow everything was overshadowed by both love and pain." Nancy continued, "I heard many voices, but felt Jack's closeness. I heard many words, but I felt his tears. Lots of hands touched me, but I felt Jack's presence. Then the pediatrician said, 'The baby has very little chance for survival. He's hydrocephalic.' He died several days later."

Nancy was moved to a private room where, for twenty hours, she received physical care and routine sedation. Twenty-four hours following delivery, she was discharged. She was advised by the staff only that she would recover faster at home than in the hospital. They believed that the hospital setting would remind her of her malformed infant and its imminent death, and thus would hamper her own recuperation. The hospital staff made this decision without consulting either Jack or Nancy. Neither did the staff make any attempt to discuss with the couple the baby's malformation or its cause. Further, neither parent was permitted to see the infant again. They were told that it was "against hospital policy," a policy which supposedly was formulated to alleviate the grief of the parents. No effort was made to secure the services of a genetic counselor or a clergyman during this critical time. Furthermore, Nancy and Jack were not even advised that services of this type were available. Thus, in the future, if they should decide to have another child, they would be unaware of, and consequently, unable to utilize such counseling.

At this point, it must be obvious to all concerned health professionals that an abrogation of responsibility and a violation of patient's rights, as illustrated by the above case history is a medical injustice.

Consider the case history of Jane and Peter E.; their experience (Case 5) will serve to exemplify the callousness and carelessness to which parents may be subjected. To be explicit, the physician and nursing staff must assume responsibility for total patient care. In addition, they must be held, at the least, morally accountable for any dereliction in that duty. It is incumbent upon all those in health care delivery systems to be aware that these responsibilities are not always met. This causes undue hardship and pain to the families involved. In the case of Jane and Peter, not only was psychological counseling necessary, but genetic counseling was indicated as well. They had suffered the trauma of a stillborn infant. Further, the child had a unilateral club foot. Incidentally, the club foot was not even mentioned to either Peter or Jane. It came to light only upon subsequent examination of the infant's medical record, which was conducted by Jane's present obstetrician. Jane was now eleven years older, and although she was past prime childbearing age, she found herself pregnant for the second time. Therefore, genetic counseling was not only appropriate, but necessary to ensure that the child of this pregnancy would not exhibit any of those defects made possible because of Jane's age.

Case 5

As indicated, Jane's first pregnancy had terminated with the birth of a stillborn infant. Neither Peter nor Jane had any idea why the baby had died, even though an autopsy had been performed. Understandably, eleven years after this unhappy episode, Jane was alarmed to learn that she was pregnant. The basis for her alarm was twofold. One was the memory of that first traumatic loss and the fear that it might recur; the second was her age. She knew that women in their thirties and forties are at greater risk of having a child afflicted with Down syndrome. Jane was so upset by this unexpected pregnancy that she contemplated an abortion. Hesitantly, she discussed this possibility with Peter. Together, they agreed that as a first step they would seek the advice of the second obstetrician, at whose office the diagnostic pregnancy test had been done.

As she and Peter sat in this physician's office, Jane related her past obstetrical history. After listening to her story, her physician concluded that her first pregnancy had been essentially normal. However, during labor, she had felt a sudden, excruciating pain in her abdomen. When closely questioned, she recalled that her abdomen had remained tense, and that the pain had not diminished. Neither of these symptoms is consistent with the normal pattern of uterine contractions during labor. Altough she had been told that the pains she had felt were "normal," her present obstetrician disagreed. He believed that the sudden, sustained pain, board-like condition of the abdomen, and the absence of vaginal bleeding, were indicative of placenta abruptio (the sudden separation of the placenta from its maternal blood supply). This condition causes fetal anoxia. Indeed, Jane reported that she had become aware of a sudden cessation of movement on the part of the baby. At that point, Peter said that he had been asked to leave the labor room.

No further details concerning the remainder of Jane's labor or delivery were available to the couple. Jane had awakened hours later, unattended by either Peter or any hospital staff member. As Jane and Peter continued their narrative, it became clear to the obstetrician that they had learned of the stillbirth of their child via a series of unrelated and inhumane mishaps. Staff members had refused to answer any questions about the baby. In spite of Jane's pleas – she had not seen the baby – no one brought the baby to her. Peter was totally ignored; his requests to see Jane and his efforts to find out what had happened to their infant were fruitless. Although no information concerning the stillbirth had been given to either of the parents, the hospital pathologist had assumed that Jane had been told. He walked into her room to explain that he needed her written permission to perform an autopsy, and thus, was the first to tell her of the baby's death. Her present obstetrician was horrified by the callousness and carelessness of all the personnel involved.

This case is hard to believe or to surpass as a graphic illustration of the insensitivity with which entire situations are sometimes handled. Many parents, however, have had similar unhappy experiences. This couple was fortunate, because their second obstetrician did take the time to listen to them, and thus was able to give them the counsel they desperately needed.

IMPLICATIONS

Some of the situations in which the need for genetic counseling is evident are best exemplified in an informal study conducted (by JRC) over a period of six months. The 100 couples who participated in this study were interviewed*

---

*Interviews were conducted in: a) a family planning center, b) an obstetrical-gynecological clinic, c) a postpartum unit, d) the office of a private obstetrician, 3) the office of a Certified Nurse-Midwife.

as part of their comprehensive health history. Thirty-seven of these couples said that they were "aware of genetics," that is, they had heard the word and knew that it related to the medical profession in some way. Of these 37 , twenty-six knew of the existence of genetic counseling service. However, only 19 said that they would know where to go if they ever needed counseling. Finally, of those 19, only 9 said that they would feel comfortable seeking such help on their own.

Twenty-seven of the women who were interviewed were over the age of 31. These women were candidates for genetic assessment and counsel because the incidence of trisomy-21 increases with maternal age. Of those 27 women, 10 had been referred to a genetic counselor for help prior to the interview. One wonders why the other 17 had not been referred to a counselor so that they could be informed of the risks involved.

The questionnaires used in this study revealed that 16 couples had had a child with congenital anomalies. These 16 couples were encouraged to seek genetic counsel at the completion of the interview. Four couples indicated that they had been advised to obtain help prior to the interview by their private physicians. The other 12 couples had not been informed of the genetic implications of their situation, nor had they been advised of the necessity for and the availability of genetic counsel. Shortly thereafter, 7 of these 12 sought professional advice, which resulted in significant changes in the management of the women's obstetric care. Presented with the various genetic risks and the options available, some elected to abort the fetus, others opted for both an abortion and sterilization, and still others went on to more extensive genetic assessment, such as amniocentesis. With diagnostic methods utilizing amniocentesis, it is possible to assess the presence of chromosomal and other abnormalities in the fetus. No matter what the results of this assessment, however, the final decision as to which course to follow rests with the parents. The counselor's role is one in which care must be exerted so that the counselor's bias does not color the presentation of the options available.

It is clear that the indications for genetic counsel are manifold, and at times, quite subtle. Nine of the couples interviewed had living children with a known anomaly, such as syndactyly, phenylketonuria, and cleft palate, which can be treated either surgically or medically. One set of parents referred to their child as "normal." It was only upon close questioning that it became apparent that their "normal" child had several congenital defects which had been repaired surgically (bilateral syndactyly, hare lip, and cleft palate). At the proper time, these children should be informed of the reproductive risks they run; this should be done as part of preparation for their future. To be sure, some problems are of greater magnitude than others. Families in which Huntington disease, or Tay-Sachs syndrome exist should be carefully and fully informed of the consequences involved. A family in which the problem is of lesser severity may also need counseling. Each member of any affected family should be informed concerning the extent of the problem and how it affects each individual.

When fetal malformations can be attributed to nongenetic causes such as drugs or viral infections, the parents can be reassured that the abnormality was caused by a change in the intrauterine environment. The parents should be advised that there is no cause for concern about the outcome of any future pregnancies, since the gene complement of the affected fetus is normal. Thus, couples may be assured that they have less cause for concern than they had feared. This is a very positive aspect of genetic counseling, and it is among those which should be stressed.

SUMMARY

In this chapter, the significance of genetic counseling, and the various ways in which candidates for such counsel are found, have been illustrated via five case histories. The informal study conducted in several primary health care facilities also is indicative of the manner in which the need for this type of help is realized. In addition, classses conducted in preparation for childbirth and parenthood would be an ideal place in which to determine if any of the prospective parents are likely candidates for genetic counsel. It would be essential that the practitioner teaching the class be sensitive enough to recognize some of the more subtle signals which might indicate a need for further investigation. He or she must also be knowledge-able enough to initiate the enquiries which would elicit the responses necessary to determine if there is cause for referral to a genetic counselor, and discreet enough to inform the prospective parents with no hint of stigma. Therefore, it would be helpful if all health care practitioners were given some updated background in human genetics, as well as information about available genetic counseling resources.

The genetic counselor must be attuned to the needs of the individual in the context of his or her relationship within an entire family. In addition, the counselor must be responsive to each individual situation, exhibit competency in dispensing genetic information, and be cognizant of the scope and limitations of such information. Finally, advisors must constantly bear in mind that a handicapped child will exert a lasting effect on a family. Without prior experience, a family will have difficulty understanding the impact of this effect. The counselor will have to explain these effects with lucidity and honesty to the family involved. At the same time, the individual must be considered as a totality greater than the sum of the results of diagnostic tests which indicate that a child may be less than perfect. This is an implementation of the holistic approach. The interdisciplinary approach addresses itself to the interdependence of the various parts of the health care system; for example, there is a reciprocal relationship between the services rendered by the physician, the nurse-midwife, and the genetic counselor, among others. Therefore, these approaches should be accepted as essential elements in total health care. In this idealized situation, total health care includes genetic counseling.

ANNOTATED REFERENCES

1. Nagle J: Heredity and Human Affairs. St. Louis, C.V. Mosby, 1974.
A thorough review of information basic to human genetics. A clear exposition of the basis of some genetic defects is given. Also describes some of the clinical manifestations of these defects and how these anomalies affect the quality of life of the individuals and families involved.

2. Eggen R: Chromosome Diagnostics in Clinical Medicine. Springfield, IL, Charles C. Thomas, 1965.
A clear, basic review of facts about chromosome structure and the effects of chromosome abnormality on the individual and society. Chapter IX, Indications for Cytogenetic Testing, lists clinical applications in which these cytogenetic techniques can be used.

> Until the advent of cytogenetic techniques, the physician faced with the distressing task of assessing the outcome of future preg— nancies following the birth of a mongol or other congenitally de- formed infant was wholly dependent upon statistical analysis. Cytogenetic techniques provide a method of obtaining objective evidence upon which to base such prognoses (p. 150).

3. AAAS Committee on Scientific Freedom and Responsibility. Scientific Freedom and Responsibility. American Association for the Advancement of Science, Washington, D.C., 1975.
Espouses the legitimacy of fetal research. It is opposed to the continuation of the ban on such reserach. Without this investigation of the human fetus, major breakthroughs in clin- ical diagnosis of fetal anomalies would have been well-nigh impossible. Specific examples of these advances are found in the diagnosis and ultimate resolution of the problems of erythroblastosis fetalis and respiratory distress syndrome.

3

How Genes Are Transmitted in Families

Marian L. Rivas, PhD

INTRODUCTION

Rapid advances in clinical genetics in the past decade have been due largely to advances and breakthroughs in clinical diagnosis and to an increased awareness of the importance of genetic factors in the etiology of disease. Accurate diagnosis, proper treatment and/or management of genetic disease and correct assessment of genetic risk depend on a physician's clinical acumen; his understanding of theoretical, analytical, and applied genetics, and his ability to elicit and interpret a good family history. The complementary approaches of medicine and genetics are basic to the genetic counseling process. This chapter, deals with the fundamental concepts of gene transmission and expression, [1] and what may be called the "genetic approach" to inherited disease.

THE BASIC PRINCIPLES

Genetic Transmission and Chromosomal Behavior

Over its evolutionary history, each species has accumulated genetic information uniquely its own, packaged in a specific set of chromosomes containing all the genes in a *genome.* In man, this set consists of 23 pairs of chromosomes for a total chromosome number of 46. As shown in Figure 1, each pair is unique in size, shape, and banding pattern. Twenty-two pairs (numbers 1 through 22) are termed *autosomes;* the twenty-third is the sex chromosome pair. Except for the sex chromosomes in males (XY), members of a chromosome pair are homologous — ie, morphologically similar save for minor variations.

In the life cycle of man (or any sexually reproducing species) growth and maintenance of the organism from the single-celled zygote stage through adulthood is accomplished by coordinated multiplication, growth, and differentiation of cells derived from the zygote. For every cell division, the genetic material of the parental cell is precisely duplicated and distributed equally to the two daughter cells.

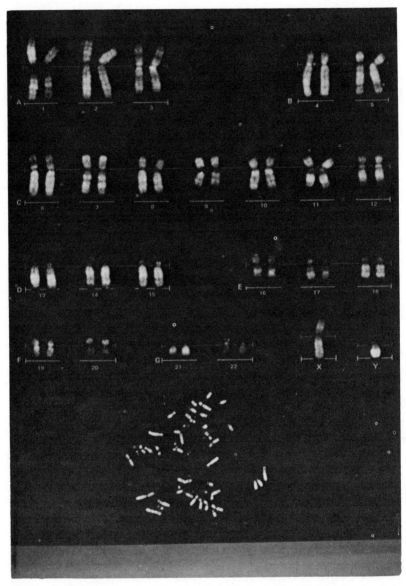

Fig. 1. Chromosomes from a normal human male by the Q-staining method revealing Q-bands as seen under a fluorescent microscope in a metaphase spread (below) and in the karyotype derived from this cell. Identification of each chromosome of the human complement is possible because of the characteristic banding pattern of each pair and the high degree of similarity between homologs. (Courtesy of Dr. R. Ellen Magenis, Univ. of Oregon Health Sciences Center).

In this way, every somatic or body cell contains the same genetic information as that originally in the zygote. However, if the same mechanisms of cell duplication were operative in the production of gametic or reproductive cells, genetic information would double each generation ad infinitum.

Thus, two types of cell division are operative during the life of an individual: 1) *mitosis*, the division process by which each daughter cell of a somatic cell retains chromosomally and genetically identical material, both qualitatively and quantitatively, and 2) *meiosis*, the reductional process that separates each member of a pair of chromosomes so that a gamete receives one-half of the "genetic packet."

As a result of meiosis, a single member of each of the 23 pairs of chromosomes is distributed to each gamete. This reduction of chromosomal (and, therefore, genetic) material by one-half is the result of an extremely precise set of divisions that guarantees that every gamete contains each of the 23 distinct chromosomes, or one *haploid set* of the genome. At the time of fertilization, when two gametes (sperm and egg) fuse, the *diploid* chromosome number (46) of the individual is restored.

As every chromosome contains thousands of genes, one can follow their transmittance and fate in relation to other genes on the basis of chromosomal behavior during cell division, particularly meiosis. Let us first consider a single gene located at a specific point — its *locus* — on an autosome. Since each autosome has a homolog, it follows that each gene A on an autosome has a counterpart A' at the corresponding or homologous locus. As shown in Figure 2a, haploid gametes contain one and only one *allele* at every locus. Since homologs separate or segregate during the first meiotic division, gametes containing A or A' occur in the ratio of 1:1. Therefore, the statement to an individual, "There is a fifty-fifty chance of your transmitting this particular gene to each offspring," has as its basis the segregation of alleles at the first meiotic division and the random involvement of a gamete bearing A or A' in fertilization.

Let us now consider the behavior of two pairs of genes, AA' and BB', located on different chromosomes (Fig 2b). The four possible genic combinations in the gametes are AB, A'B, AB' and A'B'. These combinations result from the only two possible alignments of the chromosome pairs in meiosis. If the paternal homolog of *either* pair has a 50–50 chance of being oriented toward each pole, it follows that the orientation of one chromosome pair is independent of the orientation of the other. Thus the two alignments are equally likely, with resulting gametes expected to have the four genic combinations in the ratio of 1:1:1:1. The statement, "The chance that you will transmit both genes A *and* B' to each offspring is 25%," has as its basis the independent assortment of gene pairs; ie, the 25% figure reflects the ½ chance of transmitting A (versus A') × the ½ chance of transmitting B' (versus B), since the occurrence of one event is *independent* of the occurrence of the other. If this reasoning is extended to 3 gene pairs on separate chromosomes, the number of genic combinations equals 8, (2^3); for 4 loci, the number is 16, (2^4).

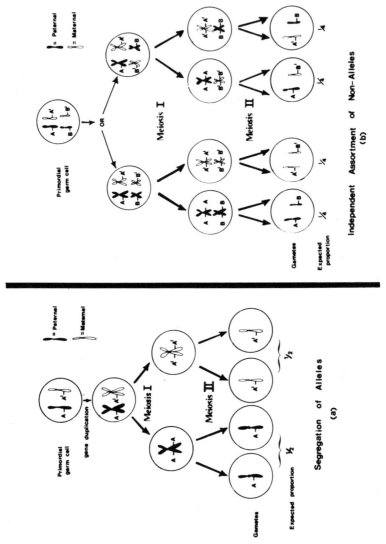

Fig. 2. Diagrammatic representation of the chromosomal bases of the Mendelian laws of segregation and independent assortment. (a) Segregation of alleles A, A' at first meiotic division and the expected 1:1 ratio of the alleles among the gametes. (b) The alternate arrangements of the maternal and parternal members of each of two chromosome pairs at meiosis I and the resulting proportion of gametes.

For 23 pairs of genes, each on a different chromosome, the probability that any gamete will contain a specific combination of chromosomes (and their genes) is $(\frac{1}{2})^{23}$, or approximately 1 in 8 million.

Independent transmission of gene pairs, however, need not hold for genes located on the same chromosome — ie, *syntenic* loci — because such genes should have a greater than random chance of being included in the same gamete. The fact that they are not always transmitted together is due to the phenomenon of crossing over, a physical exchange of chromosomal (and therefore genic) material occurring prior to the first meiotic division when each chromosome has already doubled to form two *chromatids* (gene duplication in Fig 2a).

During the alignment of homologous chromosomes in meiosis — *synapsis* — the two chromatids involved in a crossover event break at identical points and exchange segments distal to the break points (Fig 3). The parental combination of genes on one side of the break remains intact, whereas the genic material on the other side of the break is exchanged with that from the other chromatid. The frequency with which crossing over occurs is a reflection of the distance between any two loci (exceptions are known), in general, the greater the distance, the higher the crossover frequency.

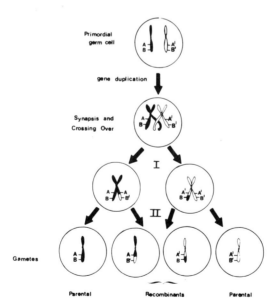

Fig. 3. Synapsis and crossing over prior to the first meiotic division. The four types of chromosomes resulting from a single crossover event are shown. The chromosomes in two of the gametes retain the parental combination of genes; the other two contain a new combination of alleles and are called *recombinants*.

From Figure 3, we see that if crossing over does not occur between the two loci — ie, the homologs are not involved in an exchange — then allele A will always travel with B, and allele A′ with B′, the ratio of the two parental combinations being 1:1 in the gametes. If, on the other hand, crossing over *does occur* between locus *A* and locus *B*, four genic (2 parental and 2 recombinant) combinations will result: AB, A′B, AB′ and A′B′ — the same four combinations expected when the two loci are on separate chromosomes (Compare with Fig 2b). However, unlike the earlier situation, the four are not equally likely. If a single crossover occurs between *A* and *B* in 10% of meiotic divisions, then 10% of all gametes produced by an individual are of the recombinant A′B, AB′ type. At a crossover frequency of 30%, 15% of the gametes will be A′B; 15%, AB′; 35% AB; and 35%, A′B′. As the crossover frequency approaches 50%, the percentage of each of the four products approaches that expected for loci assorting independently, namely, 25% AB, A′B, 25% AB′ and 25% A′B′. Therefore, syntenic loci, which are far enough apart (eg, on extreme ends of a chromosome) that crossing over is virtually certain to occur will behave as if they were on separate chromosomes. Conversely, a significant deviation from the expected 1:1:1:1 segregation ratio for two apparently independent loci is a clue to their possible syntenic relationship on a single chromosome.

The chromosomal behavior patterns that lead to segregation of alleles — ie, 1) *independent assortment* of unlinked gene pairs and 2) *recombination* of linked genes — are properties common to each meiotic event. Thus, if each meiotic process leading to a gamete is independent of that leading to every other gamete, it follows that one genic combination in a gamete will neither influence nor depend upon the combination in any other gamete. The statement, "The chance that you will transmit A′ (versus A) to each of your first two children is 25%," is based on this principle, since the probability that A′ will be involved in the first fertilization is ½ and in the second is also ½, so the chance that both will happen is $(½)^2 = ¼$. Similarly, the probability that a father will transmit both A′ and a Y-chromosome to each of two offspring is: ½ (Probability of transmitting A′) × ½ (Probability of transmitting a Y) × ½ (Probability of transmitting A′ the second time) × ½ (Probability of transmitting a Y the second time) = 1/16. In other words, the alignment of the Y-chromosome and the homolog bearing the A′ allele in the first meiotic event does not influence the way in which these two chromosomes align the second time. Thus, an individual may always, never, or occasionally transmit a particular allele or set of alleles to his offspring. On the average, given enough offspring, he will pass on any given allele 50% of the time.

Genotype—Phenotype Correlation

Even though duplication of genetic material prior to each cell division is a remarkably accurate process, errors in gene duplication, referred to as *mutations*, do occur. These changes, which take place from time to time, include 1) changes involving a single gene (point mutations) and 2) changes resulting from chromosomal changes or exchanges such as translocations, deletions, inversions, and unequal crossing over (see Chapter 4). The section that follows focuses on the former.

A *gene* or *cistron* may be defined, in the simplest of terms, as the smallest unit of genetic material – ie, the smallest portion of DNA – which determines the primary amino acid sequence of a polypeptide chain or protein. Each amino acid is designated by a triplet of nucleotide bases in the DNA chain. An alteration in a single base or group of bases may lead to an altered gene product.

An altered gene at a given locus, which codes for an altered gene product, is termed an *allele*. Whether the mutation resulting in an altered product is advantageous, neutral, or deleterious will depend on how the product deviates from the "norm." If the base changes are minor, such that the activity or function of the protein is not altered to any appreciable extent, the mutation leads to little more than a "normal" variation at that locus, which indeed may not be detectable. If, however, the mutation alters the structure of the protein so as to affect its function seriously, the consequences may be detrimental to the individual carrying it. (This is an oversimplification of the situation, to be sure, since mutations that may be deleterious under certain environmental situations may be neutral or even advantageous under different conditions. The same could be said of "neutral" genes).

Any allele is subject to error during the process of replication; ie, all alleles are liable to mutate to another form. Although mutations are relatively rare events, certain characteristic mutations recur more frequently than others. Estimates of mutation rates (μ) in man are, at best, only rough approximations, with most values falling in the range of 1×10^{-5} to 1×10^{-6} mutations per locus per generation. Mutations, therefore, introduce new gene forms into the gene pool; meiosis then disperses these forms in the population via the reshuffling of genic combinations.

The human genome is estimated to have tens of thousands of loci. Over 3,000 human genetic disorders described thus far appear to be due to mutations at single loci. Let us now consider a single autosomal locus with two alleles, A and A', each coding for qualitatively different polypeptide gene products, α_1, and α_2, respectively. Three *genotypes* (allelic combinations) are possible at this locus, namely AA, AA' and A'A'. Individuals *homozygous* for the A allele can produce only protein (or polypeptide) α_1; those homozygous for A' produce only protein α_2, and those *heterozygous* (genetically AA') produce both types of polypeptides, α_1 and α_2. If one were able to isolate or identify each of the gene products of the above locus, one could correctly infer the genotype of an individual from his *phenotype* (in this case, the presence of one or the other or both products). The genotype is said to be *expressed* by the phenotype. In this instance, the three phenotypes (α_1, $\alpha_1\alpha_2$, and α_2) would be expressions of the three genotypes at this locus.

If however, we observe the phenotype at a clinical rather than at a molecular or biochemical level — ie., we now look for the presence or absence of obvious clinical manifestations — we may not be able to detect the three genotypes.

Let us assume that allele a codes for a seriously defective protein that has little or no functional activity. A little intuition (!) will probably lead us to conclude that individuals homozygous for a (aa) would be at a serious disadvantage if this protein or enzyme played a critical role in cellular metabolism. Likewise, we would probably conclude that individuals who were homozygous for A (AA) would be compeletely normal, and that heterozygotes (Aa) may or may not manifest symptoms, depending on their capacity to handle this metabolic step with a partial enzyme complement.

If the heterozygotes manifested *some* clinical signs, then one could be reasonably certain of the genotypes of the three classes of individuals, for there would be a distinct phenotype for each genotype (assuming that AA show no symptoms and that aa are more severely affected than Aa.) If the heterozygotes show *no* symptoms, then only two phenotypes could be distinguished — normal (*AA* + *Aa*) and affected (*aa*).

It is often the case that one cannot distinguish the heterozygote from one of the homozygotes using clinical criteria alone. The phenotype, as observed at the clinical level, is often several steps removed from the state of gene action and is usually a reflection of the various effects of a mutant allele and its interactions with other gene loci. Therefore, what we observe as the phenotype may be the direct or indirect consequence of the mutant gene's effect. It is possible for the heterozygote AA′, that the product of its normal allele (protein α_1 from gene A) has sufficient activity and availability to compensate for the deficiency produced by the mutant allele A′, thereby "masking" the latter's effect at the clinical level. In general, the farther removed the phenotype is from the primary gene product, the more difficult it is to equate phenotype with a specific genotype.

Traits that are phenotypically apparent *only* in individuals homozygous for the gene are termed *recessive*. The alternate state, "absence of the trait," in such cases would be *dominant:* a single dose of a normal allele would suffice for an individual to be clinically free of symptoms. Individuals heterozygous at the locus, thus, are clinically indistinguishable from homozygous normals. When both alleles are equally manifest in a heterozygote, the traits are *codominant.*

Phenylketonuria (PKU) is an example of an autosomal recessive condition. individuals with mental retardation, fair complexion, impaired motor development, and abnormal urine phenylketones are homozygous, aa, for the mutant PKU allele a at the locus determining the enzyme phenylalanine hydroxylase and thus are incapable of converting phenylalanine to tyrosine. Parents of such individuals, who are not themselves homozygous, are clinically normal, even though genetically each must carry (mutations excluded) the mutant allele (ie, are Aa), and are heterozygous. The phenotype of PKU is recessive; the normal phenotype is dominant.

The most common form of brachydactyly, a condition characterized by short, stubby fingers with absence or underdevelopment of the phalanges, is an autosomal dominant condition. Individuals homozygous, BB, for the aberrant gene die early in infancy; heterozygotes (Bb) show various abnormalities of the hands and feet. The trait is dominant since the presence of a single dose of the B allele is sufficient for an individual to manifest the disorder. The normal phenotype in this situation is recessive, since two normal genes, bb, are required to assure freedom from this condition.

The blood groups A and B are codominant in people with type AB blood, whereas blood group O is recessive to A or B. "Dominance" and "recessiveness" are attributes of the trait and not of the gene. The condition sickle cell anemia illustrates this point well. At the clinical level, individuals presenting with retarded growth, hemolytic anemia, joint pains, and "crises" are homozygous for the β^S allele at the hemoglobin β locus. Clinically normal parents of such individuals are obligate carriers, $\beta^A\beta^S$ of the β^S gene and are phenotypically indistinguishable from homozygous normal individuals ($\beta^A\beta^A$). If samples of hemolyzed red cells from clinically normal ($\beta^A\beta^A$ and $\beta^A\beta^S$) individuals are subjected to electrophoresis, one observes two distinct results. Red cells from obligate carriers show two types of hemoglobins corresponding to the types of gene products these individuals produce, namely, HbA containing normal β^A chains and HbS containing abnormal β^S chains. Cells from homozygous normal $\beta^A\beta^A$ individuals show only a single product, HbA, upon electrophoresis. At the clinical level, the condition termed sickle cell anemia is recessive, and the normal condition is dominant; at the biochemical level, however, the phenotype "presence of sickle hemoglobin (HbS)," is dominant, since individuals with a single dose (ie., heterozygotes, $\beta^A\beta^S$) also manifest the trait. The β^S allele, in each instance, behaves exactly the same — it produces the β^S chain; our ability to detect its presence, however, depends on what we consider the phenotype to be. Relatively few genetic disorders are understood as clearly at the molecular or biochemical level as sickle cell anemia is understood.

Heterogeneity refers to the fact that certain phenotypes — eg, albinism or deafness — can have several different genetic (and nongenetic) causes [2].

Pleiotropy refers to the multiple phenotypic effects that a single gene disorder can have, eg, numerous and varied clinical manifestations of sickle cell anemia.

Distribution of Single Gene Traits in Families

Many genetic traits are distributed in families in characteristic mendelian patterns that result from 1) the segregation of alleles; 2) the location of the responsible gene on an autosome or sex chromosome; 3) the random involvement of gametes in fertilization; 4) the dominance or recessiveness of the trait.

Autosomal traits. For an autosomal locus with two alleles and three genotypes AA, Aa, and aa, there are six mating types. The genotypes of offspring expected from each of the six matings are given in Figure 4a. (Note: The relative frequency of each mating is dependent on the relative frequency of the two alleles in a population.) The proportion of each type of offspring from each mating is a consequence of the segregation of alleles in the parents and the random union of their gametes. Since any given autosomal chromosome is transmitted independently of the sex chromosomes, the distribution of genotypes is the same for male and female offspring.

What we observe in a family or pedigree, however, is not the gene(s) but the phenotype produced by the gene(s). Figure 4 illustrates the phenotypic distribution expected when the trait is dominant (Fig 4b) and when the trait is recessive (Fig 4c). Although the underlying genetic mechanisms are the same (Fig 4a), the observed phenotypic distributions differ with the expression of the gene(s).

Autosomal Dominant. The principal characteristics of autosomal dominant traits, as seen in Figure 4b, are

1) An affected person need only be heterozygous for the given allele A.
2) Every affected individual has at least one affected parent (except for mutations).
3) Male and female offspring are equally likely to be affected.
4) Individuals not manifesting the trait cannot pass on the responsible gene.
5) For rare conditions, most affected X normal matings are Aa X aa, (mating 5, Fig 4b) so that one-half of the offspring, on the average, are affected.
6) The rare AA individual may be much more severely affected than an Aa individual.

Autosomal Recessive. The distinguishing features of autosomal recessive traits, as seen in Figure 4c, are:
1) Every affected individual is homozygous for the given allele.
2) Each parent of an affected individual must carry at least one mutant allele.
3) Individuals possessing a single dose of the allele do not manifest the trait.

Fig. 4. Autosomal inheritance and patterns of transmission for allelic genes A and a at one locus. (a) The types of gametes produced by each parent and the expected genotypic proportions among offspring are given for each of the six possible matings. No distinction is made as to the sex of the parents or children, since autosomes are present in equivalent pairs in both males and females. (b) Phenotypic manifestation of a trait among parents and offspring for each mating type when the trait is dominant. Affected individuals (solid squares, males; circles, females) carry either one or two doses of the A allele. (c) Phenotypic distribution of an autosomal recessive trait among parents and offspring for each mating type. Note that only homozygous aa individuals manifest the trait and that heterozygous Aa individuals (dotted) are phenotypically normal.

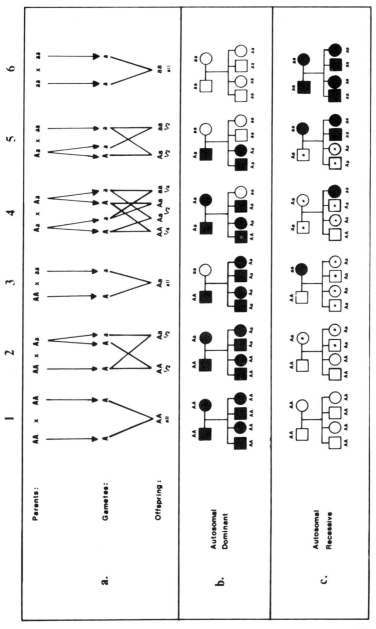

4) For rare autosomal recessive traits, most affected individuals have phenotypically normal parents (mating 4, Fig 4c).
5) On the average, the ratio of normal to affected offspring from these Aa
X Aa matings is 3:1.
6) Since relatives are more likely than non-relatives to be carriers of the same
rare mutant allele, consanguinity, the mating of relatives, is often found among
parents of individuals affected with a rare condition — the rarer the
trait, the higher the incidence of consanguineous matings among parents
of affected individuals.

X-linked Traits. Traits determined by genes on the X-chromosome are referred
to as X-linked. Although the X chromosome is involved in sex determination, most
genes on the X-chromosome have functions unrelated to sex. Colorblindness,
hemophilias A and B, G6PD (glucose-6-phosphate dehydrogenase) deficiency, Duchenne muscular dystrophy, and hypophosphatemia (vitamin D-resistant rickets)
are examples of traits determined by X-linked genes. Their expression depends on
the sex-chromosomal constitution of the individual.

For an X-linked locus with two alleles, females can be one of three genotypes,
AA, Aa, or aa. Since males have a heteromorphic XY sex chromosome pair, they
are hemizygous (carry only one allele) for each X-linked locus; thus, only two
genotypes are possible in males, A or a. (There are no proven Y-linked human disorders).

Figure 5 illustrates the segregation and transmission of alleles at an X-linked
locus for each of the six possible matings. It is apparent from this diagram that
for X-linked loci the genotype of each son is determined *solely* by the genotype
of the mother; whereas *both* parents contribute to the genotype of each daughter.

As one might expect, the phenotypic distribution of an X-linked trait in a
family depends on whether the trait is dominant or recessive in females. (These
terms have no meaning in males, since the presence of a single allele guarantees
that the phenotype must correspond to the genotype). If a single dose of the
gene is sufficient to produce the phenotypic effect in heterozygous females,
the trait is dominant; if homozygosity is required, the trait is recessive.

Fig. 5. X-linked inheritance and patterns of transmission. (a) The types of gametes with respect
to the X-chromosome produced by each parent and the expected proportion of genotypes
among male and female offspring are given for each of the six possible matings. Parental sex,
for each mating, is male (left) X female (right). (b) Phenotypic manifestation of an X-linked
recessive trait, among parents and offspring for each mating situation. Affected males are
hemizygous and affected females are homozygous for the a allele. Carrier females (dotted)
are genetically heterozygous Aa but, in general, phenotypically normal. (c) Phenotypic
distribution of an X-linked dominant trait. Hemizygous (A) males and homozygous (AA) or
heterozygous (Aa) females manifest the condition.

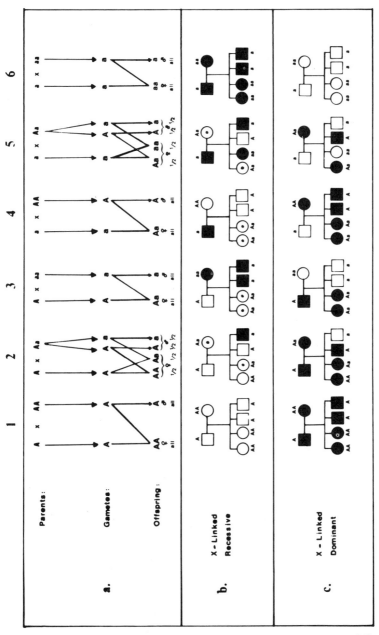

Correlation of genotype and phenotype for X-linked recessive and X-linked dominant traits can be seen in Figure 5.

X-linked Recessive. It should be noted that for X-linked recessive traits (Fig 5b):
1) more males than females express the trait;
2) heterozygous or carrier Aa females, do not express the trait (occasionally they do, but this is due to *lyonization,* or *random inactivation* of the X chromosome with variability of expression);
3) affected females (except for lyonization) are homozygous (aa); their mothers are carriers, and their fathers are affected;
4) affected males transmit their mutant allele to *each* of their daughters and *none* of their sons (the father and son involvement observed in Figure 5b, matings 5 and 6, is not an exception. The allele in the affected sons is of *maternal* origin);
5) on the average, heterozygous females transmit the recessive allele to one-half their offspring, regardless of sex.

The first three features are distinguishing features of X-linked recessive transmission; the last two are characteristics of X-chromosomal transmission and are, therefore, common also to X-linked dominant conditions.

X-linked Dominant. Since heterozygous females manifest X-linked dominant traits, more affected females are observed than for X-linked recessive conditions (contrast Fig 5c with 5b). Other distinguishing points of X-linked dominant traits follow:
1) On the average, one-half of the offspring of heterozygous female X normal male matings are affected regardless of sex. All of the offspring of homozygous female X normal male matings are affected regardless of sex.
2) *All* of the daughters and *none* of the sons of affected males are affected (the affected males in Fig. 5c, matings 1 and 2 received the A allele from their mothers).
3) On the average, the ratio of affected females to affected males is 2:1 for rare X-linked dominant traits, although the heterozygous females tend to be less severely affected than the hemizygous males.

Patterns of transmission in families. An understanding of inherent differences between autosomal and X-linked transmission and the correlation of genotype and phenotype often allows one to deduce the genetic nature of a trait in a family. Pedigrees representative of each major pattern of transmission are given in Figure 6.

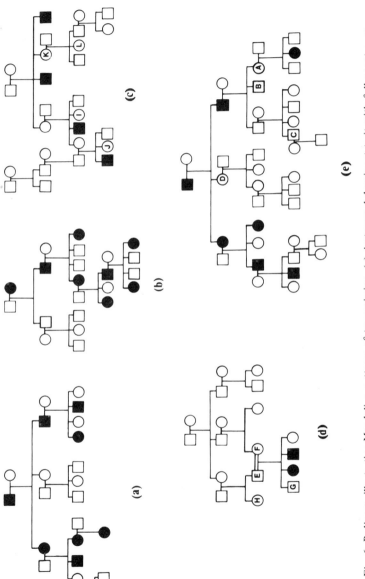

Fig. 6. Pedigrees illustrating Mendelian patterns of transmission. (a) Autosomal dominant trait with full penetrance. (b) X-linked dominant trait. (c) X-linked recessive trait. (d) Autosomal recessive trait. The double marriage bar joining E and F indicates consanguinity. (e) Autosomal dominant trait with reduced penetrance. Individuals A – L are discussed in the text.

Vertical transmission is a characteristic of dominant conditions since every affected person has at least one affected parent. One would suspect from Figure 6 that the traits in families a, b, and e are dominant. The observation of male-to-male transmission in families a and e rules out the possibility of X-linked transmission. The observation that all of the daughters and none of the sons of affected males are affected in family b makes X-linked dominant transmission likely. This type of inheritance pattern in a single family can be very difficult to distinguish from the autosomal dominant pattern. (Compare Fig 4b with Fig 5c and note the similarities and differences).

Oblique transmission is characteristic of an X-linked recessive condition. Note the positive maternal and negative paternal history of the *proband* (the affected person through whom the family was ascertained) and the excess of affected males in family c. The trait appears to skip generations, affected males being related to one another through phenotypically normal females.

Horizontal transmission, however, alerts one to the possibility of an autosomal recessive trait, as illustrated by the essentially negative family history of individuals E and F in family d, and the aggregation of affected individuals in sibships ("horizontal" pattern) rather than in parents and children ("vertical" pattern). The finding of consanguinity between the parents makes this conclusion even more likely. Autosomal recessive inheritance is generally the most difficult to prove in a single pedigree, even with the presence of consanguinity. Sporadic cases due to dominant or X-linked recessive mutations, phenocopies (environmentally caused disorders mimicking one with a genetic basis), and multifactorial traits (see below) often show a similarly negative family history.

Penetrance and variable expression. The typical patterns of transmission displayed by single gene traits are based on the assumption that an individual always manifests the trait determined by his genotype, and that every individual of a given genotype manifests the trait to the same degree. As stated above, the phenotype is the sum total of genetic, environmental and interactive factors. Since the genetic context (the composite of all loci in a genome) and the biological environment in which a gene acts differ from individual to individual, it should come as no surprise that persons will show variability in their phenotypic expression. Combinations of factors may be such that the expression of a mutant gene is so reduced in some individuals carrying the gene(s) that they cannot be distinguished from those who carry the normal allele(s). When this occurs, the trait is said not to be expressed in some individuals or to be incompletely *penetrant.*

Pedigrees of autosomal dominant traits with incomplete penetrance often show irregularities in the pattern of transmission; the trait appears to *skip* a generation as shown in Figure 6e. It is sometimes possible to identify an individual possessing the gene even though the trait is not manifested as in the case of individual A. We are certain of her genotype because of an affected parent and child, but we cannot be certain that individuals B, C and D, who are free of symptoms, are also free of the mutant gene. Incomplete penetrance, therefore, poses special problems in genetic diagnosis of relatives at risk and prognosis of genetically affected individuals.

A number of factors may influence the penetrance of a trait: environment, sex, age, gene interaction, and clinical acumen. Pseudocholinesterase (autosomal recessive) and G6PD (X-linked recessive) deficiencies are genetic disorders in which the gene(s) may not be expressed unless the individual is subjected to a specific stress situation or exposed to a toxic substance. In Huntington disease, an autosomal dominant condition with variable age of onset, its expression is a function of age, such that it is not evident at birth, but becomes fully penetrant by age 80. Transverse vaginal septum, an autosomal recessive, *sex-limited* condition, is fully penetrant in homozygous females and, for obvious reasons, not expressed in homozygous males. The environmental and genetic background of an individual may be important factors in the expression of the genes determining autosomal dominant disorders such as familial polyposis or retinoblastoma. Failure of penetrance in an individual may also be a function of the thoroughness of the physical or clinical examination. A low serum phosphate level in a clinically normal daughter of a man with classical hypophosphatemia, vitamin D-resistant rickets (an X-linked dominant condition), signals the presence of the gene. On the basis of clinical findings, the trait seems to be nonpenetrant; at the biochemical level, however, gene expression is clearly detectable.

Thus penetrance, like phenotype, is a function of our level of observation and, therefore, an attribute of the trait and not of the gene. The closer the phenotype is to the primary site of gene action, the greater the correlation between genotype and phenotype.

Multifactorial Inheritance

Complex traits that have physical, behavioral, or quantitative attributes, such as longevity, stature, intelligence, and certain behavior patterns, are much more difficult to study and analyze than single-gene traits. No gene acts alone – ie., independently of other genes in the genome – both gene–gene and gene–environment interactions contribute to the expression in every phenotype. Thus, in a sense, all traits are *multifactorial*.

However, not all genes contribute equally to the phenotype; some have more of an impact than others. What we observe phenotypically in the common mendelian patterns of inheritance is the expression of alleles at a single major locus. *Polygenic* traits, determined by a number of more less equally contributory loci, are not as conducive to pedigree analysis as are single gene traits; the phenotype observed is under the control of several loci, each producing a relatively minor effect. As a result, quantitative traits that are polygenic show *continuous varia-tion* among individuals in the population, rather than the more discrete qualita-tive phenotypes determined by single major genes.

Let us assume that several loci contribute equally to a phentoype, that at each locus there are two alleles, one with a positive effect and one with a negative ef-fect on the phenotype, and that the effects of the loci are additive (no dominance). The phenotypic variation of this trait in the population would approximate a nor-mal or Gaussian bell-shaped curve. Most individuals will show the usual or "average" phenotype. Few will manifest an extreme phenotype, since it is less likely that an individual will possess a large number of allelic factors all acting in the same direc-tion.

In this example, the variation in the population is postulated to result from genetic factors alone. For most multifactorial traits, variability is due to both gene-tic and environmental factors. *Heritability* is an estimate of the proportion of total variation resulting from genetic factors alone. In practice, it is difficult to separate genetic and environmental components of variability. Some multifactorial traits, such as fingerprint ridge patterns, have a large genetic component that is easily measured. For other traits such as height, intelligence, or blood pressure, it is much more diffi-cult to partition the observed variability into genetic and environmental components.

The threshold model. In contrast to polygenic traits showing continuous varia-tion, a number of complex traits with polygenic basis show *discontinuous varia-tion*. Congenital defects (such as club foot, pyloric stenosis, cleft lip and/or palate, and spina bifida) and some other common disorders such as diabetes, schizophrenia, and atherosclerosis are examples of polygenic discontinuous traits. They each have a relatively strong genetic component (increased risk or susceptibility among first-degree relatives and a higher degree of concordance in monozygous identical twins, versus dizygous fraternal twins), do not appear to be transmitted in simple men-delian fashion, yet show discrete (discontinuous) phenotypes – namely, presence or absence of the condition.

The *threshold model* of genetic liability has been used to explain the apparently discontinuous phenotypes of these conditions. Under the assumption that a num-ber of loci contribute equally to the phenotype and that a critical number or com-bination of alleles at the loci is required to manifest the trait, the distribution of "liability" (based on genetic factors) in the population approximates a bell-shaped normal curve (see Fig 7). Most individuals possess an "average" number of causa-tive alleles; a few individuals possess such a large number of liability genes as to place them beyond the threshold level and thus, they manifest the trait. The higher sus-ceptibility in first or second-degree relatives can be explained on the basis that close relatives are more likely to have more of these alleles in common than more distantly related or unrelated individuals. In Figure 7, the liability distribution for first-degree relatives of an affected individual is shifted to the right, with the mean of their distribution midway between the mean of the population and that of the affected probands. Therefore, compared to the population at large, a greater proportion of first-degree relatives falls beyond the threshold level. Hence they have a higher risk for a given disorder than individuals from the general population. The risk is proportionately lower in second-degree relatives, since they share only ¼ of their genes in common with the index case. The distribution of liability for these individuals lies midway between the population mean and the mean for first-degree relatives. The more distantly related a group of individuals is from the proband, the closer their mean liability is to that of the general population.

The incidence of some common congenital malformations is higher in one sex [3] . Among these is pyloric stenosis, a disorder whose incidence is 5 times greater among males. If the liability model is applied to this condition, a lower threshold for males could account for the observed excess of affected males (see Fig. 7b). Although fewer females are affected, those who manifest the condition would carry more "risk genes" than their male counterparts. It follows, then, that first-degree relatives of affected females have proportionately more risk genes than first-degree relatives of affected males and thus run a higher risk of being affected. It also follows that because of their lower threshold, first-degree *male* relatives carry a higher risk of manifesting the disorder, regardless of the sex of the affected proband. The basic assumption that there is an underlying continuous distribution of liability for this malformation appears to be reasonable on the basis of a study of congenital pyloric stenosis in English families by Carter and Evans in 1969 [3] .

Another phenomenon included in this model is the higher recurrence risk for relatives of more severely affected individuals. In Hirschsprung disease, (failure of nerve cells to innervate the colon), patients with a large portion of their colon affected appear to have more affected relatives.

Although this theoretical model of genetic liability does not explain all the observed facts and fails to predict recurrence risks accurately for many conditions, a rough approximation of recurrence in first-degree relatives is that the incidence in them would be the square root of the population incidence. For instance, if the incidence of congenital dislocation of the hip in a population were about 1 in 2,500 (disregarding the higher incidence in females), the risk for first-degree relatives would be approximately 1 in 50.

GENETIC PREDICTION – ESTIMATION OF GENETIC RISK

"What are the chances that we will have an affected child?" "What is the probability that I am a carrier of this gene?" These are probably the two most frequently asked questions in a genetic counseling setting. Provided there is no doubt as to the clinical and genetic diagnosis of the problem, the answers follow from an understanding of the basic laws of heredity and the mode of transmission of the disorder [1, 5–10] .

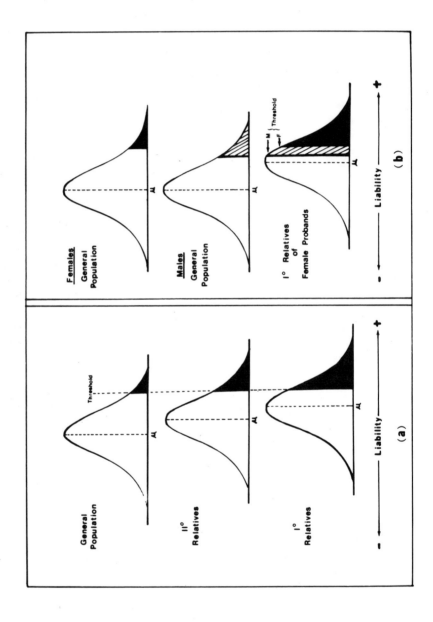

Mendelian Traits

Simple mendelian traits. The probability of a particular genotype or phenotype of an individual is calculated on the basis of the genotype(s) of his parents and/or that of the most closely related affected person in his family. For simple mendelian traits, it is often possible to deduce the appropriate probability from considerations of underlying genetic mechanism (Fig 4a or Fig 5a).

For example, the trait in family d, Figure 6, is autosomal recessive. Given that individuals E and F have had two affected children, the probability that they are each heterozygous is 1. (A probability of 1 denotes certainty, ie, they are *obligate* heterozygotes). Their risk of having a similarly affected offspring is ¼ for each subsequent pregnancy. The trait segregating in family c, Figure 6, is X-linked recessive. The probability that individual I is a carrier is 0.5, because her mother is an obligate heterozygote; ie, the probability the mother transmitted the a allele to her daughter, individual I, is ½ (review mating 2, Figs 5a and 5b). The probability is also 0.5 that individual J in this family is heterozygous since she, too, is the daughter of an obligate carrier.

For other genetic situations, probabilities can be derived from the expected genetic ratios given in Figures 4 and 5. To illustrate this point further, let us consider the probability that individual G in Figure 6d is a carrier. Since he is phenotypically normal, his genotype must be either AA or Aa. Given that both parents are heterozygotes, the probability of their having an Aa offspring is 0.5 and of having a phenotypically normal offspring is 0.75 (refer to Figs 4a and 4c, mating 4). Therefore, the probability that individual G is a carrier, given that he is phenotypically normal is 0.5/0.75 = 2/3, or 0.67.

Another example based on deductive genetic reasoning is the situation involving individual H, family d, Figure 6. The probability she is a carrier depends on the genotypes of her parents. We have already ascertained that her brother, E, is a heterozygote. Referring to Figure 4c, we find that the only two matings in which normal parents produce heterozygous offspring are matings 2 and 4. If the recessive condition is rare in the population, the more likely of the two parental matings

---

Fig. 7. Distribution of liability to a disorder in the general population and in blood relatives of affected individuals. "Threshold" represents a limit above which an individual with high (+) liability manifests the condition (shaded area). (a) Comparision of the liability distributions of first (I°) and second (II°) degree relatives of affected individuals with that of the general population when the threshold is the same for males and females. Note the shift of the mean (μ) to the right as one increases the degree of relatedness to an affected individual and the resulting increase in the proportion of individuals falling beyond the threshold. (b) Comparison of the liability distribution in first-degree relatives of affected females with that of the general population when the threshold is lower for males than for females (compare top and middle distributions). The shift of the bottom curve to the right results in a greater proportion of affected individuals. Note that more male I° relatives are affected.

is Aa × AA. Thus, the probability that individual H is a carrier is 0.5. (Note: When the frequency of the recessive allele is relatively high in a population, the increased possibility of an Aa × Aa parental mating becomes an important factor and should be taken into account in the assessment of risk).

Consanguinity. Let us now consider the consanguineous mating between first cousins, E and F (Fig 6d). On the basis of their two affected children, we are certain that each is a carrier of the recessive allele; so, the risk of an aa offspring in each subsequent pregnancy is ¼. Had they asked about their risk of having an affected child *prior* to their having had any children, the estimated risk would have been quite different from ¼, since their family history contained no clues of their carrier status.

Assessment of risk in situations involving consanguineous matings depends on the mode of transmission of the condition under consideration and the presence or absence of a positive family history. Every person is a carrier of some three to five potentially deleterious alleles. In the absence of an affected offspring or relative or accurate carrier detection tests, it is virtually impossible to be aware of the few specific recessive deleterious alleles that each of us almost certainly carries among the thousands that are known.

Suppose individual E (Fig 6d) is an unsuspecting carrier of the PKU allele. His risk of having a child with PKU will depend on the genotype of his wife. If she is AA, their risk would be 0 (their children can be only AA or Aa). If she is Aa, their risk would be ¼. First-, second- and third-degree relatives, respectively, share 1/2, 1/4, and 1/8 of their genes in common. Since the frequency of the PKU allele is low in the population, it follows that there is a greater chance of heterozygosity in a spouse if he(she) is related than if he(she) is not. Given that individual E is Aa, the probability that his wife, F, is also Aa, is 1/8 (by virtue of their common ancestry). Since the frequency of PKU carriers in the general population is about 1 in 70, the risk to this couple of an affected PKU offspring is approximately 9 times greater than for couples who are unrelated.

As shown in Table I, the amount by which the risk of having an affected offspring is increased in consanguineous matings is a function of both the degree of relatedness of the parents and the frequency of heterozygotes in the population. For relatively rare autosomal recessive conditions, such as PKU and most types of albinism, the incidence of consanguineous marriages among parents of affected children is relatively high. For more common autosomal recessive conditions such as Tay-Sachs disease, cystic fibrosis, and sickle cell anemia, with carrier frequencies of 1/30 in Ashkenazic Jews, 1/20 in Western Europeans, and 1/10 in American blacks, respectively, consanguinity becomes less of a factor.

Thus far, our discussion regarding risk in consanguineous situations has been limited to consideration of a *single* autosomal locus. We estimated the risk to

TABLE I. Risk for a Homozygous Offspring From Consanguineous Matings When One Parent Is Heterozygous

	Relationship of parents	Proportion of genes shared in common	Relative increase in risk* Carrier frequency in the population				
			1/50	1/40	1/30	1/20	1/10
First-degree	Parent–child, sib–sib	1/2	25	20	15	10	5
Second-degree	Uncle – niece, aunt – nephew, grandparent – grandchild	1/4	13	10	8	5	3
Third-degree	First cousins	1/8	6	5	4	3	>1
Fourth-degree	First cousins once removed	1/16	3	3	2	>1	none
Fifth-degree	Second cousins	1/32	2	>1	none	none	none

*Relative to that when parents are unrelated.

couple E X F of having a child with PKU as 3% if E is a carrier. This figure, however, does not reflect the couple's *total* risk of having an offspring with any recessive disorder, because the possibility also exists of heterozygosity at other
loci.

A precise estimate of the total risk would be difficult to assign without knowledge of the number or specificity of the loci at which each parent is heterozygous. Consanguinity has been empirically observed to result in slightly higher
risks of multifactorial conditions, too, such as congenital malformations and mental retardation [8] . In the absence of a specific risk estimate, an approach that
could be taken in counseling consanguineous couples is to emphasize that, although their risk of an affected offspring is increased, and by no means negligible, the probability of their having a normal offspring is appreciably higher.
Incest, however, may impose grave threats to offspring (see Chapter 4).

Mendelian traits with reduced penetrance. Not all mendelian traits present as
cleanly as the above situations imply. Environmental and other genetic factors
often modify phenotypic expression of a gene so as to obscure an individual's
genotype. Estimation of risk in such situations is possible [5, 9] , but it is a more
difficult task. This is particularly true of genetic disorders that are not fully penetrant or are characterized by a variable age of onset.

When dealing with genetic disorders with reduced or incomplete penetrance,
one cannot be certain of the genotype of a clinically normal individual. As the
degree of penetrance decreases, it becomes increasingly difficult to determine
whether a phenotypically normal offspring of an Aa X aa mating is genetically
Aa or aa (see Fig 8).

To illustrate how one estimates risk in such situations, let us calculate the
probability of genotype Aa for individuals B, C and D in Family e (Fig 6). Let us
assume that the trait that is segregating in this family is autosomal dominant with
80% penetrance. (Note: % penetrance is the proportion of persons of a given genotype who manifest the trait.) Individuals B and D each have, a priori, a 50–50
chance of having inherited the A allele from his or her affected parent. Since each
is phenotypically normal and the trait has a high degree of penetrance (80%),
one has the intuitive feeling that the likelihood of their being aa is greater. To confirm this suspicion, refer to Figure 8. We see that when the penetrance of the
trait is 80%, 20% of Aa (area a) and 100% of aa (area b) offspring are phenotypically normal. Since are b is 5 times greater than area a, we can conclude that,
given a normal phenotype, the probability that individual B (and likewise D)
is genetically Aa is 1/6 and of being aa is 5/6. (Our suspicion was correct!)
Had the trait been 50% penetrant, their probability of being Aa would have been
higher, namely, 1/3.

Predicting the genotype of individual C in this family is somewhat more difficult. He could not be Aa unless his unaffected father were also Aa; ie, his probability is *conditional* on the genotype of his father. Since the probability of geno-

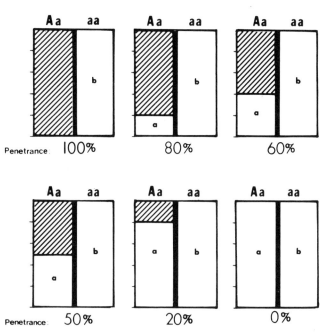

Fig. 8. Manifestation of a trait as a function of penetrance among offspring of a Aa × aa mating when the trait is autosomal dominant. For each level of penetrance a large box is divided into two equal parts to demonstrate the equal probability of each type of offspring; the left half represents the Aa and the right half, the aa offspring of the above mating. Shaded areas = proportion of Aa offspring manifesting the trait. Open area a = proportion of Aa, and open area b = the proportion of aa offspring *not* manifesting the trait. Units of measurement to the left of each box are arbitrary and are for reference only; the total area under Aa = 5; the total area under aa = 5; total area = 10. As the % penetrance decreases, area a increases. When a trait is 50% penetrant, one-half of those carrying gene Aa show the trait, so one-half of the area under Aa is shaded. Thus, the probability that a phenotypically normal offspring of a Aa × aa mating is genetically Aa, is $a/a + b$ or $2.5/2.5 + 5.0 = 1/3$ when the penetrance is 50%.

type Aa is 1/6 for his father (assuming 80% penetrance), the *a priori* probability that C is Aa is $1/6 \times 1/2$ (probability of the father transmitting the A allele to his son) = 1/12 or 8.3%. The fact that individual C is phenotypically normal further reduces his risk of heterozygosity to a level of approximately 2%.

Calculations such as these utilize *Bayesian conditional probability;* a description of the precise methodology is beyond the scope of this chapter (see Murphy and Chase [5] for a thorough treatment of this subject). Complexity of calculation, however, should not deter one from applying such reasoning whenever it is found to be appropriate. Risk figures for specific genetic situations are available in tabular or graphic form, thereby eliminating the need for lengthy calculations [2, 9, 10]. As an example, the probabilities of genotype Aa in individuals

B, C, and D can be easily ascertained from Figure 9. When the penetrance is 80%, the probability is 0.17 (1/6) for individuals B and D and 0.02 for individual C. (Note: The probability for individual C is, in fact, much lower than this estimate when one takes into account the normal offspring and siblings of C and his father.)

   Mendelian traits with variable age of onset. The phenomenon of "variable age of onset" is simply age-dependent penetrance. The proportion of persons carrying the gene who manifest the trait at a given age is equivalent to the % penetrance of that trait at that age.

   Huntington disease is a well-documented autosomal dominant condition with variable age of onset. The *cumulative* proportion of individuals carrying the dominant allele who manifest clinical symptoms by age 20, 30, 40, 45, 50, 60, and 70 is approximately 2.5%, 10%, 33%, 50%, 60%, 93%, and 99%, respectively. Since the penetrance of the disorder at age 30 is 10%, the probability that a clinically normal 30-year-old offspring of an affected individual has inherited the mutant allele is 0.47 (from Fig 9a). If he were 50 years old and clinically normal, his probability would be much lower, namely, 0.28. He would have to be symptom-free until over age 70 to be virtually certain of not having inherited the gene.

   When the individual at risk is two generations removed from a known affected individual (eg, a clinically normal grandchild of an affected person), one must take into account the ages both of the individual at risk and of his unaffected parent. Since the ages of the two persons are different, one cannot use Figure 9b to arrive at an estimate of risk (Figure 9 assumes that penetrance is the same for each generation). Calculations based on Bayesian reasoning are required [5, 9, 10]. A computer program PEDIG that utilizes the Bayesian method to calculate the genotype probabilities for any given individual in a pedigree is available [11, 12].

Multifactorial Traits

   It is known that inheritance is a major factor in the etiology of many common congenital malformations. However, the precise underlying genetic mechanism(s) of each defect remains obscure. Without a conceptual genetic model, we cannot assess probability or risk as we have done for situations involving mendelian traits. Instead, we must rely on our previous experience with the disorder (or the experience of others) and our observations of its occurrence and/or recurrence in other comparable family situations. Estimates based on observation and experience rather than theory are referred to as *empiric risks* or empiric risk figures.

   Empiric risk estimates have their limitations. They are subject to change since they are based on available data. Their validity or reliability depends on the manner in which the data were collected and analyzed, the confidence limits of the estimates, and the criteria on which the diagnosis was based.

   Before applying such estimates to a specific familial problem, one must keep in mind the characteristics of the population from which the estimates were drawn.

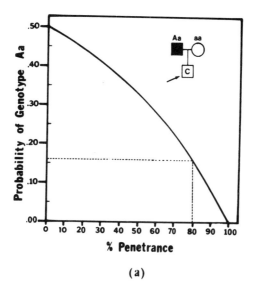

(a)

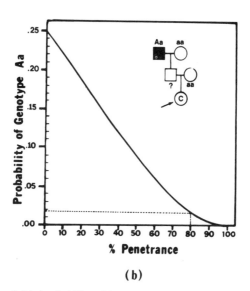

(b)

Fig. 9. Distribution of risk (probability of Aa genotype) as a function of penetrance of an autosomal dominant condition — (a) when the consultand (C) is the phenotypically normal offspring of an affected individual, and (b) when the phenotypically normal consultand (C) has phenotypically normal parents, no siblings and an affected grandparent. If the trait under consideration is 80% penetrant, the probability that the consultand is genetically Aa is 0.16 for situation a and 0.02 for situation b. NOTE: Graph (b) assumes that the level of penetrance remains constant for each generation and thus does not apply to situations in which the penetrance is age-dependent.

For example, empiric risks based on Caucasians of North European extraction may not be applicable to individuals of Black African ancestry. Likewise, risks based on families of one socioeconomic class may not apply to all. Unfortunately, good empiric data are available for only relatively few disorders, and one is often tempted to extrapolate to other conditions or genetic situations whenever information is scanty or simply not available. Despite these limitations, empiric risks, if used wisely, are approximations that can be very helpful in counseling situations.

Risk figures are available for congenital disorders such as congenital heart disease, [13] pyloric stenosis, cleft lip with or without cleft palate, club foot, and congenital dislocation of the hip [3, 4], and for conditions such as diabetes, schizophrenia, and essential hypertension. A computer program has been developed to estimate risks for families with multifactorial genetic disorders [14, 15]. Although it is not possible to list empiric information for each of these conditions, some conclusions drawn from published reports can be listed.

In general, the following are valid:

1) The risk of recurrence increases with the number of affected, and decreases with the number of normal first-degree relatives.

2) Risk may be influenced by the sex of the affected individual(s) in the family, especially for disorders with an unequal sex incidence.

3) The number of affected or unaffected second-degree relatives does not seem to affect risk appreciably.

4) An increase in risk is observed whenever affected persons are found in both the paternal and maternal branches of a family.

5) Recurrence risk appears to be influenced by the severity of the condition in the family.

6) Recurrence risk is generally lower than that for single-gene conditions.

For specific estimates of risk, one should consult appropriate sources [3, 4, 13].

Modification of Genetic Risk

As pointed out above, the best estimate of risk is that which is based on maximal utilization of available information. At times, this has meant application of empiric risks from the literature; at other times, utilization of information about the condition itself (eg, penetrance, age of onset) or its phenotypic expression in a given individual. Other, perhaps less obvious (but no less important), sources of information include the number of normal offspring of an individual at risk, the results of a carrier detection test, and the linkage relationship of the disease locus.

Modification based on family information. To illustrate the point, let us consider individuals I, J, K, and L in family c, Figure 6. All are at risk for being carriers of the X-linked recessive gene. Individuals I and J, however, have a higher risk than K. All three are daughters of an obligate heterozygote. Why then are their risks different? In the case of individual K, the fact that she has had two normal sons makes the possibility of her being AA more likely. In other words, her chances of being Aa or AA are no longer 50–50 but < 50—> 50. By how much has her risk been modified? When the prior probability of being a carrier of an X-linked recessive allele is ½, as in this case, the probability of heterozygosity given n normal sons is $1/(2^n + 1)$. Thus, the probability that K is a carrier is $1/(2^2 + 1) = 1/5$ as compared to ½ if such information were either not available or not utilized.

Since individual L cannot be Aa unless her mother were a carrier, her risk is conditional on the probability that her mother is a carrier. Thus, the probability that L is Aa is $1/5 \times 1/2 = 1/10$, or 10%. Had she had normal sons, incorporation of this additional information would have reduced her risk further.

Table II summarizes the risk of heterozygosity at an X-linked locus for a woman who has no affected brothers or sons but whose grandmother is an obligate carrier. The probability that L is a carrier can be read directly from the table. Since she has two normal brothers (n_2=2) and does not have children (n_1 = 0), her risk is 10%. If she had two normal sons, her risk of being a carrier would be only 3%. In the latter case, the probability that her next son will be affected would be 0.03 × 1/2, or only 1.5%

Modification based on carrier test results. Carrier detection tests are available for a limited number of genetic disorders; some discriminate better than others

TABLE II. Probability of a Woman's Heterozygosity for an X-Linked Recessive Gene When She Has no Affected Brothers or Sons, but her Grandmother is an Obligate Carrier

Number of normal sons (n_1)	Number of normal brothers (n_2)					
	0	1	2	3	4	5
0	0.25	0.17	0.10	0.06	0.03	0.02
1	0.14	0.09	0.05	0.03	0.02	
2	0.08	0.05	0.03	0.02		
3	0.04	0.02	0.01			
4	0.02	0.01				
5	0.01					

between carriers and genetically normal persons [16, 17]. Even if imperfect, information from carrier detection tests, when coupled with information regarding the genetic transmission of the disorder, can significantly alter the risk figure quoted an individual at risk.

Figure 10 shows a hypothetical distribution of test values for nomal and obligate heterozygotes. The overlap of the two distributions may prevent one, on the basis of only the test result, from assigning with certainty the genotype of an individual. It is obvious from these distributions that the probability of heterozygosity decreases with decreasing test value. Fewer carriers have a value of 50 than of 60. By utilizing the proportion of carriers and controls having a given lab value one can estimate the relative likelihood of a genotype given a specific test result. This information could then be used to modify (either increase or decrease) the risk estimate given an individual.

Modifications based on linkage information. The linkage relationship of a disease locus is still another important but often neglected source of pertinent information in counseling situations [18, 19]. Although subject to inherent limitations of precision and applicability, linkage is potentially useful in 1) determining the

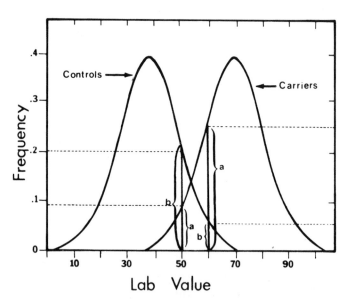

Fig. 10. Hypothetical distribution of test values in control populations (left) and obligate heterozygous or carrier (right) individuals. Overlap of the two distributions denotes the less than perfect resolution of genotypes on the basis of a laboratory test value. a = proportion of known carriers with a given lab value; b = proportion of control individuals with the same lab value.

parental origin of a new mutant allele; 2) demonstrating genetic heterogeneity; 3) indirectly diagnosing genetic disorders in utero-and 4) improving risk estimates.

The last is of special interest to us. If the linkage relationship of the locus determining Huntington disease (HD) were known, this information could be used to refine further an individual's risk. Let us assume that the *HD* locus is linked for example to the *ABO* locus (there is no evidence that they are linked). If a woman's affected parent were blood type A and her unaffected parent type O, we could predict, on the basis of her ABO blood type, the probability that she had inherited the HD allele. Let us assume that her affected grandparent was type A and her other grandparent, type O. Her affected parent, then, must have received both the HD and A alleles from his affected parent. If the woman at risk were type A, and the HD and ABO loci were 5 map units* apart, there would be a 95% chance that she also inherited the HD gene; if she were type O, she would have a 95% chance of *not* having inherited the HD allele. The prediction is not 100% accurate because of the 5% possibility of crossing over between the loci.

By utilizing the information gained from linkage to modify her current risk (based on her age), one could provide her with a more precise estimate of her chance of carrying the HD gene. If her prior risk was 0.40, and she was type 0, one could assure her that the probability that she has inherited the HD allele is 0.03. In other words, her risk would now be comparable to that of a phenotypically normal 60-year-old with an affected parent, and hence would place her at a lower risk group for having a child with Huntington disease. It would be the rare individual who would not react differently to the two estimates of risk!

THE FAMILY HISTORY

The collection and recording of family data are not limited to clinical genetic activities. For centuries religious and/or social groups and individuals interested in genealogy have been gathering and recording family information. What differentiates this type of family history from that elicited by a clinical geneticist is the manner in which it is approached. Approach, in turn, is based on intent.

In the nonclinical situation, the goal is to record familial lineage – ie, the genealogical relationship of individuals in a kindred – with some vital statistics, such as names, birthdates, deathdates, place of birth, etc, on each person. In clinical genetics, the "pedigree" and "genetic" approaches become synonymous. The goal is to gather pertinent family information in the hope that it will provide clues to the genetic (or nongenetic) nature of the disorder under consideration; that it will serve to confirm, reject, or formulate a tentative diagnosis; and that it will be useful in the assessment of genetic risk for individual members of the family [20] .

---

*The unit of map distance, called a Morgan (M), is defined as the length of chromosomal segment which, on the average, experiences one exchange per strand (chromatid). For short intervals the frequency of recombination will be directly proportional to the map interval since double crossovers will be negligible.

If the family history is elicited properly, the pedigree becomes much more than a diagrammatic representation of familial relationship.

The family history centers around the proband or index case. In most cases, this is the affected individual who brought a family to the attention of the physician. This person, however, is not always affected. Unaffected married first cousins with a negative family history who express concern about their possibly increased genetic risk, and the fetus (of a 40-year-old woman) at risk for Down syndrome, may also be index cases. Designation of the proband or index case is important since it allows one to correct for possible biases in ascertainment when evaluating pooled family data [1, 5, 6]. More importantly (in the present context), it focuses attention on the reason for a genetic evaluation, and this, in turn, provides one with the framework in which to proceed.

The nature of the problem and the question(s) to be answered will necessarily dictate the extent of the family history. Information on the proband's parents, siblings, children, grandchildren, aunts, uncles, first cousins, and grandparents is usually considered adequate for most situations. Family information is best corroborated by other family members. Often an older relative will remember critical information if consulted. Genetic counselees will come better prepared if forewarned of the need for detailed family information about their relatives as well as themselves.

Family Information

Name and sex. The full legal name (eg., Elizabeth Ann Jones, née Smith, not "Liz") and sex of each individual. This facilitates tracing of medical records and permits record linkage with other families previously ascertained (see below). The maiden name of females may be a clue to possible consanguinity in the family.

Age (date of birth). This may be essential for identification of individuals, especially those with like-named relatives. For disorders with variable age of onset, age may be a clue to an individual's risk or liability to genetic disease. An unaffected 12-year-old brother of a proband with Duchenne muscular dystrophy is unlikely ever to develop the disorder. On the other hand, a 3-year-old brother of a 12-year-old boy with retinitis pigmentosa is still at risk for developing the condition. A clinically normal 75-year-old man at risk for Huntington disease is certainly "free" of the gene, and his offspring would not be at risk for the condition.

Date and cause of death. Age at the time of death may provide a clue to the presence or absence of a trait in an individual. A family history of early death from "heart disease" in several family members may be important in determining the genetic nature of the clinical problem in a proband with hypertension. Also, whether autopsy studies were performed will indicate potential sources of valuable corroborative data.

Reproductive history. Information on the number and sequence (birth order) of livebirths, stillbirths, miscarriages, spontaneous and induced abortions should be recorded for the present and previous marriages of each individual, with clear indication of who the other parent was for each pregnancy. Pregnancy outcomes of previous marriages may give an insight into whether either branch of the family warrants closer scrutiny. A positive family history of miscarriages and/or stillbirths alerts one to the possibility of a segregating chromosomal abnormality; a number of unaffected siblings of a proband may modify the genetic interpretation of recurrence risks; a number of unaffected offspring and grandchildren of an individual at risk for an autosomal dominant disorder with reduced penetrance decreases the possibility in this person of the Aa genotype; likewise, the number of normal sons of a potential carrier of an X-linked recessive disorder determines the amount by which her risk is reduced.

Pregnancy history. Unusual conditions during pregnancy and/or labor such as infections, malnutrition, irradiation, use of drugs, anoxia, difficult delivery, etc may reveal environmental factors contributing directly or indirectly to an infant's condition. Multiple miscarriages may be indicative of increased risks for genetic disorders; previous premature births may be from uterine abnormalities; excessive birth weights of other children may mean maternal prediabetes, with increased risks of miscarriages, prematurity, and congenital malformations.

Ethnic background and/or race. Racial and ethnic background of individuals, especially grandparents, may provide a useful clue when establishing or confirming a tentative diagnosis. Many single-gene or multifactorial traits that appear to be rare in the general population have a much higher incidence in people of specific ethnic extractions. For example, Tay-Sachs disease, familial dysautonomia, Niemann-Pick disease and hypercholesterolemia have a relatively high frequency in Ashkenazic Jews; the incidence of β-thalassemia, G6PD deficiency (Mediterranean type) and familial Mediterranean fever is high among individuals of Mediterranean background; sickle cell anemia, hemoglobin disease, β-thalassemia and hereditary persistence of fetal hemoglobin are relatively common disorders among Blacks. Among French-Canadians, albinism, hereditary tyrosinemia, oculopharyngeal muscular dystrophy, von-Willebrand disease, and Morquio disease have a relatively high incidence and show regional distribution due to local gene pools.

Medical history and health status. Details concerning the present and past health status of each individual should be recorded. Specific questions about disease or clinical manifestations related to the patient's problem should be asked about *each* individual and not simply as "Has anyone in your family had. . . . " The latter approach, although easier and certainly quicker, is not likely to produce specific answers since the patient is unaware, in most instances, of what can be clinically or genetically significant. By asking specific questions focused on an individual (ie, providing name, age, etc), one can be more directive in the questioning, and thus be in a better position to elicit precise information. For example, a positive answer to a query such as "Did he or she have jaundice?" may lead to recognizing

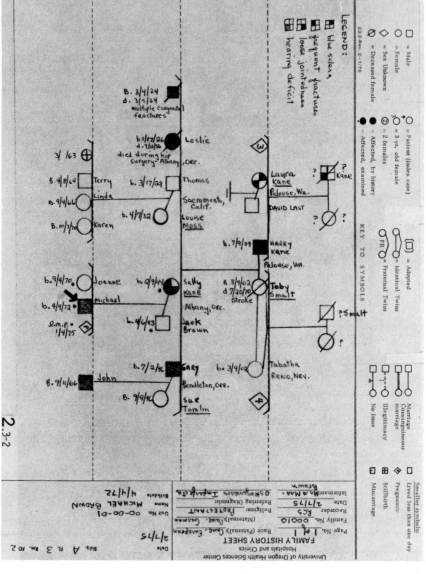

Fig. 11. Pedigree form with simulated family data, used at University of Oregon for inclusion in patient records. (Courtesy of Division of Medical Genetics.)

hemolytic anemia, even if a negative response is obtained when just asking whether anyone in the family had hemolytic anemia.

Medical records. Correct diagnosis and delineation of the genetic nature of a disorder depends on *reliable* information; eg, it is often necessary to substantiate the fact that the patient's apparently normal father who died at age 45 was actually free of findings attributable to Huntington disease. Or it may be important to determine whether a proband's first cousin, who is mentally retarded, indeed does have Down syndrome, as reported by the family; or whether a critical individual, on whom a genetic conclusion rests, shows any signs diagnostic of the disorder. The recording of physician's name, place(s) of hospitalizations or institutionalization, etc will facilitate tracing of pertinent information.

The information obtained from the family history (which can be quite lengthy!) can be concisely summarized in the form of a pedigree. Figure 11 illustrates a simulated pedigree recorded on a standard family history form and retained as part of an individual's medical record. Information regarding age, sex, name, birth and death dates, birth order, reproductive history, relationship to the proband, and any manifestation of disease is recorded directly on this sheet. Other pertinent information, such as physician's name, place and dates of hospitalization, and additional comments, is recorded on the reverse side. Since the findings of a genetic evaluation become a part of an individual's medical history, they are available for the purposes of reference, updating, and/or reevaluation at a later date.

The taking of a complete, accurate, and detailed family history is not a guarantee that the genetic or nongenetic nature of the problem will become clear. The history often is negative, leaving doubt as to the reason for or cause of the condition or disorder. One should not be discouraged by this, however. The family history remains the single most important tool for the clinical geneticist and genetic counselor since it is often impossible to determine, before recording it, what may or may not prove relevant to the case in question. For that matter, it is impossible to predict what may *become* relevant in the future as a result of acquired knowledge and new insights.

ACKNOWLEDGMENTS

Many of the ideas incorporated in this chapter were developed during 1971– 1976. I am indebted to the graduate students of the Rutgers University Human Genetics program and the medical students of the University of Oregon Medical School for helping me crystallize my thoughts on the subject. Drs. Robert D. Koler, Everett W. Lovrien and R. Ellen Magenis graciously consented to review this chapter and offered valuable suggestions for its improvement. I would especially like to express my thanks to Robin C. Schwartz, MS, for the assistance given me during the preparation of this manuscript.

ANNOTATED REFERENCES

1. Sutton HE: "An Introduction to Human Genetics." 2nd ed, New York: Holt, Rinehart & Winston, 1975.
   An excellent comprehensive up-to-date text on human genetics for medical students and graduate students in genetics.
2. Childs B, der Kaloustian V: Genetic heterogeneity. N Engl J Med 279:1205, 1970.
   A discussion of the importance of determining genetic heterogeneity.
3. Carter CO, Evans KA: Inheritance of congenital pyloric stenosis J Med Genet 6:233, 1969.
   Detailed treatment of empiric data for a multifactorial disorder with unbalanced sex distribution.
4. Bonaite-Pellie C, Smith C: Risk tables for genetic counseling in some common congenital malformations. J Med Genet 11:374, 1974.
5. Murphy FA, Chase GA: "Principles of Genetic Counseling." Chicago, Yearbook Medical Publishers, 1975.
   A crisp exhaustive presentation of the logical and mathematical analysis of risks for genetic counseling situations, by two leading mathematical geneticists.
6. Emery AEH: Methodology in medical genetics: "An Introduction to Statistical Method." Edinburgh, Churchill-Livingstone, 1976.
   A more concise treatment of the mathematical and statistical techniques used in medical genetics, by a leading medical geneticist.
7. Maag UR, Gold RJM: A simple combinatorial method for calculating genetic risks. Clin Genet 7:361, 1975.
   A simplified approach for estimating recurrence risks.
8. Fraser FC, Biddle CJ: Estimating the risks for offspring of first-cousin matings: An approach. Am J Hum Genet 28:522, 1976.
   Brief article pointing out the uncertainty of current data on risks to offspring of consanguineous matings.
9. Bolling DR, Chase GA, Murphy EA: A matrix method for calculating recurrence risks of unilocal disorders for genetic counseling. Ann Hum Genet 40:25, 1976.
   A proposal for a simplified approach for estimating recurrence risks.
10. Murphy EA: The rationale of genetic counseling. J Pediatr 72:121, 1968.
    Article explaining the Bayesian approach to physicians.
11. Heuch I, Li FHF: PEDIG - a computer program for calculation of genotype probabilities using phenotype information. Clin Genet 3:501, 1972.
12. Conneally PM, Heuch I: A computer program to determine genetic risks: a simplified version of PEDIG. Am J Hum Genet 26:773, 1974.
13. Neill CA: Genetics of congenital heart disease. Ann Rev Med 24:61, 1973.
    A critical discussion of the concept of multifactorial inheritance as based on empiric data.
14. Smith C: Computer programme to estimate recurrence risks for multifactorial family disease. Bri Med J 1:495, 1972.
15. Smith C, Mendell NR: Recurrence risks from family history and metric traits. Am Hum Genet 37:275, 1974.
16. Merritt AD: Population genetics and hemophilia – implications of mutations and carrier recognition. Ann NY Acad Sci 240:121, 1975.
    A discussion of carrier detection and its limitations in an X-linked disorder.
17. Thompson MW, Murphy EG, McAlpine PJ: An assessment of the creatine kinase test in the detection of carriers in Duchenne muscular dystrophy. J Pediatr 71:82, 1971.
    A discussion of the limits of carrier detection tests in an X-linked disorder.

18. Rivas ML, Conneally PM: Application and significance of linkage in the detection and prevention of genetic disease. "Genetic Counseling." Edited by H Lubs, F de la Cruz. New York: Plenum Press, 1977.
A theoretical treatment of the practicality of using linkage information in assessment of genetic risk.
19. Schrott HG, Karp L, Omenn GS: Prenatal prediction in myotonic dystrophy: guidelines for genetic counseling. Clin Genet 4:38, 1973.
An example of the use of linkage data in prenatal diagnosis.
20. Fraser FC: Taking the family history. Am J Med 34:585, 1963.

4

Genetic Problems Related to Reproduction

Orlando J. Miller, MD

INTRODUCTION

Genetics and reproduction are inextricably intertwined. Birth occurs only after the very important period of intrauterine development. Normal development requires two complete sets of chromosomes, one contributed by the gamete from each parent. One or both of these chromosome sets must carry a normally functioning copy of each of the thousands of genes involved in the anatomical, biochemical, and physiological processes required for normal embryogenesis [1] (See Chapter 3). Development can go wrong if there is a gross chromosome abnormality, a mutant gene, or abnormal environmental factors, which can be physical (elevated temperature, reduced pO_2, ionizing radiation), chemical (pollutants, drugs, hormones), or infectious [2, 3]. Similarly, acquired or inherited abnormalities in the mother, leading to an inhospitable intrauterine environment, can also cause abnormalities of fetal development.

Abnormal pregnancy outcome is always a distressing experience. Parents, quite naturally, worry about possible causes and risks of recurrence. The task of explaining whatever is known about causes and risks falls within the purview of genetic counseling. The challenge of explaining complex medical probabilities to concerned parents is the same, whether a particular problem has a nongenetic, genetic, or unknown cause.

SEXUAL MATURATION

Normal Maturation

The age of menarche has been steadily falling, over the last century, from roughly 17 years to 12 years in the technologically more advanced countries of the world, paralleling improvements in nutrition and health. There has been an even more striking recent increase in sexual activity among young teenage individuals, with a concomitant rise in teenage pregnancies. Because of the *social* immaturity of teenagers in our society — most are still being educated for a career in adult society, have not yet begun their careers, and have not established a nuclear family of their own — pregnancies in this group of individuals present particular hazards in addition to those due to the incomplete physical maturity of the young teenaged parent. Counseling is a very important part of the management of these pregnancies.

Who gets pregnant? Increasingly, teenage sexual activity is found among all groups in our society, not just those lower in the socioeconomic scale. Pregnancy can be deliberate or accidental (including forcible rape). Its incidence is inversely related to the availability of contraceptive knowledge and techniques, but it is also influenced by the attitudes of the teenager, who may reject contraceptive precautions and may view sexual activity, or even pregnancy, as a sign of successful rebellion against society or its representatives in her own family. (See Chapters 8, 9.)

What are the resources for coping with pregnancy in a teenager? One must consider the emotional resources of the pregnant girl herself, and the role of the male partner. Is he supportive, or does he feel trapped and want nothing to do with childrearing? Does the pregnant girl look forward to her pregnancy and to being a mother, or is she frightened and "turned off" by the whole thing? Is the girl's family supportive? What is their view of the pregnancy? Will they care for the baby or help their daughter do so? What financial resources are available?

The physician needs to have psychosocial information to assess the risks of pregnancy in a particular teenage girl. It is important to know when sexual activity is correlated with recreational drug use, especially since sex is sometimes used as a source of money to buy illicit drugs. The need here, as with every pregnant patient, is to obtain a history of any exposure to agents that might be teratogenic [2, 3].

Identity of the putative father may have great genetic implications, particularly for out-of-wedlock pregnancies in teenagers. Any deleterious gene carried by either parent may be relevant; especially important is consanguinity or incest, which markedly increases the danger that an unborn child may have serious genetic handicaps. For example, it has been estimated that up to 50% of the progeny from a father-daughter mating have malformations or mental retardation [4].

Another aspect of this problem is that a proportion of individuals have repeated pregnancies while still in their teens. This means that the physician who sees such a patient during her first pregnancy has the opportunity, and responsibility, of ensuring that faulty sex education or inadequate contraceptive advice does not result in another, possibly unwanted, pregnancy.

Genetic Causes of Abnormal Sexual Maturation

Precocious sexual maturation sometimes begins in children just a few years of age. The causes of precocious puberty, in all its forms, are dealt with in textbooks of endocrinology [5, 6]. They include a number of genetic factors. Congenital adrenal hyperplasia (autosomal recessive) can lead to precocious sexual maturation in males. A tumor in the region of the pineal, hypothalamus, or pituitary glands can have the same effect in both males and females. Such tumors can be genetically caused – eg, as a complication of dominantly inherited neurofibromatosis – which has implications for counseling.

Delayed or absent sexual maturation may also have genetic causes, and the latter condition is responsible for a small proportion of cases of infertility [7, 8]. Either the sexual infantilism or the infertility may bring the patient to a physician, who should keep in mind the possibility that there may be affected relatives (eg, sisters and maternal aunts or cousins in the testicular feminization syndromes, Table I).

FERTILITY

Normal Fertility

Conception requires the formation of normal male and female gametes, as well as normal structure and function of the male and female reproductive tracts, so that sperm and ovum can meet in the uterine tube and the fertilized egg can implant in the physiologically prepared uterine wall. Contraceptive methods are based on preventing fertilization or implantation by imposing temporal, physical, chemical, or physiological blocks to one or another of these processes in the male or female. For cultural reasons, more attention has been paid to the female in developing contraceptive methods, but there is no scientific basis for this emphasis. Contraceptive methods are described in detail in textbooks of reproductive medicine [7, 8]. The genetic counselor should be aware of the types and effectiveness of the various contraceptive methods, keeping in mind that some of his patients who are at high risk of having an abnormal child may elect to have no more children rather than to use prenatal diagnosis (and selective abortion) or donor insemination as means of preventing the birth of a child with a specific genetic disorder [9, 10].

Infertility and Sterility

Nearly 15% of couples are unable to have children [11]. Among these infertile couples, one can sometimes demonstrate that one or the other person has an absolute block to normal reproductive performance. A number of genetic as well as nongenetic causes of sterility and infertility are known – some involving the male, others the female.

Causes of infertility. *Nongenetic Causes of Infertility – Female.* Structural abnormalities of the female geneital tract can prevent conception. An imperforate

TABLE I. Genetic Causes of Pseudohermaphroditism

Type	Type of Recessive Inheritance	
	Autosomal	X-linked
I. Male pseudohermaphroditism		
A. Defective androgen synthesis: deficiency of		
1. 20,22-desmolase	+	
2. 3-β-hydroxysteroid dehydrogenase	+	
3. 17-hydroxylase	+	
4. testicular 17-ketosteroid reductase	+	
5. testicular 17,20-desmolase		+
B. Reduced response to androgen		
1. Complete: testicular feminization		+
2. Incomplete, type I		
Lubs syndrome		+
Gilbert-Dreyfus syndrome		+
Reifenstein syndrome		+
Rosewater syndrome		+
3. Incomplete, type II		
PPSH,* 5-α-reductase deficiency	+	
C. Persistence of Mullerian duct: hernia uteri inguinale	+	
II. Female pseudohermaphroditism		
A. Excessive adrenal androgens secondary to deficiency of		
1. 21-hydroxylase	+	
2. 11-hydroxylase	+	

* Pseudovaginal perineoscrotal hypospadias.

hymen is one that is correctable. Congenital absence of the vagina and the uterus cannot be corrected, but if the uterus is intact, surgical construction of an artificial vagina may restore fertility. Blocked fimbriated ends of the uterine tubes, usually the result of venereal or tubercular salpingitis, is a common cause of infertility. Surgical correction of the block does not usually result in normal fertility, presumably because the function of the tubes is still abnormal, as a result of changes induced by the earlier infection.

Functional abnormalities, such as anovulation with polycystic ovaries, seen in the Stein-Leventhal syndrome, can also cause infertility, as can structural abnormalities of the uterus; also, a bicornuate or unicornuate uterus can produce fetal deformations by restricting fetal movements or growth, resulting in joint contractures or distorted head growth.

Nongenetic Causes of Infertility — Male. Structural abnormalities in the male sometimes cause infertility or sterility. In some cases, there is congenital anorchism, with a complete lack of secondary sexual maturation and sometimes incomplete or absent male sexual differentiation. Testicular damage at any time after birth can lead to infertility.

Functional abnormalities in the male are also known causes of infertility. Undescended testicles fail to produce sperm, presumably because the higher intraabdominal temperature has an inhibitory effect upon germ cells and spermatogenesis. Malformations or acquired lesions in the male duct system can also lead to infertility.

In many cases it may be unclear whether the cause(s) of infertility in a given couple can be pinpointed and whether they are genetic or nongenetic. Genetic evaluation can be of use in these cases. Sometimes the presence of a condition that will produce sterility can be detected in childhood, or even at birth. Diagnostic work-up may be imperative in terms of assigning a genetic role in the rare case, since other relatives may be affected. The parents can be counseled promptly so they can prepare their child for the realities of unattainable fertility, but the affected individual should be counseled again much later, when the information can be grasped more fully and its implications more readily understood.

Genetic Causes of Infertility — Single Gene Effects. There are numerous genetic and chromosomal causes of infertility. Single gene disorders may act at the level of the central nervous system, hypothalamus, or pituitary gland to block the production of the gonadotrophic hormones that are essential for ovarian and testicular function (Table II). Cryptorchidism can be caused by mutation of either autosomal or X-linked genes.

A series of genes are known which control enzymes essential for normal adrenal cortical function [5]. Homozygous mutant genes at these loci can lead to absence of a functional enzyme and a metabolic block in the production of an adrenal hormone (Table I). The lack of this hormone leads to overproduction of pituitary adrenocorticotropic hormone, and the resultant overstimulation of the adrenal glands leads to the production of adrenal androgen and some degree of masculinization of the female fetus. These anatomical changes can be corrected surgically, and replacement therapy can prevent the continued overproduction of adrenal androgens and resultant precocious puberty, enabling these females to enjoy normal reproductive lives.

Inherited absence or defect of an end-organ receptor for testosterone is found in externally normal females with absent uterus, testicular gonads, and XY chromosomes (Table I). These individuals are infertile. Since the mutant gene is on the X chromosome, and only XY individuals are affected, the inheritance pattern is X-linked recessive, but affected individuals are phenotypically female rather than male. These individuals have additional health hazards, because their gonads may undergo malignant change after puberty.

Other genes are known to have products that are essential for androgenic hormone synthesis or tissue response to them (Table I). All lead to male pseudohermaphroditism and are discussed in a later section of this chapter. Males with cystic fibrosis, a disease affecting exocrine gland function, are infertile due to obstructive degenerative changes in the transport ducts of the vas deferens. Females

TABLE II. Genetic Causes of Hypogonadotrophic Hypogonadism (hh)

Disorder	Type of Recessive Inheritance	
	Autosomal	X-linked
Panhypopituitarism	+	
Isolated hh	+	
hh with microcephaly and syndactyly	+	
Kallman syndrome: hh with anosmia		+
hh with ataxia		+
Laurence-Moon syndrome*: hh with spastic paraplegia	+	
Biedl-Bardet syndrome*: hh	+	
Biemond syndrome II*: hh with coloboma	+	

* Mental retardation and pigmentary retinopathy present in all three disorders; obesity and polydactyly only in the last two.

with cystic fibrosis may also be infertile, presumably because of the altered characteristics of the cervical mucus [5] .

Genetic Causes of Infertility — Chromosome Disorders. Infertility is associated in many patients with a sex chromosome abnormality (Table III). Usually the phenotypes seen are the Turner syndrome in females with streak gonads and consequent sexual infantilism, or Klinefelter syndrome in males who usually show an absence of spermatogenesis and elevated gonadotropic hormone level.

Chromosome abnormalities other than these involving sex chromosomes are not usually associated with structural or functional abnormalities of the reproductive system, unless cryptorchidism, hypospadias, or other malformations are present. Thus, many of these individuals — eg, females with Down syndrome (21 -trisomy) — are capable of reproducing. Their chances of bearing a child with a chromosome abnormality is much increased. The risk of their becoming pregnant are also increased, now that so many of these individuals live at home or in a community setting rather than in an institution for the mentally retarded. The physician should be prepared to provide the family with information on the potential fertility of these individuals and their high risk of producing abnormal children.

Management of infertility. Treatment of infertility requires, first, accurate diagnosis. Certain conditions are amenable to surgical correction or hormonal therapy. For example, the pseudohermaphroditism that occurs in females with congenital adrenal hyperplasia due to an 11-hydroxylase or 21-hydroxylase defect can be corrected by relatively minor surgery and adrenal hormone replacement therapy. Pregnancy has occurred in individuals so treated, and there is little evidence that they need suffer any ill-effects related to their disease. The risk that their children will be affected with the same genetic disorder is very small (say, 1 in 400 or less), unless the affected individual, who is homozygous for the mutant gene, marries a

Table III. Sex Chromosome Causes of Infertility

A. In females, usually due to presence of streak gonads
 1. 45,X (XO)
 2. 45,X/46,XX mosaicism
 3. 45,X/46,XY mosaicism
 4. other mosaics
 5. 46,X,iso(Xq) – isochromosome for X long arm
 6. 46,X,iso(Yq) – isochromosome for Y long arm
 7. 46,X,Yp – deletion of Y short arm
B. In males with Klinefelter syndrome
 1. 47,XXY and mosaics with a 47,XXY cell line
 2. 48,XXYY*
 3. 48,XXXY*
 4. 49,XXXYY*
 5. 49,XXXXY*
 6. 46,X,t(X;Y) – X-Y translocation
C. In other males
 1. 46,X,t(A;Y) – autosome-Y translocation

---

* Mental retardation is usually a more serious finding in these cases.

relative. Since a first cousin would have a 1 in 4 chance of carrying the same mutant gene, with a 1 in 2 probability of each child being homozygously affected, the overall risk if an affected person married a first cousin would be 1 in 8. The responsibility of counseling should include educating both the individuals affected by a recessive disorder and their unaffected siblings, who have 2 chances in 3 of being heterozygous carriers, concerning the markedly increased risk, for them, of consanguinous matings. (See Chapter 3.)

When a male is infertile or carries a high risk of having genetically handicapped children, he and his marriage partner should be informed about the option of artificial insemination by donor, which is generally safe and effective when acceptable to a couple [12].

Some forms of infertility are associated with a lack of ovulation, the mechanism of action of "the pill." This kind of infertility can be overcome by inducing ovulation by hormonal means. It has been suggested that ovulation inducers, including stopping the pill, raise the incidence of triploid or otherwise chromosomally abnormal conceptuses. The evidence for this effect is weak, and the collection of more data is essential to resolve this issue. The effect, if present at all, appears to be slight, certainly not large enough to deter a relatively infertile couple for whom having a baby is of prime importance. But the effect is large enough to warrant warning the couple about the risks, particularly of multiple births, after hormone stimulation of ovulation. It is equally prudent to advise avoiding pregnancy for 3 to 6 months after discontinuing the pill [3, 8].

Fecundity

Virtually no human population in advanced countries, with the exception of small isolates like the Hutterites, has as many children as the reproductive potential, or fecundity, or women would permit. In technologically advanced countries, birth rates have fallen markedly, in a few countries reaching a point at which zero population growth has been achieved. With smaller family size has come a greater concern to utilize whatever means are available to assure the highest possible standards of health for the children who are born, and this has led to increased emphasis on improved antenatal and perinatal care. In this context, consideration of any risks of genetic disease has an important place. (See Chapters 8, 9.)

PREGNANCY

Maternal Genetic Disorders in Pregnancy

The obstetrician is well aware of the importance of genetic disease in pregnancy, particularly through his involvement in the management of Rh and ABO blood group incompatibilities and diabetes mellitus [13]. There are many other genetic disorders that are sometimes important. Although individually rare, in toto they constitute a complicating factor in a significant proportion of pregnancies, and an understanding of them is important in assessing maternal risks throughout the pregnancy and postpartum period, as well as risks to fetal well-being.

Bleeding disorders. The obstetrician is heavily attuned to the danger signal of intrapartum bleeding, a sign of possible premature separation of the placenta or placenta previa. Rarely, a known or potential heterozygous carrier of either X-linked hemophilia A or B requires management of the pregnancy. Sometimes prenatal sex diagnosis is decided upon because the risk to the offspring is asymmetrically distributed, with virtually no risk for daughters but a 50% risk for sons. Bleeding and spontaneous abortion have been reported following amniocentesis in such females. It is conceivable this was the result of uncontrolled retroplacental bleeding in an affected male pregnancy, but no proof exists that female carriers do not have intrinsic susceptibility to retroplacental bleeding. Additional problems might arise in bleeding disorders due to other mutant genes (Table IV). The autosomal dominant von Willebrand's disease, like classical hemophilia leads to a reduced level of antihemophilic globulin and the possibility of bleeding problems in an affected woman, such as severe intrapartum or postpartum bleeding as well as risks of fetal bleeding after amniocentesis. Afibrinogenemia, a cause of severe intrapartum bleeding, is an acquired disorder, not to be confused with congenital hypofibrinogenemia, a factor I deficiency, which is a genetic disease and is not usually found in women of childbearing age.

TABLE IV. Genetic Causes of Coagulation Defects

| | | Type of Inheritance | | |
| | | Recessive | | Dominant |
Factor	Deficiency State	Autosomal	X-linked	Autosomal
I	Congenital hypofibrinogenemia	+		
II	Hypoprothrombinemia	+		
III	Antithrombin deficiency			+
V	Congenital parahemophilia	+		
VII	Hypoproconvertinemia	+		
VIII	Hemophilia A		+	
VIII	von Willebrand disease			+
IX	Hemophilia B		+	
X	Stuart-Prower factor deficiency	+		
XI	Plasma thromboplastin antecedent deficiency	+		
XII	Hageman factor deficiency	+		
XIII	Fibrin stabilizing factor deficiency			+

Chondrodystrophies. Classical achondroplasia and the other chondrodystrophies pose obstetrical hazards because of the small and abnormally shaped pelvis in affected women. Cesarean section is generally required for delivery in these cases. Achondroplasia is an autosomal dominant disorder, and the affected individual has a 50-50 chance of transmitting the mutant gene to the fetus, even where there is no prior family history of the disease other than the affected parent. Usually, no special measures are necessary for the delivery of a chondrodystrophic fetus. In the case of an affected infant, however, close pediatric observation is essential, because many of the infants have severe respiratory problems at birth, a tendency toward internal hydrocephalus, and increased susceptibility to inner ear infections, as well as instability of spinal and other joints. [5] .

Connective tissue disorders. Ehlers-Danlos syndrome is a group of rare, variously inherited disorders in which there is hyperelastic skin, loose-jointedness, and skin fragility [14]. There appear to be at least seven different genes involved; four have dominant expression, but mutation of three of the genes has been shown to result in recessively expressed deficiency of a specific enzyme involved in collagen biosynthesis: lysyl oxidase (X-linked), collagen lysyl hydroxylase, or procollagen peptidase (both autosomal). The genetic heterogeneity is reflected in clinical heterogeneity. During pregnancy, patients with Ehlers-Danlos syndrome are at increased risk of developing varicose veins, hernias, osteoporosis, dislocated joints and pubic symphysis, rupture of the uterus, premature delivery, perineal tears and postpartum hemorrhage. Later, menorrhagia and uterine prolapse are common.

For the dominant forms, if either parent is affected there is a 50-50 risk that a child will be affected. It is worth noting that the fetus with Ehlers-Danlos syndrome is very likely to be born prematurely because of premature rupture of the membranes. Since, on the average, one-half of the siblings of an affected child will also be affected, a recurrence of premature delivery is common in affected women.

Marfan syndrome is an autosomal dominant disorder in which very long fingers and toes (arachnodactyly) are found in association with dislocation of the lens, high myopia, spontaneous retinal detachment, kyphoscoliosis and loose joints, inguinal hernia, and lung cysts. Aortic dilatation and aneurysm are common; rupture of such an aneurysm is a catastrophic complication of pregnancy, of which more than a dozen cases have been reported [14].

Hemoglobinopathies. Sickle cell (SS) anemia can lead to severe complications of pregnancy, with sickle cell crises being particularly important as intravascular sickling may lead to pulmonary and other emboli. The anemia, too, can be a problem; folic acid therapy is valuable, and avoidance of anoxia, acidosis, or dehydration is critical. Cesarean section prior to labor has been advocated to minimize the risks of dehydration and anoxia while allowing more controlled anesthesia. Combined hemoglobin S-hemoglobin C (SC) disease, while generally less severe, also constitutes a hazard during pregnancy, and requires similar management. Sickle cell heterozygotes (SA) have a higher risk of urinary tract infection during pregnancy but otherwise present no special problems.

The thalassemias are an even graver health hazard to the mother. Although few homozygous individuals have survived to reproduce, with more effective treatment, many obstetricians may be faced in the future with the problem of pregnancy management in these patients.

Phenylketonuria. This autosomal recessive disorder presents a very special fetal hazard in the pregnant phenylketonuric woman, because of the enormously high frequency of microcephaly and other birth defects. (This will be dealt with later in this chapter.) The disorder presents no special obstetrical problem, except that the extremely restrictive diet control required during pregnancy complicates provision of balanced nutrition for the mother as well as the fetus.

Porphyria. Acute intermittent porphyria is an autosomal dominant disorder in which there is an increased level of delta-amino-levulinic acid synthetase and a decreased level of porphobilinogen deaminase [5, 13]. Severe attacks of neurologic dysfunction can be precipitated by a variety of agents, including barbiturates, sulfonamides, estrogens, anticonvulsants, ergot, some tranquilizers, aspirin, infections, and dieting or fasting. In 10-20% of women the attacks are cyclical, related to the menstrual cycle. The effect of pregnancy is unpredictable, but attacks can recur during pregnancy and especially in the postpartum period. An attack may consist merely of abdominal pain with constipation, but may include signs of automatic neuropathy, peripheral neuropathy with back or leg pain, paresthesia, respiratory paralysis, and death. Brain involvement may lead to seizures, psychotic episodes, and coma. The importance of accurate diagnosis is obvious, and the avoidance of precipitating factors a paramount concern.

Seizure disorders. Epilepsy has always been a special problem during pregnancy, because the anoxia sometimes associated with a seizure poses a threat to the fetus. Some of the anticonvulsive drugs – eg, trimethadione and diphenylhydantoin – are teratogenic (see below) [15]. It seems worthwhile to avoid such drugs during early pregnancy, the critical period for embryonic development, if clinically possible. Phenobarbitol appears to have a lower teratogenic effect. If its use in a particular patient is sufficient to prevent seizures, it should be used in place of diphenylhydantoin or similar anticonvulsants.

Maternal-fetal blood group incompatibility. Erythroblastosis fetalis arises from destruction of fetal red blood cells by maternal antibodies to a paternally derived blood group antigen not present in the mother. Rh blood incompatibilities are responsible for most of the serious cases of erythroblastosis, in which red cell destruction is so profound during pregnancy that fetal hydrops and death occur. Intrauterine transfusion can be of help in some (the less severe) of these advanced cases. Fortunately, within the past decade or so, antibody injection of Rh negative women soon after delivery or abortion has been shown to prevent development of active immunity to fetal Rh D antigen. It has therefore become standard practice to use Rhogam or similar anti-Rh D gammaglobulin, and this has markedly reduced the incidence of Rh-sensitized women.

ABO incompatibility is responsible for a generally milder form of erythroblastosis which can almost always be managed effectively using measures no more heroic than phototherapy or exchange transfusion, and even the latter is rarely necessary.

Vitamin D-responsive genetic disorders. Autosomal dominant, autosomal recessive, and the more common X-linked dominant forms of hypophosphatemia and rickets, responsive to large doses of vitamin D, have all been observed [5]. Early diagnosis and institution of therapy may be helpful in preventing the typical rachitic bony changes. Affected females may require cesarean section because of the pelvic deformities. The risk of having an affected child is 50% in each pregnancy in the autosomal dominant form and the X-linked dominant form when the pregnant female is affected; when the male partner is affected, 100% of the daughters will receive the mutant gene, but none of the sons will. (See Chapter 3.)

Fetal Wastage

Conceptuses and abortuses. Studies in experimental animals as well as the human suggest that about a third of fertilized eggs never implant. Conception begins with implantation and only some time after this event can pregnancy be diagnosed. At least one-sixth of all conceptions terminate in spontaneous abortions. The known causes of abortion include external and maternal environmental factors as well as gene and chromosomal factors, with chromosomal abnormalities being by far the single most important factor.

Chromosomal aneuploidy in abortuses. About 40-50% of spontaneous abortions are associated with a chromosomal imbalance in the conceptus [16] usually involving an increase in the number of chromosomes. About a fifth of the chromosomally abnormal abortuses are triploid, with three complete sets of chromosomes, $3n = 69$, instead of the usual two sets, $2n = 46$. Triploidy is almost always an embryonic lethal factor, leading to abortion. It is extremely rare in full-term pregnancies, being associated with multiple malformations leading to stillbirth or neonatal death. Some two-fifths of the chromosomally abnormal abortuses are trisomic, $2n + 1 = 47$. Trisomies of virtually every autosome, 2 through 22, have been found among abortuses, but almost all of them are embryonic lethals; the exceptions that appear in liveborn populations are the well-known trisomies, 21, 18, and 13, and the less common trisomy 8, although these, too, are more likely than not to end in abortion. Autosomal monosomy, $2n-1 = 45$, is rare among abortuses, and one is tempted to speculate that, since deletions (partial monosomies) are more detrimental for embryonic development than duplications (partial trisomies), monosomy is probably a preconceptional lethal, with death of the embryo occurring prior to implantation.

Sex chromosome aneuploidy is also found among abortuses. By far the most common type is the XO (45, X) condition, which produces Turner syndrome in the adult. However, whereas the XO karyotype occurs in only about 1 in 2,500 newborn females, it accounts for about a fifth of all chromosomally abnormal abortuses. That is, XO is 99% lethal in the first trimester, a somewhat surprising finding in view of the relatively mild manifestations seen in XO newborns or adults. XXX, XXY, XYY, and more complex sex chromosome aneuploidies are relatively uncommon among abortuses in keeping with the relatively minor developmental defects seen in newborns or adults with extra sex chromosomes.

Multiple abortions. A woman who has had one spontaneous abortion has an increased risk of having a second; after two or more, this risk reaches a level twice that of a woman who has never had an abortion (30% vs 15%). Some women appear to be at even higher risk, and in some women every pregnancy has terminated in abortion. Infections, toxic factors, and gynecological abnormalities have been implicated in recurrent abortion, as have genetic and chromosomal factors. The simple numerical abnormalities, such as trisomy, have a slightly increased tendency to recur, but a much bigger risk of recurrence is associated with the presence in either parent of certain types of chromosomal rearrangement — for example, balanced translocations and inversions, where the risk of spontaneous abortion due to a chromosome imbalance may exceed 50%. When parents have had more than two spontaneous abortions, there is up to a 10% likelihood that one of the parents has a chromosomal abnormality [17].

A graver consequence of parental chromosome translocations is the high risk that a liveborn child may have chromosome imbalance with associated major malformations. Genetic counseling for couples with multiple abortions must thus include consideration of abnormal pregnancy outcome as well as increased probabilities of miscarriage.

Teratogens

Fetal development involves the interaction of many genetic and environmental factors. Birth defects can arise from the predominant effect of a single gene abnormality, a chromosomal imbalance, the interaction of two or more genes, or the effect of one or more abnormal environmental factors. The clinical geneticist's task is to evaluate the relative importance of each of these factors in an affected individual, or the risk that one or more of these factors, acting on one or the other parent, may lead to an affected child. Environmental agents can alter genes, chromosomes, or development. Thus, we can speak of environmental mutagens (changing genes), clastogens (breaking chromosomes), and teratogens (causing malformations), although some agents may have two or even all three effects. Here we shall be concerned with agents that are definitely teratogenic, or for which there is strong evidence of teratogenicity. A classification of these is given in Table V.

Environmental and occupational teratogens. *Physical and Chemical Agents.* Ionizing radiation is a well known environmental mutagen, clastogen, and teratogen. In addition to the background level provided by cosmic rays and radioactive decay in natural rocks and some building materials, there are potentially more hazardous sources (atomic bomb explosions or nuclear reactor accidents), and a variety of other sources affecting special populations such as uranium miners, X-ray staff, or radioisotope workers (eg, technicians working with radioiodine). Medical exposure is of more concern to the physician. For more than 50 years it has been known that doses of X-irradiation delivered to the pelvis for treatment of malignancy could lead to the birth of a child with microcephaly and mental retardation. (The nuclear explosions at Hiroshima and Nagasaki produced some of the same effects.) Low doses of diagnostic radiation to the pregnant mother may cause childhood cancer, which could be the result of either a cellular teratogenic or mutagenic effect [2]. Hence it is prudent to take elective X-rays in fertile women of childbearing age only during the 10 days from the onset of their last menstrual period.

Methyl mercury is the best known environmental chemical teratogen. Ingestion of contaminated fish by pregnant women in Japan led to the birth of children with microencephaly and cerebral palsy. While convincing evidence does not exist to implicate many other pollutants as human teratogens, dozens of agents (including heavy metals, pesticides, and industrial solvents) have been shown to be tera-

TABLE V. Teratogens in the Human

Environmental and occupational
  Physical and chemical
    Ionizing radiation
    Methylmercury
  Infectious
    Viral (rubella, cytomegalovirus, herpes simplex II)
    Other (syphilis, toxoplasmosis)
Maternal environment
  Phenylketonuria
  Diabetes mellitus
  Steroid hormone imbalance
  Hypothyroidism
Diet and drugs
  Alcohol
  Thalidomide
  Anticonvulsants (diphenylhydantoin)
  Folic acid antagonists (amethopterin)
  Antitumor drugs (alkylating agents)
  Vitamin K antagonists (warfarin)
  Androgenic hormones, some synthetic progestagens
  Diethylstilbestrol
  Tetracycline

---

togenic in one or more experimental animals, and it seems likely that several of these are teratogenic in the human [2].

Infectious agents – Viral. The rubella virus is a potent human teratogen, as shown by many studies since the pioneering work of Gregg in 1941. Infection during the first trimester leads to abortion or rubella syndrome in half the cases, with congenital heart disease, cataracts, microcephaly, mental retardation, and hearing loss (nerve deafness). About one in five women who sustain the infection in the second trimester also has an affected child, but after the 16th week of gestation hearing loss is usually the only feature. Since immunity to rubella is effective for many years, abortion of women who have rubella in the first half of a pregnancy is widely accepted. Rubella infection in pregnancy can also cause abnormalities of liver function and platelet function. An infected fetus may continue to excrete the rubella virus for months or even years after birth, and be a dangerous source of infection, particularly for hospital staff. It is important to document the infection since other virus infections – eg, coxsackie – produce similar but nonteratogenic fevers and rashes in pregnant women. Nasopharyngeal secretions can be cultured for the virus even several days after the rash subsides. A rising antibody titer in the maternal serum is another way to document the recent occurrence of rubella infection.

The development of an effective rubella vaccine provides a basis for eliminating rubella-induced teratogenesis. The population at highest risk are women in their reproductive years who lack rubella antibodies in their serum. Pregnancy should be avoided for several months after vaccination of such women. Immunization some years earlier would clearly be preferable.

Cytomegalovirus infection, which is very common in pregnant women (perhaps 1 in 8), has also been shown to be teratogenic. The virus can cross the placenta, infecting 1% or so of all children in some populations. A small fraction of these have hearing loss or mental retardation.

Herpes simplex type II is a third virus with a demonstrated teratogenic potential. Infection of the fetus usually leads to fetal death, but sometimes to brain damage, or grave neonatal illness.

Gonococcal infection in the mother can be transmitted to the infant during birth, and is an important cause of neonatal ophthalmitis leading to blindness. Gonococcal infection in a woman can also leave her infertile with scarred Fallopian tubes.

Infectious agents – Bacterial. The prevalence of syphilis has increased in recent years. The pregnant woman who is infected with Treponema pallidum can transmit the infection to the fetus, leading usually to stillbirth but sometimes to the birth of a child with characteristic lesions of skin, skeleton, and viscera. Spirochetes can be recovered from such lesions, and therapy, usually with penicillin, is imperative to prevent progression of the disease.

Infectious agents – Protozoal. Genital infection by Toxoplasma gondii during pregnancy can lead to stillbirth or premature birth. A very high percentage of fetal toxoplasmosis results in infants with microcephaly, hydrocephaly, cerebral calcification, chorioretinitis, psychomotor retardation, and growth retardation. This is the reason pregnant women are advised to refrain from fondling pet cats or cleaning up after them.

Maternal environment. Metabolic disorders in a pregnant woman can have a profound effect on the fetus. Here we will consider only four examples; phenylketonuria, diabetes mellitus, steroid hormone imbalance, and thyroid imbalance.

Phenylketonuria. Neonatal detection of phenylketonuria (PKU) and prompt initiation of a low-phenylalanine diet has practically abolished the severe mental retardation that was formerly almost invariably found in this inborn error of metabolism [5]. Consequently, a growing number of physically and intellectually normal phenylketonuric females are entering their reproductive years. Since the unpleasantly restrictive low-phenylalanine diet is not necessary for normal brain development after the first few years of life, and its use is thereafter discontinued, the phenylketonuric individual who becomes pregnant has an elevated serum phenylalanine. This, or some related factor, has a profound effect on the fetus, leading in almost every case to microcephaly, mental retardation, or a congenital heart defect. Whether a low-phenylalanine diet throughout pregnancy would prevent the abnormal fetal development is not yet known, but this is the only measure that can be offered to women with PKU who intend to have children.

Diabetes mellitus. The incidence of stillbirths, immaturity, metabolic disturbances, and congenital malformations are all increased in the children of women with diabetes, the increase being more marked in the more severe diabetics. The mechanisms of these effects are unknown. Acidosis has been implicated, as has the hypoglycemia occasionally associated with insulin therapy. Whatever the mechanism, the incidence of all types of malformations is increased.

Steroid endocrine imbalance. The presence of a virilizing ovarian or adrenal tumor in pregnancy can lead to masculinization of the external genitalia in the female fetus. Functional virilization of the mother can have the same effect.

Thyroid imbalance. Pregnancies complicated by hypothyroidism are associated with a higher incidence of spontaneous abortion, stillbirth, prematurity, and congenital malformation and mental retardation.

Hyperthyroidism is associated with reduced fertility, but when a pregnancy occurs, there is a risk that drug treatment may cause fetal malformations, and that the infant at birth will show signs of maternally transmitted hyperthyroidism.

Diet and drugs: Iatrogenic factors. Alcohol has been implicated as a teratogen [18]. Excessive intake of alcohol by pregnant women may lead to fetal loss, intrauterine growth retardation, or birth of a child with the fetal alcohol syndrome: microcephaly, telecanthus, epicanthus, small palpebral fissures, small mouth, micrognathia, palatal abnormalities, and psychomotor retardation.

Prescription drugs constitute an extremely important class of teratogens. The classic example of an iatrogenic teratogen is thalidomide, the sedative-tranquilizer that was responsible for an epidemic of phocomelia and associated anomalies [2]. No other tranquilizers have been proven to be teratogenic, although the phenothiazines are suspect. However, several anticonvulsants – eg, diphenylhydantoin – are teratogenic, leading to intrauterine growth retardation, an abnormal facies, telecanthus, epicanthus, cleft palate, terminal digital hypoplasia, and underdeveloped nails [15].

The administration of folic acid antagonists (eg, amethopterin, or other antitumor agents), to pregnant women usually leads to spontaneous abortion. However, about a fourth of the survivors have intrauterine growth retardation as well as brain, skeletal, and visceral malformations [19]. The same is probably true of the cytotoxic antitumor alkylating agents, cyclophosphamide, busulphan, and chlorambucil, although the evidence is limited.

Vitamin K antagonists – eg, warfarin (Coumadin) – can lead not only to retroplacental hemorrhage and abortion but to teratogenic effects as well [19].

Androgenic hormones or high doses of synthetic progestagens, similar in structure to methyltestosterone (pregnenolone, ethinyltestosterone, ethisterone, norethisterone, norethindrone), can produce masculinized external genitalia of the female fetus. Progestational agents, estrogens, and oral contraceptives are suspected of having teratogenic effects, but the evidence is still scanty.

Diethylstilbestrol, a potent nonsteroidal estrogen, is representative of a new class of teratogen, the transplacental carcinogens, and the only one known to produce tumors in the human [20]. Pregnant women who received diethylstilbestrol (DES) produce daughters who have a markedly increased risk of developing adenocarcinoma of the vagina in childhood or as young adults. Abnormalities of the male genital tract, including epididymal cysts, hypotrophic testes, and micropenis may occur in up to a fourth of the males born to women who took DES early in pregnancy.

The tetracyclines are antibiotics that cross the placenta, have an affinity for developing osseous and dental tissues, and lead to staining and dysplasia of the teeth of the individual so exposed. They have no known teratogenic effects other than on the teeth, although they affect skeletal development in experimental animals [2].

Heroin, lysergic acid (LSD), marijuana, and other "street" drugs have all been suspected of causing fetal malformations. Despite intensive studies, none of these has been a proven teratogen, although LSD causes miscarriages and heroin or methadone causes distressing withdrawal syndromes in the newborn infant. "Angel dust," [phencyclidine (PCP)], is thought to be a teratogen.

The risks associated with drug therapy are higher in pregnant women than in any other group because so many drugs cross the placenta to affect the fetus. Certain embryonic tissues are markedly susceptible to such exogenous agents, and the effects are often irreversible, leading to congenital malformations. Awareness of the special risks of pregnant women enables physicians, and particularly obstetricians, to play a major role in the prevention of congenital malformations.

It is important to keep in mind that nearly two-thirds of cases of congenital malformation are of unknown cause, and that it is very difficult to show whether a particular agent is teratogenic in man. Drug interactions, when multiple agents are combined, constitute another hazard that is only beginning to be understood. The best advice, in these circumstances, is to minimize the pregnant woman's exposure to all drugs, chemicals, X-rays, or other exogenous agents.

Sex Determination and Differentiation

Chromosomal. The basic chromosomal determinants of sex have been known for many years. The presence of two X chromosomes normally leads to female development, whereas the presence of an X and a Y leads to male development. Individuals with a single sex chromosome, 45,X or XO, develop as females although their streak gonads lack germ cells; XXY, XXXY, and XXXXY individuals develop as males. These observations indicate that sex differentiation is determined by the presence or absence of a Y chromosome, but that fertility in the female generally requires the presence of at least two X chromosomes.

Genetic. A male sex-determining gene has been mapped to a region near the centromere of the Y chromosome, usually on the tiny short arm. This gene is required for the production of the male-specific H-Y cell surface antigen, which appears to be involved in the initiation of testis differentiation [21]. At least five additional autosomal or X-linked genes (Table I) are involved in the production of androgenic hormones by the interstitial cells of the differentiated testes. One or more additional genes (Table I), which appear to be X-linked, are involved in the synthesis of the receptor protein required for the response of target tissues to male hormones. Estrogenic and progestational hormones also act by binding to specific receptor molecules, and one would expect mutation or deletion of the genes (s) for one of these receptors to interfere with hormone action; however, no examples of unresponsiveness to female hormones have been reported, perhaps because this responsiveness may be essential for implantation and such a mutation would thus be embryonally lethal.

Endocrine. Endogenous hormones play a major role in extra-gonadal sex differentiation [8], though other factors are important too. The fetal testes produce testosterone, which is required to stimulate the growth and differentiation of the Wolffian duct derivatives. Androgenic hormones are incapable of suppressing the continued differentiation of the Mullerian derivatives, but a (presumably polypeptide) morphogenetic factor from the fetal testis does this. Ovaries are not required for female differentiation of genital structures. In the absence of male hormone, the Wolffian ducts fail to differentiate into the male duct system. In the absence of the fetal testis morphogenetic factor, the Mullerian ducts and external genital structures differentiate in a female direction, perhaps in response to placental hormones.

Exogenous hormones can upset the normal course of sex differentiation [7, 8]. Androgenic hormones or synthetic progestagens similar in structure to methyltestosterone can masculinize the female fetus if administered during the critical period of sexual development in early pregnancy. Maternal androgenic hormones, whether the result of functional virilization during pregnancy or an endocrine tumor, can have the same relatively mild and correctable teratogenic effect.

ANTENATAL DIAGNOSIS

Antenatal diagnosis for the prevention of genetic disease began more than 20 years ago, with the utilization of sex chromatin studies on amniotic fluid cells in cases where the fetus was at a 25% risk of having a severe X-linked recessive disorder such as Duchenne muscular dystrophy. The rationale for determining the sex of the fetus was that the risk was asymmetric, with sons at 50% risk of having the disease and daughters at virtually no risk. The test was no more than 85% accurate, and the number of subjects was limited. Consequently, widespread acceptance of antenatal diagnosis of genetic and chromosomal disease had to await the demonstration, by Steele and Breg in 1966, that some of the cells in amniotic fluid could be grown in culture and chromosome preparations derived for karyotype analysis. Methods have been developed for detecting enzyme deficiencies in small numbers of cultured amniotic fluid cells, setting the stage for increasingly widespread applicability of antenatal diagnosis of genetic as well as chromosomal abnormalities [1, 9, 10].

The purpose of antenatal diagnosis is twofold. First, it allows one to detect some of the fetuses with genetic, chromosomal, or other disorders that can produce severe birth defects or postnatal disease, and to do so in time to terminate the pregnancy when this is requested by the parents. Second, and in a far greater percentage of cases, it enables one to reassure certain couples that this pregnancy is not going to produce a child with the specific disorder for which they are at high risk. In view of this second goal, it seems unwarranted to refuse antenatal diagnosis to a couple who do not plan to abort an abnormal fetus. Furthermore, the attitude of such a couple may change if they find themselves no longer in the position that they can hope to be lucky — after all, the odds are, say 50:1 in their favor — but instead are faced with the virtual certainty that this pregnancy, if continued, will produce a child with, say Down syndrome.

Techniques

In this new field, the range of procedures used is limited, but increasing efforts are being made to develop new approaches. Here we shall deal only with the most commonly used procedures [1, 9, 10, 22–35].

Amniocentesis. Transabdominal needling of the pregnant uterus to withdraw a sample of amniotic fluid was developed as an aid in the management of severe erythroblastosis due to Rh incompatibility. This procedure, amniocentesis, has been carried out as early as the first trimester, when it is used for the replacement of amniotic fluid by hypertonic saline to induce abortion. For most antenatal diagnostic studies (other than those for assessing fetal lung maturity or erythroblastosis), amniocentesis is carried out between the 16th and 19th weeks of pregnancy, counting from the onset of the last menstrual period. Verification of the gestational age by ultrasound is now a routine in many centers, where this technique is also used to localize the placenta [24]. Since the cells in the amniotic fluid tend to settle quickly, it is necessary to avoid tapping a woman who has been lying in the same position for some time. She should move about shortly before the procedure, perhaps rolling from side to side, and should have an empty bladder at the time of amniocentesis. Using sterile technique and under local skin anesthesia, a spinal needle is inserted, two or three samples of fluid are removed and each is transferred to a sterile container. If the initial few milliliters of fluid are grossly bloody, it is usual to switch to another syringe before removing more fluid, to minimize the amount of blood in the later samples. The samples should be transported to the laboratory as expeditiously as possible.

Amniotic fluid cell culture is performed in a relatively small number of laboratories, and the number of samples each can handle is limited. It is therefore important that arrangements be made well ahead of time for the processing of a given sample. This is essential when a test other than karyotype analysis is called for. Virtually every laboratory that is able to culture amniotic fluid cells successfully has some capability for chromosome studies, but only a handful of laboratories in the country perform certain biochemical tests.

Amniotic fluid. The volume of amniotic fluid is very small in early pregnancy. It increases rapidly from about the 14th week of gestation, when fetal urine begins to to make a major contribution to the total volume. The amniotic fluid also contains other components, including a transudate of maternal serum containing small molecules and even some proteins. Most of the chemical components of amniotic fluid (other than hemoglobin breakdown products, which are elevated in severe erythroblastosis) have been of little use in antenatal diagnosis, but α-fetoprotein is a noteworthy exception [22].

Alpha-fetoprotein (AFP) is a product of the fetal liver. In mid-trimester it reaches a peak level of 2,000-3,000 μgm/ml in the fetal serum. AFP is present in the amniotic fluid in much smaller amounts, reaching a peak level of 10-20 μg/ml. Fetal AFP also reaches the maternal serum, where it shows far lower peak values. The fetal cerebrospinal fluid (CSF) has a high AFP level, and in the presence of open neural tube defects (anencephaly and spina bifida) leakage of AFP from the CSF raises the level in the amniotic fluid and secondarily in the maternal serum. The level in amniotic fluid and maternal serum may also be raised to some extent in threatened abortion, fetal distress, placental insufficiency, twin pregnancy, congenital nephrosis, and certain other conditions. Nevertheless, determination of amniotic fluid AFP levels, especially from the 16th-22nd week of gestation, provides a method for detecting a large proportion of open neural tube defects.

The concentration of α-2-macroglobulin (mol wt 850,000) can also be of value in diagnosing these conditions. Normally, amniotic fluid contains only very low concentrations of such high molecular weight substances, but a neural tube defect allows passage of quite large molecules into the fluid. There are even fetal macrophages in the fluid in some cases of anencephaly and spina bifida but this is not as useful a parameter because of its occurrence in some other situations as well.

Amniotic cells. The number of cells in the amniotic fluid increases markedly after about 14 weeks of gestation, perhaps because many of them are shed by the fetal urinary tract and this is the time that fetal urine begins to contribute largely to amniotic fluid. A small proportion of these cells are able to divide and grow into colonies of cells. It is these whose chromosomes can be studied during cell division. The quality of metaphase spreads obtained from cultured amniotic fluid cells is as high as that obtained from any other material, and any chromosome abnormality that can be detected in cultured leukocytes, skin fibroblasts, or other tissues can be diagnosed in utero. Viable cells are scarce before 16 weeks of gestation, and many people feel that 17 weeks is the optimal time for obtaining amniotic fluid for culturing the cells. The cells which grow are fetal in origin perhaps coming primarily from the urinary tract. These cells express a limited range of their genetic content, and the absence of a particular protein or enzyme (eg, hemoglobin [23, 25]) may thus be due to the state of differentiation of the cells rather than to a genetic defect. Studies of cultured amniotic fluid cells from controls are essential to determine which enzyme defects can be detected antenatally. For the thalassemias, where the genes for a hemoglobin polypeptide are missing, chemical detection of these genes in these amniotic cells (by DNA hybridization) is possible [23].

Amniocentesis in the 16th-19th week of pregnancy provides a basis for determining the chromosome constitution, or karyotype, of the fetus, and this is its major use [10, 35]. Cultured amniotic fluid cells can also be used for diagnosing inborn errors of metabolism. More than 60 such disorders can be diagnosed antenatally at this time.

At amniocentesis the amniotic fluid is frequently bloody. The red blood cells are usually of maternal, but sometimes of fetal, origin. The presence of fetal blood in the amniotic fluid can markedly elevate the AFP level. Avoidance of damage to the placenta at amniocentesis by the use of ultrasound for location of the placenta can reduce the incidence of bloody taps [24].

Ultrasound and X-ray. The method of choice in indirect imaging of the fetus is ultrasound. This source of energy appears to be relatively harmless, and the image resolution possible with the method is sufficiently great to permit accurate estimation of the biparietal diameter of the fetal head from about the 12th-13th week, and for detection of anencephaly or encephalocele not much later. Intrauterine growth retardation can be detected well before the 28th week by sequential untrasonic evaluation.

Ultrasound provides an effective means of localizing the placenta and diagnosing multiple pregnancies [24]. In twin pregnancies it is possible to needle the two amniotic cavities independently, using dye infusion into the first compartment to verify that at the second amniocentesis the needle is not in the same sac. There is now sufficient data from measurement of fetal limb dimensions by ultrasound to show that diagnosis of the short-limbed dwarfism syndromes is possible in midpregnancy. Furthermore, the volume of the fetal bladder can be calculated from ultrasound measurements, and this can be used to derive estimates of fetal renal excretion rates in utero. This allows detection of renal agenesis and related disorders by the 20th week of pregnancy.

Routine use of X-rays to the pelvis should be avoided during pregnancy because of the mutagenic effect of ionizing radiation. There are, however, some conditions in which radiographic diagnosis is indicated. For example, when an elevated AFP level is found, and ultrasound does not reveal anencephaly, one can look for spina bifida by amniography. A lipophilic radio-opaque substance which has an affinity for the vernix caseosa is instilled into the amniotic fluid on the fetal skin and the fetal surface is studied. As better resolution becomes possible with ultrasound, the advantages of amniography may be lessened. However, newer radiographic techniques may become useful. One of these is low-dose computerized axial tomography (CAT) scanning, which, like ultrasound, gives a cross-sectional view through any tissue and might aid in the diagnosis of some malformations of internal organs – eg, polycystic kidneys. It is unfortunate that X-ray diagnosis of bony abnormalities – eg, osteogenesis imperfecta – is not reliable before about the 24th week of gestation because of the limited calcification of long bones earlier in pregnancy.

Fetoscopy. Direct visualization of the fetus has been achieved by the use of endoscopes. Initially these were introduced through the cervix, but this has been discontinued because it produced a high incidence of leakage of amniotic fluid, infection, and subsequent abortion. The transabdominal approach has been used with more success, although here, too, the use of an instrument 5-10 mm in diameter is associated with a high risk of fetal death. Improvements in design – eg, the introduction of fiberoptic systems – have made it possible to develop instruments no larger than 2.2-2.7 mm in diameter, and these are tolerated much better than the larger ones [25]. Nevertheless, in view of the size of the probe, and the necessity to introduce it with a sharp trocar, it is important to avoid injuring the placenta with it. Therefore, ultrasound is used to localize the placenta and fetus, and to monitor the depth of penetration of the amnioscope.

What can be learned by fetoscopy? This depends upon luck as well as the experience of the operator. The field of view is narrow, and only a small portion of the fetus can be visualized at one time – eg, a hand or the lip region. Furthermore, if there is blood or meconium in the amniotic fluid, visibility can be very poor. In favorable circumstances, one may be able to visualize a malformation of an extremity, an encephalocele, a cleft lip or other gross change. Perhaps more important is the ability to obtain a fetal blood sample through a tiny sampling needle under direct visualization of a placental vessel, or even a skin biopsy by inserting biopsy forceps through the cannula in place of the endoscope. The biopsy constitutes a source of fetal cells that can be studied directly or grown in culture. The blood sample contains fetal blood (unfortunately, usually contaminated by maternal blood, sometimes to an extent that raises doubts about the validity of such samples for diagnosis of fetal blood components). Adequate numbers of dividing cells can be obtained in 2-3 days from blood leukocytes, rather than the 2-3 weeks often required with amniotic fluid cells; if contamination by maternal blood were not a problem, the time advantage would strongly favor this approach. Blood samples obtained by fetoscopy have been used to diagnose β-thalassemia, and should be useful in diagnosing sickle cell anemia, other hemoglobinopathies, and blood clotting defects [25, 27].

Recently, fetal blood samples have been used to measure fetal blood creatine phosphokinase levels, which are abnormally high in patients with Duchenne muscular dystrophy. But this means has proven inconsistent for diagnosis of this problem.

Indications for Antenatal Tests

Antenatal tests for genetic, chromosomal, or other abnormalities are too expensive and the number of trained personnel too limited for these procedures to be offered to every pregnant woman. Their employment should therefore be considered in relation to the level of risk of an affected child to a specific couple or in a particular population, also keeping in mind the nature and severity of the projected disorder and what can be done about it. For example, cystic fibrosis cannot yet be diagnosed antenatally. Sickle cell disease can be detectable, but one method used − fetoscopy, obtaining a blood sample from a placental vessel, and measuring the synthesis of Hb-S − poses grave technical limitations since fetoscopy must still be regarded as moderately dangerous for the fetus [25]. Another more promising sophisticated gene-linkage technique may prove more widely applicable [29].

Maternal screening. Some disorders occur at relatively high frequency in specific populations (sickle cell anemia in Africans and Afro-Americans, Tay-Sachs disease in Ashkenazi Jews, and open neural tube defects in the Irish and Welsh). In view of this high incidence of serious disease, it may be feasible to screen these populations in order to identify the individuals who are at high risk of having an affected child.

Screening for sickle cell and Tay-Sachs heterozygotes is similar in the sense that one is examining a healthy population who have no reason to question their own state of health. The difference is that it is relatively straightforward to prevent the birth of a child who will develop Tay-Sachs disease, but more difficult to do the same for sickle cell disease, because the hexoseaminidase deficiency responsible for Tay-Sachs disease is readily detectable in cultured amniotic fluid cells, whereas the restriction enzyme degradation and electrophoretic analysis of fetal DNA is technically more difficult [29]. Because of the difference in the options open to carriers, it is not surprising that screening to identify heterozygous carriers of the gene for Tay-Sachs disease is enthusiastically espoused by

Jewish groups, while screening for sickle cell hemoglobin carrier status has far fewer proponents among potential carriers. Nevertheless, the physician should be aware of the nature of the problem in these cases and the various options by which the birth of an affected child can be prevented, including donor insemination by a noncarrier.

Neural tube defects, hydrocephaly, anencephaly, and spina bifida, are three times commoner in some populations, especially people of Irish or Welsh descent, than in others. Their incidence in most populations, one per 500 to 600 births, is high enough to warrant general use of an easy and simple maternal screening test, such as the immunological assay for AFP [22]. The AFP level is increased in the maternal serum in the majority of pregnancies involving an open neural tube defect. However, the magnitude of the increase is limited, so that while an AFP greater than 2 standard deviations above the mean occurs in over seven-eighths of anencephalic pregnancies, such a high level is seen in no more than two-thirds of spina bifida pregnancies. Thus, if one used maternal serum AFP values as the screen, nearly one-third of the cases of spina bifida would be missed [30]. The way this situation is handled at present is to identify couples at increased risk of having a child with a neural tube defect and to use more realiable antenatal tests in these cases (see below).

Maternal age. For many years the exponential rise in the incidence of Down syndrome with increasing maternal age (but not paternal age) has been known [10, 31]. Earlier risk figures were based on estimates of the incidence of Down syndrome diagnosed clinically. Since the introduction of antenatal diagnostic studies in which chromosome studies are carried out, it has become clear that the earlier incidence figures were underestimates and that while an exponential increase in risk is clearly correct, the magnitude of the risk is severalfold greater than expected — eg, more than 1% at age 35, and perhaps 10% above age 45, rather than 0.5% and 2%, as previously believed, at mid pregnancy [32].

Increasing maternal age affects the risk for trisomy of any chromosome, not just number 21. Most trisomic fetuses will probably abort spontaneously prior to the 17th week of pregnancy, but not all will [32].

Pregnancies at Risk for Specific Disorders

Neural tube defects. A woman who has given birth to a child with anencephaly, hydrocephaly, or spina bifida has an increased risk (3–5%) of having a similarly affected child in any future pregnancy. In view of this high risk, these women should be screened for an elevated AFP in the amniotic fluid. Determination of maternal serum AFP level is no substitute in this high-risk population because of its lesser reliability.

Chromosomal translocation or inversion. When either the male or female partner has a structural chromosome rearrangement, say a translocation or inversion, their fetus has an increased risk of carrying an unbalanced chromosome complement. In such cases, amniocentesis and karyotype analysis of cultured amniotic fluid cells are strongly indicated.

Previous birth of a trisomic child. The risk of recurrence is over 1%, so that antenatal diagnosis is fully warranted [32].

Hazards of antenatal tests

Thousands of mid trimester amniocenteses have been performed in the past 10 years, most of them in the past 3 years. The best estimate of the hazards of this procedure has come from collaborative studies of several thousand pregnancies in which this procedure was carried out in collaborating major medical centers [33, 34]. The conclusion that can be drawn from these studies, and observations at a number of other centers [35], is that the procedure is sufficiently safe to warrant its continued application in pregnancies with a risk of at least 1 in 200 of producing a seriously abnormal child.

To mother. *Physical.* No maternal deaths or other serious maternal complications have been reported in association with amniocentesis for antenatal diagnosis. Saline-induced abortion has, on occasion, led to a maternal death, and for this reason some centers prefer to terminate mid-trimester pregnancies with the safer prostaglandins rather than using hypertonic saline or resorting to hysterotomy [36].

Infection is an infrequent complication of amniocentesis, related either to an exogenous source of contamination, or rarely, to perforation of the bowel. Intraperitoneal bleeding, performation of the bladder, a broken needle, and other complications are uncommon but do occur.

Spontaneous abortion within several weeks following amniocentesis has been reported in 3–4% of cases. However, this is not a significantly higher incidence of abortion than occurs ordinarily between the 14th and 19th weeks of pregnancy, and is considerably lower than the incidence of spontaneous abortion in the 3 weeks prior to a scheduled amniocentesis. Thus, although about three-fourths of spontaneous abortions occur in the first trimester, enough occur in the second trimester, specifically after the 16th-19th week of gestation, to provide a high "noise" level that makes it difficult to determine whether amniocentesis has much of an effect. On the basis of existing data, amniocentesis may lead to as many as 0.5% more abortions or as few as virtually zero additional abortions [30, 33–35].

Feto-maternal transplacental bleeding as a result of amniocentesis could lead to maternal isoimmunization. The presence of a positive Kleihauer test in a Rh-

negative mother following amniocentesis is considered an indication for administration of anti-Rh D serum in some centers. This would not, of course, prevent
isoimmunization to antigens other than Rh D, but this appears to be no more than
a rare complication.

Psychological. For couples at increased risk of having an abnormal child,
especially those who already have one so affected, pregnancy engenders considerable stress [30]. We have found that genetic counseling sessions are helpful to
many of these couples, frequently giving them a more realistic estimate of their
risk and an optimistic appraisal of what antenatal diagnosis can do in their case.
In addition, a session with a counselor who is expert in eliciting relevant family
history information sometimes reveals that a particular couple is at an increased
risk of having a child with an additional unsuspected disorder — eg, Tay-Sachs
disease, muscular dystrophy, neural tube defect, type II hyperlipidemia, or osteogenesis imperfecta.

The diagnosis of an abnormality confronts some couples with a situation in
which several of their values are in sharp conflict. Genetic counseling can
help here, especially if there has been prior contact so that the counselor is not a
stranger. Ideally, the counselor can put the couple in touch with a variety of sources
of further information or support — eg, parents of children affected with the same
disorder or, for some, a priest, minister, or rabbi [37].

To fetus. There is little evidence that a normal fetus is harmed by amniocentesis.
Direct damage from a needle impaling a vital part of the fetus appears to be rare.
Damage to the placenta, with bleeding, is more common, but this usually has no
measurable deleterious effect. A possible exception is the rather frequent occurrence of abortion following amniocentesis in known carriers of hemophilia. It is
possible that abortion in these cases occurred because the fetus was hemophilic
and placental bleeding was thus excessive. Fetal death secondary to infection or
placental separation may also occur, but the frequency of such complications
appears to be low [33–35].

The diagnostic limitations of all the tests that are now possible still cannot
guarantee detection of all fetal abnormalities. No known cause has been found for
many disorders, which altogether affect almost one of every 30 pregnancies unpredictably.

SUMMARY AND CONCLUSIONS

Pregnancy and birth are critical events in the life of a family or an individual.
Medical and physical problems related to these events can be very stressful, particularly if they are not readily treatable.

Families with such problems often are concerned about possible implications for future childbearing, so the diagnosis, interpretation of cause, and explanation of implications for progeny can be beneficial to many of these families. Furthermore, certain inherited problems of reproduction may affect other relatives, who might benefit from identification, preventive treatment, and counseling.

These problems include disorders of sexual maturation, infertility, and inherited disorders with special hazards for pregnancy. In addition, genetic, chromosomal, and environmental factors all can play a role in fetal maldevelopment. It is often possible, by evaluating the past medical and family history of a couple, and pregnancy experience of an expectant mother, to detect couples who are at an increased risk of having an abnormal child.

Appropriate treatment for many disorders of sexual maturation or fertility is dependent on timely detection and early therapy. Pregnancies for women with certain inherited diseases should be planned and managed, to maximize the safety for the mother and to optimize normal outcome for the fetus. Agents which are potentially toxic to a fetus should be avoided.

A growing number of antenatal diagnostic tests have been developed for accurately identifying an affected fetus. Thus more and more disorders, especially those with a genetic or chromosomal basis, are becoming preventable, if only by termination of the pregnancies in which they occur. Furthermore, in the great majority of cases the couple can be assured that the particular fetus does not have the specific disorder for which there was great concern. The net effect of the introduction of such antenatal diagnostic testing is a reduction in the incidence of induced abortion, greater freedom for couples in reproductive planning, and the allaying of much anxiety in families concerned about the outcome of this or any future pregnancies.

Genetic counseling may be appropriately sought by all families with a problem related to reproduction. Understanding of the genetic basis of a problem may help motivate a family to comply with a difficult treatment regimen. The availability of fetal diagnostic tests, even with their present limitations, helps many families make difficult decisions about future children; and in those cases where a family can be assured that their problem is not genetic, the counseling will have had a beneficial effect, alleviating fears and helping the family cope with their specific problem.

ANNOTATED REFERENCES

1. Riccardi VM: "The Genetic Approach to Human Disease." New York: Oxford University Press, 1977.
   An excellent synthesis of genetics and medicine at an easily readable level.
2. Wilson JG: "Environment and Birth Defects." New York: Academic Press, 1973.
   A comprehensive discussion of teratogenesis.
3. Heinonen OP, Slone D, Shapiro S (eds): "Birth Defects and Drugs in Pregnancy." Publishing Sci: Littleton, Mass., 1977.
   A useful tabulation of birth outcome and drug exposure in more than 50,000 pregnancies followed prospectively.

4. Adams MS: Incest: Genetic considerations. Am J Dis Child 132:124, 1978.
5. Gardner L (ed): "Endocrine and Genetic Diseases of Childhood and Adolescence" (2nd ed). Philadelphia, W.B. Saunders, 1976.
6. Williams RH (ed): "Textbook of Endocrinology" (5th ed.). Philadelphia: W.B. Saunders, 1974.
7. Novak ER, Jones GS, Jones HW: "Gynecology, (9th ed)." Baltimore: Williams & Wilkins, 1975.
8. Hafez ESE, Evans TN (eds): "Human Reproduction: Conception and Contraception", Hagerstown, Md: Harper & Row, 1973.
9. Lubs HA, de la Cruz F (eds): "Genetic Counseling." New York: Raven Press, 1977. Proceedings of a workshop on genetic counseling and its assessment. Several chapters deal with reproductive aspects, especially antenatal diagnosis.
10. Milunsky A (ed): "The Prevention of Genetic Disease and Mental Retardation." Philadelphia: W.B. Saunders, 1975. Useful chapters on screening and various aspects of antenatal diagnosis.
11. Bergsma D (ed): "Genetic Forms of Hypogonadism." Birth Defects: Original Article Series 11:(4), 1975.
12. Curie-Cohen M, Lutrell L, Shapiro S: Artificial insemination by donor in the United States. New Engl J Med 300:619, 1979.
13. Burrow GN, Ferris TF (eds): "Medical Complications During Pregnancy." Philadelphia: W.B. Saunders, 1975.
14. McKusick VA: "Heritable Disorders of Connective Tissue" (4th edition). St. Louis: C.V. Mosby, 1972.
15. Smith DW: Teratogenicity of anticonvulsive medications. Am J Dis Child 131:1337, 1978.
16. De Grouchy J, Turleau C: "The Clinical Atlas of Human Chromosomes." New York: Wiley, 1977.
17. Kim HJ, Hsu LYF, Paciuc S, Christian S, Quintana A, Hirschhorn K: Cytogenetics of fetal wastage. N Engl J Med 293:844, 1975.
18. Hanson JW, Streissguth AP, Smith DW: The effects of moderate alcohol consumption during pregnancy on fetal growth and morphogenesis J Pediatr 92:457, 1978.
19. Smith DW: "Recognizable Patterns of Human Malformation" (2nd ed). Philadelphia: W.B. Saunders, 1976. An extremely valuable systematic compendium of malformation syndromes.
20. Herbst AL, Kurman RJ, Scully RE, Poskanzer DC: Clear cell adenocarcinoma of the genital tract in young females. N Engl J Med 287:1259, 1972.
21. Wachtel SS, Koo GC, Breg WR, Thaler HT, Dillard GM, Rosenthal IM, Dosik H, Gerald PS, Saenger P, New M, Lieber E, Miller OJ: Serologic detection of a Y-linked gene in XX males and XX true hermaphrodites, N Engl J Med 295:750, 1976.
22. Brock DJH: Biochemical and cytological methods in the diagnosis of neural tube defects. Prog Med Genet, 2:1, 1977. A recent review of maternal serum and amniotic fluid tests.
23. Wong V, Ma HK, Todd D, Golbus MS, Dozy AM, Kan YW: Diagnosis of homozygous α-thalassemia in cultured amniotic-fluid fibroblasts. N Engl J Med 298:669, 1978.
24. Kerenyi TD, Walker B: The preventability of "bloody taps" in second trimester amniocentesis by ultrasound scanning. Obstet Gynecol 50:61, 1977.
25. Alter BP, Modell CB, Fairweather D, Hobbins JC, Mahoney MJ, Frigoletto FD, Sherman AS, Nathan DG: Prenatal diagnosis of hemoglobinopathies: A review of 15 cases. N Engl J Med 295:1437, 1976.
26. Bove A (ed): "Prenatal Diagnosis. Proceedings of an INSERM symposium." Paris Inst National de la Santé et de la Recherche Médicale, 1976.

27. Firshein SI, Hoyer LW, Lazarchick J, Forget BG, Hobbins JC, Clyne LP, Pitlick FA, Muir WA, Merkatz IR, Mahoney MJ: Prenatal diagnosis of classic hemophilia. N Engl J Med 300:937–941, 1979.
28. Golbus MS, Stephens JD, Mahoney MJ, Hobbins JC, Haseltine FP, Caskey CT, Banker BQ: Failure of fetal creatine phosphokinase as a diagnosictic indicator of Duchenne muscular dystrophy. N Engl J Med 300:860–861, 1979.
29. Kan YW, Dozy AM: Antenatal diagnosis of sickle-cell anaemia by D.N.A. analysis for neuralniotic-fluid cells. Lancet 2:910–912, 1978.
30. Chamberlain J: Human benefits and costs of a national screening programme for neuraltube defects. Lancet 2:1293–1296, 1978.
31. Holmes LB: Genetic counseling for the older pregnant woman: New data and questions. N Engl J Med 298:1419–1421, 1978.
32. Hook EB: Spontaneous deaths of fetuses with chromosomal abnormalities diagnosed prenatally. N Engl J Med 299:1036–1038, 1978.
33. NICHD National Registry for Amniocentesis Study Group: Midtrimester amniocentesis for prenatal diagnosis: safety and accuracy. JAMA 236:1471, 1976.
34. Simpson NE, Dallaire L, Miller JR, Siminovich L, Hamerton JL, Miller J, McKeen C: Prenatal diagnosis of genetic disease in Canada: Report of a collaborative study. Canad MAJ 115:739–746, 1976.
35. Golbus MS, Loughman WD, Epstein CJ, Halbasch G, Stephens JD, Hall BD: Prenatal genetic diagnosis in 3000 amniocenteses. N Engl J Med 300: 157–163, 1979.
36. Osofsky HJ, Osofsky JD (eds): "The Abortion Experience." Hagerstown, Md: Harper & Row, 1973.
   Several useful chapters on the biology, pharmacology and sociopsychology of abortion.
37. Fletcher J: The brink: The parent-child bond in the genetic revolution. Theol Stud 33:457, 1972.
   In-depth interviews of several couples undergoing amniocentesis, reported by a sensitive thoughtful ethicist.
38. Blumberg BD, Golbus MS, Hanson KH: The psychological sequelae of abortion performed for a genetic indication. Am J Obstet Gynecol 122:799–808, 1975.

5
Genetic Problems Affecting Infants

Barbara R. Migeon, MD

INTRODUCTION

Incidence of Congenital Diseases

As the frequency of infectious diseases and malnutrition decreases, the incidence of congenital abnormalities becomes more prominent. About 30% of admissions to children's hospitals in recent years have been for complications of congenital malformations and inborn errors of metabolism [1, 2]. The true incidence is unknown because many fetuses with abnormalities do not survive the strong selection pressure in utero [3]. Many of these congenital disorders, tend to aggregate in families. Among the aims of genetic counseling are identifying and informing those families who have a *significant* risk of recurrence, and reassuring those families who do not.

Heterogeneity of Etiology

For inborn errors and those congenital malformations that have genetic components, the probability of repetition is high; whereas, for those attributable mainly to an environmental agent, the problem may never recur. Since information regarding recurrence is essential for genetic counseling, it is important to distinguish between the alternative etiologies. This may not be easy to do. The underlying basis for most congenital malformations, including those most commonly referred for genetic counseling, is not yet known. Furthermore, the means of discovering the etiology are not readily available. One of the important problems in this regard is the relative inaccessibility of the fetus as it develops in utero, making it impossible to demonstrate defects that may occur in developmental processes. Furthermore, there is considerable overlap between the clinical appearance (phenotype) of disorders that are genetically determined and those that have major environmental determinants. For example, the association of deafness with mental retardation and heart defects in the "rubella syndrome" — resulting from a viral infection in the fetus — may occur also in disorders attributable to a single defective gene and in those caused by chromosomal tri-

111   © 1979 Alan R. Liss, Inc.

somy. Even if an anomaly can be attributed to a genetic cause, it is often difficult to determine, on the basis of clinical phenotype, if it has been transmitted as a point mutation or as a result of a chromosomal abnormality. The
phenotype resulting from trisomy for chromosome 13 is identical to that of
Smith-Lemli-Opitz syndrome [4] attributable to a point mutation transmitted
recessively.

Because the causes of malformations and metabolic errors are so heterogeneous, it is important to obtain as specific a diagnosis of the disorder as possible. In recent years, a variety of gene-determined congenital disorders have been
sorted from diseases previously considered single entities. Presently, we can identify at least seven varieties of defects that lead to an accumulation of mucopoly-
saccharides [5], as well as many forms of chondrodystrophies [6]. The naive
assumption that all achondroplasia is attributable to the same single dominantly
inherited mutation has lead to erroneous predictions regarding the prognosis and
recurrence risks. For many disorders attributable to single gene mutations one
needs to distinguish forms that are X-linked from those that are autosomal and
those that are dominant from those that are recessive, because the risk of
recurrence is dependent upon the mode of transmission.

Disorders for Which Genetic Counseling Is Appropriate

Genetic counseling is appropriate for a variety of disorders, ranging from those
for which the genetic basis is known to those associated with exposure to environmental agents. For the former, accurate estimates of the probability of reccur-
rence can usually be determined; for the latter, there is reassurance that the risk
of recurrence is relatively small.

INBORN ERRORS OF METABOLISM

In general, inborn errors of metabolism are single-gene-determined. Most of
these are transmitted as autosomal or X-linked recessives, although a few dominantly transmitted metabolic disorders are known. The clinical abnormalities are
caused by an absent or defective enzyme or other protein.

Enzymes are proteins that serve to speed up these reactions and are necessary
for normal function and differentiation of cells. Metabolic pathways depend on
the coordinated activities of several enzymes that act sequentially to form a
specific product or to degrade complex molecules. Abnormalities of an enzyme
may produce deleterious effects similar to the effects of mutations affecting
other enzymes in the pathway. Clinical abnormalities that result from defective
enzymes are often attributable either to reduced formation of an essential product or to acculumation of toxic precursors as a result of the metabolic block.

If the abnormal enzyme is involved in processing constituents of food, such as galactose in galactosemia and phenylalanine in phenylketonuria (PKU), the inherited abnormality is aggravated by the presence of that constituent in the diet and can be ameliorated by dietary restriction [7].

In some inborn errors, the defective protein is not an enzyme but a protein necessary to maintain the structure of the cell; in others, the mutation may affect proteins that transport products from one cell to another or from one part of the cell to another. Inherited deficiencies of hormones, blood-clotting factors, antibodies, and hemoglobin are also included among the inborn errors of metabolism.

Although each metabolic error is unique with regard to its underlying cause, it is often difficult to distinguish one inborn error from the other on the basis of clinical appearance alone. Clinically similar symptoms may result from a variety of gene mutations. For instance, two distinct defects have been found in infants born with a clinically similar degenerative disease of the nervous system: the more common Tay-Sachs disease occurs primarily among Ashkenazi Jews, where as Sandhoff disease is rarer and occurs in non-Jews. Although the same enzyme is defective in the two disorders, the mutations involve different genetic loci.

Metabolic Disorders Presenting in the Newborn

Infants with inherited metabolic disturbances usually have normal organogenesis and most often show no physical malformations at birth. Their abnormal metabolism, manifested postnatally, may present no problem in utero, either because the mother carries out this function for her fetus, or because an abnormality is not harmful until after birth or after feeding has started. However, in infants with deficiencies of thyroid hormone production or of galactose metabolism, growth and development of the fetal nervous system may be impaired, so that at birth some irreversible brain damage has *already* occurred [9].

It is likely that *other* inborn errors cause severe disturbances in *fetal* metabolism and development. Such errors may be responsible for fetal death and subsequent miscarriage, and certainly for some malformations. In fact, some inborn errors *are* associated with congenital malformations. Inherited abnormalities affecting sex hormone metabolism, such as in the adrenogenital syndromes, characteristically produce abnormal development of external genitalia [10]. Unfortunately, many of the inborn errors leading to abnormalities in fetal development remain undefined because the defective protein is essential at a time when the fetus is inaccessible for study.

On the other hand, for many of the inborn errors presenting in infancy, the defect in metabolism is known and can be demonstrated in cells cultured from an affected individual. This makes it possible to detect an affected fetus. See Prenatal Diagnosis chapter.

Metabolic Disorders Not Associated With Congenital Diseases

Inborn errors of metabolism may lead to diseases that appear after infancy. Some of these may not be expressed until later life. Such disorders may originate as a point mutation or may be multifactorial. β-lipoproteinemia and the hyper-cholesterolemias, α_1-antitrypsin deficiency, many of the myopathies, and diabetes are examples of these disorders (see Chapter 7).

CONGENITAL MALFORMATIONS

The word "congenital" means "at birth," but does not necessarily imply a hereditary cause. Many congenital malformations are genetic, and perhaps all malformations have at least some predisposing genetic determinants. [14]. Some congenital malformations recur in families with frequencies indicating that the abnormal phenotype is due to point mutations acting in single or double dose according to Mendelian patterns of inheritance (see Chapter 3). Many other congenital malformations, such as cleft lip, congenital dislocation of the hips, and neural tube defects like spina bifida, are found more frequently among relatives than in the general population, suggesting some genetic component. Although a small number of these cases may be attributable to single gene defects, a larger number of these malformations are no doubt attributable to the effect of genes at more than one loci, each of the multiple loci having a small but cumulative effect. Examples of this type have not yet been documented in human populations, but they can be expected based on our knowledge of human biology and pathogenesis of disease.

Disorders Associated With Chromosomal Imbalance

A large number of congenital malformations are associated with the presence of gross chromosomal abnormalities. Substantial gains and losses of genetic material lead usually to a pleiotropic effect — ie, result in multiple rather than single abnormalities. Frequently, cardiac malformations occur along with renal abnormalities, and these are often accompanied by bone and joint deformities and brain maldevelopment as well.

It must be remembered that the presence of multiple congenital malformations does not exclude the possibility of a single gene aberration causing a specific defect at an early stage of morphogenesis. Single defects of this kind can disturb the subsequent development of many apparently unrelated structures, that happen to have a common derivation.

Therefore, chromosomal abnormalities may be phenocopies of single gene disorder or may mimic syndromes produced by environmental teratogens — that cause malformations.

Disorders Due to Environmental Teratogens

Exposure of the fetus to a host of exogeneous factors can result in congenital malformations. Such disorders are often difficult to distinguish from those of genetic etiology. Cells and tissues have a limited number of ways to respond to a variety of insults; therefore, environmental agents can alter the phenotype in the same way a mutant gene can. Estimating the time in development when the "injury" occurred may be helpful in excluding some environmental teratogens. For example, no teratogenic factor (genetic or environmental) can produce cleft palate or spina bifida after fusion of the normal palate or spine has been completed by the fourth month of gestation. However, ascertaining the time at which the defect was first detectable may not discriminate between environmental and genetic teratogens. Among the agents implicated as teratogens have been infectious organisms such as rubella virus, physical agents such as X rays, which can damage the parental germ cells or the fetus in utero, and chemicals or drugs such as thalidomide, cortisone, and even alcohol when the intake is excessive.

Maternal Factors

Maternal diseases such as phenylketonuria (PKU), diabetes, hyperthyroidism, and tuberculosis have been associated with an increased frequency of congenital abnormalities in the fetus [1]. Frequently, mothers with abnormal metabolism have more than one affected infant. Therefore, congenital disorders, even when found in members of the same family, do not necessarily indicate a genetic abnormality in the fetus itself. Instead the problem may lie in an abnormal *maternal environment*. When the mother has PKU, her fetus may be adversely affected by the high level of phenylalanine in the maternal blood. In the case of tuberculosis, the causative agent seems to be the antituberculosis medication taken by the mother rather than the tubercle bacillus itself.

Interaction Between Environment and Genetic Factors

The majority of congenital malformations probably result from interaction between the individual's genotype and his environment. Even those that seem purely environmentally determined may have genetic components that influence susceptibility; one fetus may be more susceptible to damage than another exposed to the same infectious agent or abnormal chemical environment. It is known that synthetic progesterone administered to the mother may masculinize the genitalia of her female fetus [10]. Yet, although many women have been treated with synthetic progesterone early in pregnancy, only a few of the infants resulting from these pregnancies have been masculinized as a result of the treatment. Differences in the way these compounds are metabolized may explain the variable susceptibility.

Another example of interaction between environmental and genetic factors is the case of erythroblastosis, where the expression of the abnormality is dependent not only upon the maternal and fetal Rh genotypes, but also upon the maternal and fetal ABO blood group antigens (genetic factors) and whether fetal cells enter the maternal circulation in significant numbers (environmental factor) [11]. Only if fetal cells leaked across the placenta into the maternal circulation during delivery of a previous incompatible offspring is the fetus at risk of the disorder, as it is the exposure of fetal cells to maternal ones that leads to the production of harmful antibodies. Environmental factors may also play a role in the production of some congenital malformations, as spina bifida and cleft palate, which are familial but do not follow the usual Mendelian ratios observed for single gene mutations.

Among the cancers occurring in early childhood, there are several that occur in members of the same family. Underlying these recurrences seems to be a genetic predisposition carried in the germ line of the parent. These germinal mutations transmitted from the parent, in combination with somatic mutations induced by multiple environmental agents after birth, have been implicated as etiologic agents [12].

Disorders Associated Wtih Mental Retardation

Families of children with mental retardation frequently seek genetic counseling. Unfortunately, when the occurrence is sporadic rather than familial, it is difficult to determine if the cause is genetic. This is especially true when the clinical abnormalities are common or ill defined. It is important that the proband have a diagnostic evaluation to determine whenever possible the cause of the retardation. The work-up should include a careful history of events during the pregnancy to ascertain if there was maternal illness or birth injury. Amino acid screening of the urine for abnormal metabolites should be carried out. If warranted on the basis of the physical examination, chromosome studies should be obtained. Unfortunately, the presence of small chromosomal abnormalities in the retarded individual is often difficult to interpret, as these may be common and harmless population variations (or polymorphism) rather than pathological rearrangements. At least 3% of normal individuals have morphological alterations of a chromosome, evident on microscopic examination but not related to disease. Studies of the chromosomes of the parents and normal sibs are often needed to discriminate between polymorphism and disease-related abnormalities.

OTHER DIAGNOSTIC CONSIDERATIONS

As a rule, it is easy enough to identify an inborn error or a congenital malformation of genetic etiology if the diagnosis has been made previously on another member of the family. Being forewarned, it is customary to search for evidence of abnormal metabolism in the infant at risk as soon as he is born, or even pre-natally. If there is no previously affected child, it may be difficult to recognize the abnormality before irreversible damage has occurred. For many of the in-born errors, as PKU or maple syrup urine disease, it is important to identify an affected infant very early so that proper dietary regimens may be established in order to prevent the irreversible damage to the brain and other complications. New-born screening programs have been established for several diseases and have iden-tified many families for counseling purposes [13] (see Chapter 13). Screening programs of this type are intended for diseases for which treatment is available, ie, PKU, maple syrup urine disease. In these cases, there is a need to identify in-fants for early treatment to prevent irreversible pathology.

For some inborn errors of metabolism leading to diseases for which treatment is not available, programs have been instituted to screen for the carrier of the disease, ie, to screen parents who may be at risk for having a child with the dis-ease [14]. In this case, screening is carried out for disorders where prenatal diag-nosis is possible. The screening strategy is based on the expectation that mem-bers of the population that will be screened have a significant risk of carrying the pertinent abnormal gene.

When an inborn error has been identified, the possibility that the infant has a variation of the disorder should be considered. There are multiple forms of many metabolic disorders, including mucopolysaccharidosis, achondroplasia, or elip-tocytosis; the heterogeneity is due to genocopies, ie, genes that mimic one another. Some forms may be determined by an X chromosome locus, in which case the risk to the sibs of the affected child is greater than when the gene is an autosomal one. Different mutations have been found to underly the clinically similar forms of disorders of mucopolysaccharide metabolism known as Hurler and Hunter syn-dromes [5]. The former, transmitted as an autosomal recessive, carries little risk that sibs of affected individuals will have abnormal offspring; yet the latter, trans-mitted as an X-recessive, carries with it a significant risk that clinically unaffect-ed female sibs will transmit the disease to their offspring. It seems important to encourage research that will identify heterogeneous forms in new disorders so that the accuracy of diagnosis can be improved and counseling can be more appropriate.

Many families consult the genetic counselor concerned that the disorder lead-ing to the death of their child in early infancy may recur in future offspring. It is helpful when postmortem studies of the affected child have been carried out. Too often, this information is not available, nor is there even a clue as to cause of death. Postmortem studies should be obtained whenever possible, as a means of establishing the cause of the lethal disorder. Sometime in the future, perhaps, tissues from these infants may be cultured routinely and stored for future reference.

To identify an unknown disorder as one with genetic components, the first step is a careful history, with attention to diseases that may be found in the family. For diseases that are transmitted as autosomal recessives, a positive family history is frequently not obtained, but a history of similar disorders among other members of the family may be an important clue to disorders that are transmitted as dominants or as chromosomal variants. The history of consanguinity is frequently found in cases of rare diseases transmitted as autosomal recessives (see Chapter 3). Details of pregnancy and the birth process are often helpful in determining if obstetrical factors might account for the phenotype of the affected child. Whether the mother had any particular deficiency in her diet or was taking medications during pregnancy should be noted since nutritional deficiencies, as well as drugs, may be teratogenic. Eliciting a careful history of the child's developmental progress will help determine when the abnormality was expressed for the first time.

If there is an affected living infant, clinical laboratory tests may aid in establishing the diagnosis. Xrays of bones and internal organs may reveal abnormalities not detectable by physical examination. Blood and urine analysis for the presence of abnormal metabolites may be in order, and can be carried out at most major medical centers. Furthermore, it is sometimes appropriate to obtain a sample of skin cells and to prepare cell cultures that can subsequently be analyzed for enzymes relevant to the infant's symptoms. Unfortunately, it is not yet practical to run a battery of *screening* tests for a large number of rare inherited disorders. It is feasible, however, to obtain chromosome studies whenever indicated.

INDICATIONS FOR CHROMOSOME STUDIES

Chromosome studies are indicated for all infants with multiple congenital malformations. Chromosomal deletions or duplications large enough to be obvious under the ordinary microscope usually involve many genetic loci, so that the imbalance often leads to multiple abnormalities in the developing embryo. Infants who are small for their developmental age, both in length and in weight, are especially suspect, since chromosomal errors lead to intrauterine growth retardation.

As carried out presently, chromosome studies may not always reveal even significantly large alterations in the genetic material, although the newer banding techniques may demonstrate abnormalities not detectable by standard staining procedures.

Karyotyping is also indicated for infants with Down syndrome or other known trisomy syndromes to determine if the extra chromosomal material responsible for the abnormality is transmitted as a chromosomal rearrangement involving more than one chromosome (a translocation chromosome). In the case in which a translocation has occurred, there is some risk that one of the parents carries the rearranged chromosome in a *balanced* form. Although such a parent is usually clinically normal, he (or she) has a significant risk of transmitting that chromosomal rearrangement (translocation chromosome) in an *unbalanced* form to offspring, and hence the chance for other affected infants. Therefore, whenever a variant chromosome *is* found in a child, it is customary to examine the parental karyotypes to determine the mode of transmission and risk of recurrence. If one parent does carry an abnormal chromosome, then it is usually a good idea to karyo-type all other members of the family who may have the abnormal chromosome, because they also are at risk of having an infant with the same abnormality. For further discussion, see Chapter 4.

OTHER CONCERNS OF PEDIATRICIANS

Parents who have given birth to a less than normal child often have tremendous emotional reactions to that discovery, and are not usually prepared, at that time, to consider their reproductive future [15] (see also Chapter 11, this volume). Therefore, an extended course of counseling is usually indicated. The primary emphasis should be on the affected child, his prognosis and possible treatment. Gradually, information regarding what is known of the etiology is in order, as well as reassurance, whenever possible, that parental thoughts and deeds had little to do with the production of the abnormality; this is especially appropriate for disorders with genetic components. It may take several months before information regarding future offspring is *perceived,* many of those parents to whom such information was given too early deny ever having *heard* it [16].

For disorders where members of the extended family may carry the pertinent mutation or translocation chromosome, testing of all relatives at risk should be encouraged to prevent a needless second tragedy in the same kindred.

CONCLUSION

Disorders in infancy for which genetic counseling is appropriate are abundant and include those attributable to point mutations, chromosomal abnormalities, and genetic susceptibility to environmental teratogens. Congenital abnormalities, including inborn errors with vastly different causes, may appear clinically similar, making predictions of the probability of recurrence difficult. The closer one comes to pinpointing the specific defect responsible for the clinical phenotype, and its mode of transmission, the more reliable will be estimates of recurrence.

REFERENCES

1. Warkany J: "Congenital Malformations." Chicago: Year Book Medical Publishers, 1971.
2. Childs B, Miller SM, Bearn AG: Gene mutation as a cause of human disease. In Sutton HE, Harris MI (eds): "Mutagenic Effects of Environmental Contaminants." New York: Academic Press, 1972, p. 3.
   Note: Childs and colleagues found that 7% of 9,352 hospitalized pediatric patients had either a single gene defect or chromosomal abnormality, 16% had malformations including cardiac abnormalities, and 4% had unclassified central nervous system malfunctions.

3. Creasy MR, Crolla JA, Alberman ED: A cytogenetic study of human spontaneous abortions using banding techniques. Hum Genet 31:177, 1976.
4. Smith DW, Lemli L, Opitz JM: A new syndrome of congenital anomalies, J Pediat 64:212, 1964.
5. Neufeld EF: Mucopolysaccharidosis: The biochemical approach in medical genetics. In McKusick VA, Clarborne R (eds): "Medical Genetics." New York: HP Publishing Company, 1973.
6. Rimoin DL: The chondrodystrophies. "Advances in Medical Genetics." In Harris H, Hirshborn (eds): New York: Plenum Press, 1975, vol 5, pp 1-118.
7. Hsia YE: Treatment in genetic diseases, In Milunsky A (ed): "The Prevention of Genetic Disease and Mental Retardation." Philadelphia: Saunders 1973, pp 277-305.
8. Srivastava SK, Beutler E: Studies on human B-D-N-acetylhexosaminidases. III. Biochemical genetics of Tay-Sachs and Sandhoff's diseases. J Biol Chem 249:2054, 1974.
9. Gardner L (ed): "Endocrine and Genetic Diseases of Childhood and Adolescence" 2nd Ed. Philadelphia: Saunders, 1975.
10. Wilkins L: In Blizzard RM, Migeon CJ (eds): "Diagnosis and Treatment of Endocrine Disorders in Childhood and Adolescence," 3rd Ed. Springfield, Ill: Charles C Thomas, 1966.
11. Clarke CA: The prevention of Rh isoimmunization. In McKusick VA, Clarborne R (eds): "Medical Genetics." New York: HP Publishing Company, 1973, p 263.
12. Knudson AG, Strong LC, Anderson DE: Heredity and cancer in man. In (Steinberg AG, Bearn AG (eds): "Progress in Medical Genetics," vol 9. New York: Grune & Stratton, 1973, p 113.
13. Hsia DYY, Holtzman NA: A critical evaluation of PKU screening. In McKusick VA, Clarborne R (eds): "Medical Genetics." New York: HP Publishing Company, 1973, p 237.
14. Kaback MM, O'Brien JS: Tay-Sachs: Prototype for prevention of genetic disease. In McKusick VA, Clarborne R (eds): "Medical Genetics." New York: HP Publishing Company, 1973, p 253.
15. Breg R. Family counseling in Downs syndrome. Ann N Y Acad Sci 171:645, 1970.
16. Leonard CO, Chase GA, Childs B: Genetic counseling: A consumer's view. New Eng J Med 287:433, 1972.

6

Genetic Counseling for Problems Affecting Older Children and Adults

Robin J. Caldwell, PhD, and Walter E. Nance, MD, PhD

INTRODUCTION

Genetic counseling has suddenly become the vogue. Counseling is now an articulated career goal of many graduate students entering the field of human genetics. Special programs have been established to train paraprofessional personnel to assist in the collection of genetic data and the provision of genetics services [1]. Scholarly geneticists who have never themselves been directly involved in counseling programs heatedly debate the relative merits of alternative counseling strategies on the pages of our scientific journals [2–4]. Doubtless there are many reasons for this awakening interest. The dramatic advances in genetics and molecular biology during the 1950s and 1960s have increased public awareness of the frightening potential of science to modify human evolution. In amniocentesis, human cytogenetics, and the diagnosis and treament of metabolic diseases, basic research has yielded knowledge that can be of great practical value in improving the human condition. Finally, as human families have begun to decrease precipitously in size, parents are becoming increasingly concerned that their one or two children be wellborn. Nonetheless, these factors cannot adequately account for the current interest in genetic counseling or for the mystique that is growing up around this process.

In our opinion, genetic counseling does not differ qualitatively from many other aspects of medical practice. The physician-counselor usually is a specialist in rare diseases. Differential diagnosis is one of the most important activities that occurs in many general genetic counseling clinics [5]. The communications skills required to elicit and provide information during a genetic counseling session do not differ substantially from those used by any effective physician. Genetic counseling, however, is a time-consuming process. If the time required to assemble and analyze the family history is included, genetic counseling sessions can seldom be completed in less than an hour. One reason why physician-counselors may do a better job of genetic counseling than can practicing clinicians is that most of them do not earn a living by counseling. If they did, they probably could not afford to spend very much time with each family.

A major difference between medical advice and genetic counseling is that the physician customarily acts as an advocate in giving medical advice for the course of treatment he has selected. Most genetic counselors, on the other hand, strongly support the concept of nondirective counseling [5a]. Cynics have argued that there is no such thing as nondirective counseling, and that the counselor always conveys his prejudices—nonverbally, if not overtly. Even if this criticism were true, it would still be important to promote nondirective counseling as an explicit ideal. Society has little to fear from the application of foreseeable advances in genetic technology to individuals in the population as long as the decision about whether to use the technology is made by the individual consumers. There is potential for great mischief only when decisions of this type are made arbitrarily by physicians, philosophers, sociologists, theologians, committees, governments, or genetic counselors, without consulting the consumers. There are few specialties in medicine that deal with such diverse problems as does human genetics. This chapter reviews some of the problems that frequently recur in genetic counseling.

The challenge, as illustrated by the areas discussed, is to identify patients who have genetic problems.

Medical Diagnosis

Many genetic disorders of later presentation have an insidious onset. The medical diagnosis of some of these, such as the muscular dystrophies, is notoriously difficult until the condition has become quite advanced. Often the patient and relatives are aware that something is wrong for years before a correct medical diagnosis is made (see Chapter 15). In such circumstances knowledge that a known genetic disease has affected family members can greatly simplify and accelerate the diagnostic process. Without this information, a mysterious ailment can be referred to many physicians with different subspecialty experiences before a genetic basis is considered. An equally unsatisfactory experience is when a more common diagnosis is mistakenly applied, after which much time may be spent on inappropriate treatment before the true diagnosis is recognized.

An illustrative example is Wilson disease, which in the adolescent often mimicks subacute hepatitis, sometimes complicated by a transient hemolytic anemia, and in the young adult may present as an extrapyramidal neurological disease resembling multiple sclerosis, or as a psychiatric disturbance, occasionally accompanied by intellectual disintegration. If recognized, prompt diagnosis could lead to effective treatment for this abnormality of copper metabolism, which would otherwise continue to cause progressive liver and brain damage.

The vast number of rare genetic disorders, including many as yet unrecognized, should not lead to despair or denial, but rather to a flexible readiness to challenge an unconfirmed diagnosis, and to an awareness that genetic possibilities have to be considered in the differential diagnosis of virtually any medical condition.

The potential benefit of a correct medical diagnosis is not only for *genetic counseling* of relatives at risk, but also for case-finding by *detecting* relatives at risk [5b], so that timely preventive treatment can be initiated.

Genetic Diagnosis

Standard textbooks and subspeciality monographs used to contain vague statements about a given condition being "genetic." This type of imprecision is disappearing with better general understanding of the *different* genetic patterns of inheritance (see Chapter 3) and better appreciation of the need for a *precise* genetic diagnosis.

Familial does not equal genetic. Obviously there are many bases for concurrence of medical conditions in a family other than genetic ones. Nonetheless, the recurrence of a condition among close relatives is a powerful reason to examine whether there is a genetic predisposition to that condition within the family. To conclude that there is a genetic basis, however, demands the fulfillment of stringent criteria, because a careless asumption can have unwarranted implications for other relatives, or for other families with the same condition.

A medical diagnosis can include several genetic possibilities. Even for apparently well-defined disorders such as hemophilia, tests can distinguish factor VIII deficiency from the somewhat milder factor IX deficiency, both of which are X-linked recessive, and other tests will distinguish factor VIII deficiency due to von Willebrand disease, which is autosomal dominant, or the rarer deficiencies of other factors, which are autosomal recessive. For the muscular dystrophies, where definitive chemical diagnoses still elude the medical scientist, there are autosomal recessive conditions that resemble X-linked recessive conditions, and sometimes dominantly inherited conditions are medically indistinguishable from phenocopies that are recessively inherited. Furthermore, some of these are much milder than others, which is information of intense interest to affected families. Because of these uncertainties, a correct medical diagnosis does not necessarily equal a correct genetic diagnosis, and critical information may be provided by family information about who is *not* affected as well as who *is* affected.

Genetic counseling for conditions affecting older children and adults, therefore, is critically dependent both on a correct medical diagnosis and on a correct genetic diagnosis. The following sections provide examples from various types of medical conditions to illustrate these points.

SELECTED DISEASES OF LATE ONSET

Genetic diseases that become manifest in older children may cause several problems for the genetic counselor. First, because these diseases are not apparent at birth, individuals with a positive family history may seek genetic counseling to learn if they themselves are affected. If a diagnosis cannot be made readily, repeated medical visits and consultations may be required thus creating or aggravating possibly groundless anxieties about a disease.

Variability in severity or expression of genetic diseases is an important problem. For instance, autosomal dominant neurofibromatosis may never produce more than a few skin blemishes and nodules in one person, whereas an affected relative can have brain impairment, serious nerve damage or body deformities, grotesque marring of facial features, or even malignant degeneration arising as early as the second decade of life. This poses a dilemma for the genetic counselor: to explain and warn an affected family without arousing excessive fears about complications that may never occur.

Another type of problem is genetic heterogeneity — the fact that a disorder can arise from several unrelated genetic causes. Many genetic syndromes such as diabetes mellitus [6], the mucopolysaccharidoses, the glycogen storage diseases, and the hyperlipidemias [7] have all been subdivided into diseases caused by mutations at different loci even though the clinical manifestations within each syndrome are very similar.

Multifactorial Diseases

Diabetes. The recognized variants of diabetes mellitus constitute an excellent example of genetic heterogeneity. Rimoin and his colleagues have tabulated 32 genetic diseases in which overt diabetes or at least some abnormality in glucose metabolism may be an integral component [6]. Some of these diseases are clearly defined, monogenic traits. On the other hand, the recent twin studies of Tattersall and Pyke have clearly shown that, although concordance is the rule among identical twins with maturity-onset diabetes, in juvenile diabetes about 30% of monozygotic twin pairs appear to remain discordant, a fact that suggests that some cases are mainly environmental in etiology [8]. The recent demonstration of an association between juvenile-onset diabetes and HL-A type [9] as well as the demonstration of the possible role of viral infections in precipitating diabetes [10], have indicated plausible specific pathogenic mechanisms that could explain the interaction between genetic and environmental factors in some cases of diabetes.

What does the genetic counselor actually have to offer in this situation? Familiarity with the rare monogenic syndromes that are commonly associated with diabetes could lead to the idea of an unexpected diagnosis. Assuming these syndromes have been excluded, twin and family studies still provide clear evidence for a gene-

TABLE I. Relative Risk of Diabetes for Relatives of Affected Probands *

	Onset < 20 years of age			Onset ≥ 20 years of age		
	Parents	Sibs	Offspring	Parents	Sibs	Offspring
Proband (juvenile onset)	× 5	× 15	× 22	× 2	× 8	No data
Proband (adult onset)	No data	× 7	× 5	× 2	× 3	× 2

* Adapted from Simpson [11]. Frequency of diabetes in the control population is assumed to be 0.128 for males in the 10– 19–year–old age group and 0.150 for females in the same age group. Frequency of the disease increases with age.

tic component among remaining cases. Empiric risk figures suggest that the incidence of diabetes among the offspring of a juvenile diabetic is 22 times that observed in the general population (Table I). Although these data provide impressive evidence for familial aggregation, the absolute risk of 2.8-3.3% is still fairly low [11]. However, until the basic defect in diabetes is understood, genetic counseling for the disease is likely to remain imprecise. Many patients with latent diabetes can be detected through the use of provocative tests, and perhaps the most important consequence of a genetic approach to this disease is that knowledge of the familial nature of the disease in many families can lead to the diagnosis of affected individuals.

Mental illness. Mental illness is another example of a highly heterogeneous condition for which there is evidence of familial aggregation. Moreover, mental illness poses even greater variation in diagnostic criteria and more disagreement about etiology and nosology than does diabetes. Contributing environmental factors such as culture, education, and psychologic stress are undoubtedly of great importance in determining the nature and severity of psychiatric illness. At the same time, these are environmental variables that are difficult to isolate and characterize by objective parameters, which, although suggestive, may or may not be appropriate to the individual case. Fischer's data indicate that the risk of developing schizophrenia for the first-degree relatives of a schizophrenic is about 10% [12]. Karlsson's extensive studies on inheritance of schizophrenia suggest that first-and second-degree relatives of schizophrenics may have a threefold to fivefold increase in risk above that of the general population (Table II) [13]. It may be that a more balanced presentation of these risk figures would be appropriate in managing families with psychiatric illness, with equal emphasis on the likelihood that close relatives will be normal. A supportive approach of this type would be particularly ap-

TABLE II. Relative Risk of Schizophrenia for Relatives of Affected Proband in Iceland.

Relationship	Relative Risk of Schizophrenia
First-degree relatives	
Parents	X 3.8
Sibs	X 5.0
Offspring	X 4.4
Second-degree relatives	
Uncles, aunts	X 2.9
Nephews, nieces	X 4.1
Third-degree relatives	
First cousins	X 1.6

* Adapted from Karlsson [13]. The life-time risk of developing schizophrenia for the general Icelandic population was assumed to be 0.73%.

propriate for patients seeking counseling who have already completed their families.

Heart disease. Several well-defined chromosomal and monogenic syndromes are associated with structural anomalies of the heart. Marfan syndrome is an excellent example of a monogenic trait that presents many challenges for the genetic counselor because of the generally ominous, but highly variable prognosis. Besides cardiac abnormalities, Marfan syndrome is associated with characteristic skeletal abnormalities and ectopia lentis. Although dissecting aneurysm is a common cause of death in Marfan syndrome, not all affected individuals will die from cardiac disease, and those who do may succumb at widely varying ages. Although patients with Marfan syndrome are often aware of several relatives who died from "heart attacks," they may be unprepared to relate this to themselves. In the absence of any effective preventive therapy, the rather grim prognosis of a dissecting aneurysm should not be starkly outlined without due consideration of the possible psychological reactions of the patient. On the other hand, patients, and particularly other family members, may well need to be informed of the possibility of cardiac involvement so that they can adapt their plans and life-styles accordingly. A patient with pseudoxanthoma elasticum diagnosed in his late 20s, for example, may benefit considerably from knowing that both he and his family doctor are alert to any early signs of cardiac involvement, so that appropriate treatment may be initiated promptly.

Certain of the familial hyperlipoproteinemias show highly significant risk factors for myocardial infarction. In addition to families in which major genes for hyperlipoproteinemia appear to be segregating, studies of quantitative inheritance suggest that both genetic and environmental factors contribute to the determination of lipoprotein values that exceed the "normal" range. Coronary artery disease is clearly the end result of many factors, including diet, exercise, cigarette smoking, body weight, and psychological stress. The recognition of these multiple environmental hazards has led to the proposal and initiation of costly intervention trials to modify the life-styles of affected probands or other people found to have a high risk for developing coronary artery disease. However, efforts to modify the smoking habits of potentially affected individuals are frequently doomed to failure when they are extended from symptomatic to presymptomatic patients. Full utilization of the family history as a risk factor offers a strategic alternative to bypass this dilemma. Rather than attempting to alter the diet habits of the entire nation (laudable though this goal might be), it might be more effective to attempt to identify the 0.5%-1.0% of the population who, because of their family history and other factors, have the highest risk of developing coronary artery disease. These patients, with their nuclear families, could be enrolled in an intensive intervention program designed to prevent the development of heart disease, and the personal knowledge of affected family members with coronary artery disease would constitute a strong motivation for compliance with treatment.

Cancer. Approximately one-half of all cancer mortality is caused by malignancies in three sites: the lung, the large intestine, and the breast. Earlier epidemiological studies concentrated on identifying causal environmental agents, with reasonable success. Linking cigarette smoking to lung cancer, high-meat and low-cereal diets to intestinal cancer, and reproductive history to breast cancer has offered some hope for reducing cancer incidence rates in the susceptible population. However, the implication of environmental agents in carcinogenesis does not rule out underlying genetic factors that may contribute to the susceptibility to cancer. Identification of these genetic factors would enhance the effectiveness of cancer-screening programs. Not only would screening programs for use on genetically predisposed individuals be far less expensive, but also earlier diagnosis would be more likely if only a particularly susceptible segment of the population needed to be screened. For example, there is considerable uncertainty about cost and risk of mammography screening programs for breast cancer in relation to the benefits. However, the cost-benefit analysis would be dramatically altered if a program concentrated on women who were first-degree relatives of patients with breast cancer. Of course, at the most elementary level, all cancers arise from genetic factors since almost all theories of malignancy postulate some loss or alteration in gene control or gene structure.

Certain rare inherited diseases are associated with a clearly increased risk of malignancy. Xeroderma pigmentosum is one such disease. Most commonly inherited as an autosomal recessive trait, xeroderma pigmentosum has also been observed to behave as an autosomal dominant disease with a milder expression

[14]. The disease is heterogeneous and is caused by a deficiency in one of
several enzymes normally required to repair the DNA damage caused by ultraviolet irradiation of the skin. This leads to the development of multiple skin cancers
as well as other malignancies. Some affected children reportedly have fared fairly
well when "raised in the dark," that is, kept entirely away from any ultraviolet
light exposure. The difficulties inherent in this kind of upbringing are obvious.
Still, it is the best treatment now available for a condition with a grim prognosis.

Other inherited diseases that lead to chromosome instability and a predisposition to cancer include Bloom syndrome, Fanconi anemia, and ataxia-telangiec-
tasia — all autosomal recessive traits. Although the presenting symptoms differ in
these diseases, they are all associated with an increased risk of lymphoreticular
malignancies in affected individuals and possibly in carriers as well. Often the
parents, aware of leukemia in family members, are not surprised at the genetic
associations. Occasionally, however, the associated risk of malignancy is unknown
to them, and the counselor must be prepared to deal with the psychological trauma
that often results from mentioning the possibility of cancer.

Adenocarcinoma of the intestine occurs in 50% of patients with the autosomal
dominant condition, familial polyposis coli, by 30 years of age. This association
is well recognized, and the genetic counselor should emphasize the importance of
regular examinations of family members. Often prophylactic colectomy is advised.

Certain common cancers show some degree of familial predilection, but even
these may often be due to shared environmental experiences. As with other multifactorial diseases, the genetic counselor can only rely on empiric risk data in
cases where a specific cancer-prone syndrome cannot be diagnosed. Several of the
more common cancers, including carcinomas of the breast, prostate, colon-rectum,
stomach, and endometrium, show a site-specific threefold increase in risk for first-
degree relatives of cancer probands [15]. The fact that different types of cancer
may occur frequently in the same family suggests that, whatever the underlying
genetic causal factors may be, they operate in several types of malignancies.

Of the common cancers, the one best known to cluster in families is cancer
of the breast. Several risk factors have been found to be associated with breast
cancer, including age at first pregnancy, age at menopause, and also bilateral
involvement in close relatives. Particularly in high-risk groups, thermography can
lead to early diagnosis. It is interesting that two of the most common cancers,
breast and colon cancer, have significantly increased coexistence among relatives
of cancer probands. Other reports have documented the concurrence of breast
and ovarian cancers in several family members.

Ulcerative colitis, which has a tendency to be familial, can also lead to the development of cancer. Patients with localized ulcerative colitis probably have no
greater risk for cancer than the general population; however, if there is total or
near-total involvement of the colon, the risk is very much higher and seems to be
directly related to the duration of the colitis. Genetic factors are implicated by

data from several concordant monozygotic twin sets. Ulcerative colitis has never been reported in only one member of a monozygotic twin pair. Family and population studies indicate that environmental factors are not the sole causal agents. Practical information the genetic counselor should provide would include the increased empiric risk for family members and the importance of frequent physical examinations [16].

One of the hindrances in convincing people that cigarette smoking causes lung cancer is that almost everyone knows someone who "smoked two packs a day and lived to be 95." It is conceivable that the differences between smokers who develop lung cancer and those who do not may have a genetic basis. Unsubstantiated evidence has suggested that smokers in whom high levels of the enzyme aryl hydrocarbon hydroxylase can be induced have an increased risk of developing lung cancer [17]. If true, these observations would be of great importance as an example of genetic and environmental interaction in the etiology of disease and could have important implications for screening to identify a high-risk population and focusing educational campaigns on those individuals in the population who are most likely to benefit.

Deafness. Genetic heterogeneity is perhaps nowhere so manifest as in the inherited syndromes involving deafness. There are more than 100 recognized genetic diseases that may cause some degree of hearing loss, either conductive or sensorineural, as one of the primary effects, and they may variously involve dominant, recessive, or X-linked inheritance. Many of the mutant genes for deafness have pleiotropic (ie, multiple apparently unrelated) effects, and the evidence of these associations can alert physicians to the cause of hearing loss. For example, autosomal dominant Waardenberg syndrome is characterized by heterochromia iridium (different colored irises), white forelock, dystopia canthorum (wide-set inner canthi of the eyes), and a low-set hairline. About 20% of these patients show unilateral or bilateral sensorineural hearing loss, which is often profound and usually present at birth. Most affected patients do not show all the cardinal features of this condition.

Treacher-Collins syndrome, also autosomal dominant, involves a conductive hearing loss. However, in this syndrome, half the affected individuals have a negative family history. The implication is that a significant proportion of cases probably represent new mutations. The condition thus persists, despite fewer affected individuals having progeny than do their normal siblings, so that the observed incidence of cases reflects a balance between the introduction of new genes into the population by mutation and their removal by natural selection.

Usher syndrome, a recessive trait involving both deafness and retinitis pigmentosa leading to blindness, is upsetting information for the patient seeking counseling. Since no effective medical treatment is available, the appropriate time for establishing a diagnosis is open to debate. Most educators believe that the years when relatively normal vision is retained could be put to better use if the diagnosis were established early. On the other hand, it is a matter of common knowledge that it is difficult if not impossible to motivate patients with progressive loss of vision to prepare for blindness before it occurs.

A very good argument, however, can be made for early diagnosis of Jervell–Lang-Nielson syndrome, an autosomal recessive disease. This condition involves a congenital sensorineural hearing loss that is associated with a prolonged QT interval on the electrocardiogram. Myocardial repolarization is abnormal, leading to cardiac arrhythmias and fainting. About 20–30% of patients affected with this syndrome die by 20 years of age. Since effective pharmacologic or surgical treatment is available for this condition, early diagnosis can allow improved chances for survival.

About 60% of all deafness is hereditary. Because most of the genetic cases are probably simple Mendelian dominant, recessive, or X-linked traits, the genetic counselor should be able to offer precise estimates of recurrence risk. Unfortunately, there may be no history of affected relatives in recessive cases or in the many dominant cases of deafness that show variable expression. Consequently, in the absence of a recognizable syndrome or a "positive" family history, it may be difficult if not impossible to identify genetic cases with certainty. In this situation, empiric risk figures are again the only recourse.

SPECIAL PROBLEMS OF GENETIC COUNSELING

Multifactorial Inheritance

Although the threshold model of polygenic inheritance may provide a rationale for the counselor (see Chapter 3), it has been our experience that patients find the polygenic model to be a very incomprehensible explanation for their recurrence risks. Even when visual aids are used and great care is taken to explain the model to highly intelligent couples, they still seem to regard the explanation as genetic doubletalk. Implicating a large but unspecified number of genes with small deleterious effects seems more threatening than does a clear, discrete single gene mutation. A much more satisfactory method of counseling for multifactorial disease is to present the data simply as an empiric recurrence risk. We tell patients that it would be a mistake to assure them that "lightning never strikes twice," and, based on data collected from hundreds of families like themselves, we can provide a recurrence risk estimate. If they remain unconvinced by the explanation, we tell them that "in some patients the disease is caused by a single gene or genes and we have tried to exclude these rare causes. Among the remaining patients, some cases may be largely genetic, perhaps resulting from the interaction of several genes, whereas in other families environmental factors may predominate. What we know is that if a large number of families like yours is averaged, a numerical recurrence risk (in a given range) can be obtained." We usually do not attempt to explain to the parents of a single child affected with a multifactorial trait that their predicted recurrence risk will become higher if they have a second affected child. However, on occasion we have told couples that "when there has been only one affected child, we cannot be sure whether genetic or environmental factors were of greater importance, but if there have been two affected children, this does not actually increase your recurrence risk. It simply means that you had a higher risk all along, but had no way of knowing it."

Late-Onset Degenerative Diseases

Genetic diseases that have a late age of onset such as Huntington chorea (see Chapter 15) present special problems for counseling, since there may be no way to establish the diagnosis at a time when it is relevant for family planning.

Young adults in families with dominantly inherited senile macular degeneration must watch their parents and grandparents lose their vision without knowing whether they themselves carry the gene; there is a strong tendency toward fatalism in such situations, and perhaps this is a good thing. For the parent who does not know himself whether he carries a gene for a dominantly inherited disease with late onset, transmitting some of that uncertainty to a child may not be perceived as an unreasonable burden, yet families, and individuals within families, differ markedly in their reactions to this kind of uncertainty.

A major thrust of human genetics research in the future will doubtless be directed toward clarifying the genetics of the chronic and degenerative diseases of old age. We have much to learn about the medical and psychological impact of chronic diseases of late onset on the individual and the family. Only when this information is available will it be possible for the genetic counselor to give his client a balanced view of the health burden associated with specific genotypes that are not expressed until later life.

Mating

The choice of a mate is a personal one and is rarely made on the basis of who possesses which recessive genes. Apart from considerations of the undesirability of directive counseling, many individuals consider this type of advice to be an invasion of privacy. Frustrating though it may be for the genetic counselor who feels he knows better than his client the dreadful consequences of a predicted condition with its psychological and monetary costs, there are few acceptable alternatives to offer.

One of these alternatives is artificial insemination by a genetically normal donor to bypass one of the heterozygous parents. Although artificial insemination has been available for many years, in the United States it has usually been employed for male infertility rather than genetic considerations. In the genetic counseling clinic this procedure should always be presented as a viable option for couples wishing to avoid the birth of a second child affected with a recessive disease. Regrettably, in our experience most parents reject this possibility.

Where there are strong reasons for intermarriage within a racial or religious isolate, individuals may adopt one of several attitudes. One of these is the fatalistic acceptance of the recessive disease as a part of their family, even contributing to their characteristics as a unique group. A second is a denial of the existence of consanguinity, an attitude frequently encountered, for instance, by outside researchers working with American Indian groups. The question routinely asked to elicit information regarding consanguinity is, "Are your parents related in any way?" Although the answer may be "no," a carefully prepared pedigree will often reveal very high levels of consanguinity. The reasons for denial are undoubtedly varied. There may be vague uneasiness about social stigmatization if the marriage to a relative is revealed; perhaps a more likely explanation is that perceptions of relatedness differ, particularly among some American Indian groups. The misconceptions can usually be corrected if the geneticist takes time to explain what he means by "related."

Counseling strategy that can be adopted for members of an inbred isolate is to suggest that mates be sought among members of a different line of the same group. For example, Amish communities can be found not only in Pennsylvania, but also in Ohio and Indiana. Over the years, different recessive phenotypes have emerged in the subgroups. An Amish individual from Pennsylvania could reduce his genetic risk somewhat by seeking a mate from some other Amish community.

Another example of a counseling problem posed by assortative mating is that of marriages among the deaf. Because of their special educational needs many hearing-imparied individuals attend residential schools for the deaf and, consequent to the close social contact and mutual similar handicap, they often marry each other. Such marriages sometimes produce complex genetic problems that are difficult to unravel. If a parent affected with one type of recessive deafness also carries another recessive gene for deafness in the heterozygous state and marries a partner who is homozygous for the second recessive gene, half of the children would be affected with the recessive trait, and the pedigree would spuriously appear to be one of dominant deafness.

New Mutations

As mentioned previously, the existence of environmental phenocopies among all the major genetic disease of adult onset often confounds distinction between cases with a significant genetic component and those primarily environmental in origin. In addition to determining if genes are involved at all, the genetic counselor is sometimes obliged to distinguish between a new mutation and a gene that may be present in other family members. The distinction is important, because although new mutations begin a new line of inherited disease, relatives other than offspring will not be at risk.

The mutation rate in man is variously estimated as being between 1×10^{-4} and 1×10^{-6} per locus per gamete [17a]. For genetic diseases that are maintained in the population despite lowered fitness or even lethality, it is assumed that the mutation rate is in equilibrium with selection against the gene. Approximately 33% of affected hemophilic males have no family history of the disorder. These cases are presumably the result of new mutations, an assumption consistent with the inheritance of an X-linked trait when that trait has been, until recently at least, lethal in the sense that few affected males survived long enough to produce offspring. Thus, one-third of the hemophilia-bearing X chromosomes were lost to the gene pool while two-thirds remained to propagate through heterozygous female carriers. Primarily because of the availability of factor VIII concentrate, hemophilic patients now have a much better chance for an almost normal life, and many of them reach adulthood, marry and reproduce. Thus, although the proportion of cases that are new mutations will probably decrease in future, the overall incidence of hemophilia will very likely increase.

Genetic counseling for hemophilia is usually sought by female relatives of an affected male. They may be sisters, cousins, or aunts in the maternal line. Having observed the effects of the disease, they want to know their carrier status and the likelihood of producing a hemophilic male. A carrier of hemophilia has a 50% chance of passing the hemophilia-bearing X chromosome to her offspring. This probability, taken with the 50% chance of bearing a male child, leads to a 1 in 4 chance of producing a hemophilic son. Amniocentesis for hemophilia, at present, can be offered only to identify and avoid the birth of males. Few carriers, however, accept this option. Unfortunately it is much easier to identify males in utero than it is to identify carriers for hemophilia. A recently completed cooperative study for the detection of the carrier state of classic hemophilia which was conducted by the National Heart, Blood, and Lung Institute indicated that, even though carrier detection has been much improved, it is still not perfect [18].

Theoretically, carriers of hemophilia should have 50% biologically active factor VIII. The wide range of "normal" activity and the vagaries of X inactivation and genetic heterogeneity prevent the use of factor VIII levels to identify carriers with any certainty. The ability to detect factor VIII antigenic protein by a specific antibody has permitted the development of a discriminant ratio of factor VIII coagulant activity to factor-VIII-related antigen for carrier detection. The cooperative study revealed that, overall, correct classification by the ratio ranged from 72% to 94% [18].

To summarize, not all female relatives of hemophilic males have increased risks of being carriers. Indeed, pedigree analysis shows that in some families with two remotely related hemophiliacs, the presence of a substantial number of normal males may make two separate mutations a more probable explanation than inheritance of the hemophilia gene from a common ancestor. When combined with the results of carrier-detection tests, pedigree analysis can provide useful, although not necessarily absolute, information for females who may be heterozygotes.

In contrast to the importance of new mutations in hemophilia, a recent study by Francke and her co-workers [19] indicated a marked deficiency of new mutations among males for Lesch-Nyhan syndrome, another X-linked recessive disorder in which affected males have developmental retardation, spasticity, choreoathetosis, and a compulsion for self-mutilation. No patients have ever been known to reproduce; therefore, one-third of the genes coding for the defective enzyme, hypoxanthine phosphoribosyl transferase, are lost every generation. Data on 176 female relatives of 47 unrelated patients with Lesch-Nyhan disease were analyzed to determine the incidence of new mutations in probands, the incidence of new mutations among the mothers, and the presence of any heterozygote advantage. In the 47 families, only four probands appeared to represent new mutations, but for the heterozygous females, the proportion of new mutants was not significantly different from expected, which suggests that mutation rates differed for males and females. These investigators also suggested a paternal age effect on X-linked recessive mutations since the age of fathers of "new" carriers was considerably older than the mean paternal age in the general population [19]. This study has not been universally accepted because it was subject to the ascertainment bias inherent to investigations of rare biochemical disorders [20].

Genetic Variation

The recipients of genetic counseling react with a wide range of emotions, including anxiety, guilt, fatalism, and denial. A conscientious counselor must be prepared to deal with these reactions and provide explanations, responsible alternatives, and support that may go far beyond the mere citing of a recurrence risk. After the birth of a child with a congenital malformation or genetic defect, it is only natural for parents to seek a cause and to wonder whether they could somehow have prevented the abnormality. Whenever appropriate, we try to assure the parents that nothing they did or did not do after the time of conception could have influenced the outcome. For recessive traits we point out that everyone possesses several deleterious or "weak" genes, and that there is nothing at all unique or even unusual about being a carrier of a deleterious gene. In general, we explain, it is only if an individual has a double dose of the same abnormal gene that a problem may arise, and this can happen only when, by chance, both parents are carriers of the same abnormal gene. Moreover, the genetic load of abnormal genes is a burden that all members of society carry; the only difference is that after the birth of an affected child the parents know what one of their abnormal genes is and they can plan future pregnancies accordingly if they so choose. For a dominant trait, we explain that the abnormal gene a parent carries is no different from any other mutant gene, except that it happens to be a gene that is expressed in single dose. An appreciation of the universality of abnormal genes can do much to sublimate the feelings of blame, rage, shame, or guilt that the parents of an affected child might otherwise experience (see Chapter 11).

As noted previously, there is growing evidence that recessive genes may have effects in the heterozygous state by predisposing the carrier to chronic diseases in later life. Swift has estimated that as much as 5% of all cancer may occur in individuals who are heterozygous for one of four recessive genes that are associated with a high risk of malignancy in the homozygous state [21]. Pulmonary emphysema and hepatitis are recognized complications of homozygous α-1-antitrypsin deficiency and these complications are probably more common in heterozygotes as well. Finally, a variety of diseases, such as juvenile-onset diabetes and ankylosing spondylitis are associated with specific H-LA types, presumably reflecting pleiotropic effects of the alleles in question. These genetic risk factors offer many opportunities for disease detection and prevention. The role of mandatory population screening for the detection of high-risk genotypes still remains highly controversial. Screening programs for phenylketonuria (PKU) have yielded many important insights into some of the potential problems of such programs. It is now clear that a minority of infants with a positive PKU test in the neonatal period actually have a disease that should be treated with a low-phenylalanine diet. Before any screening program is initiated, an effective follow-up system for confirming testing as well as therapeutic management should be available. This problem does not arise in screening programs limited to families of an affected proband, since one can assume with high probability that a positive screening test result in a relative is from the same disease as in the affected brother or sister.

A final problem that must be confronted if genetic counseling is to become a truly effective branch of preventive medicine concerns the dissemination of genetic knowledge laterally within a pedigree and vertically across generations. To be most constructive, genetic counseling should be provided to couples at risk before the conception of an affected child. It is a sobering experience to reascertain families with serious X-linked diseases who had been given competent, careful counseling a decade before and to find that genetic information about the disease had not been transmitted, with the genes, by mothers to their carrier daughters. Similarly, our health care delivery system is not designed to facilitate the transmission of relevant genetic information to collateral relatives who may be at risk. This problem is a difficult one, particularly if the affected proband or the parents do not wish other family members to know of their potential risk. Resolution of the legal issue of whether, in this situation, the counselor has a social obligation that transcends the traditional privilege of the doctor-patient relationship would do much to clarify this murky area of medical ethics (see Chapter 14).

ACKNOWLEDGMENTS

This is paper #28 from the Department of Human Genetics of the Medical College of Virginia and was supported in part by grant #1 PO1 HD 10291-01 from the National Institutes of Health and a Clinical Service grant from the National Foundation—March of Dimes.

REFERENCES

1. Lustig L, Poskanzer L: Genetic associates. N Engl J Med 295:1436, 1976.
2. Feldman MW, Lewontin RC: The heritability hang-up. Science 190:1163, 1975.
3. Morton NE: Heritability of IQ. Science 194:9, 1976.
4. Feldman MW, Lewontin RC: Heritability of IQ. Science 194:12, 1976.
5. Nance WE, Rose S, Conneally PM, Miller J: Opportunities for genetic counseling through institutional ascertainment of affected probands. In Lubs HA, de la Cruz F (eds): "Genetic Counseling." New York: Raven Press, 1977, pp 307–331.
5a. Hsia YE: The genetic counselor as information giver. In Capron A, Lappe M, Murray RF, Powledge TM, Twiss SB (eds): "Genetic Counseling, Facts, Values and Norms." BDOAS XV (2). New York: Alan R. Liss for The National Foundation – March of Dimes.
5b. Crane RJ: The case of the illegitimate gene. Postgrad Med J 51:637–642, 1975.
6. Rimoin DL, Schimke RM (eds): "Genetic Disorders of the Endocrine Glands." St. Louis: CV Mosby, 1971.
7. Nyhan WL, Sakati NO (eds): "Genetic and Malformation Syndromes in Clinical Medicine." Chicago: Year Book Publishers, 1976.
8. Tattersall RB, Pyke DA: Diabetes in identical twins. Lancet 2:1120, 1976.
9. Cudworth AG, Woodrow JC: HL-A antigens and diabetes mellitus. Lancet 2:1153, 1974.
10. Gamble DR: A possible virus etiology for juvenile diabetes. In Creutzfeldt W, Köbberling J, Neel JV (eds): "The Genetics of Diabetes Mellitus." New York: Springer-Verlag, 1976, pp 95–105.
11. Simpson NE: Diabetes in the families of diabetics. Can Med Assoc J 98:427, 1968.
12. Fischer M, Harvald B, Hauge M: A Danish twin study of schizophrenia. Br J Psychiatry 115:981, 1969.
13. Karlsson JL: Inheritance of schizophrenia. Acta Psychiatr Scand Suppl 247, 1974.
14. Anderson TE, Begg M: Xeroderma pigmentosum of mild type. Br J Dermatol 62:402, 1950.
15. Lynch HT (ed): "Cancer Genetics." Springfield, Illinois: Charles C Thomas, 1976.
16. Lynch HT, Lynch J, Guirgis H: Heredity and colon cancer. In Lynch HT (ed): "Cancer Genetics;" Springfield; Charles C Thomas, 1976, pp 326–354.
17. Kellermann G, Shaw CR, Luyten-Kellerman M: Aryl hydro-carbon hydroxylase inducibility and bronchogenic carcinoma. N Engl J Med 289:934, 1973.
17a. Lubs HA: Frequency of genetic disease. In Lubs HA, de la Cruz F (eds): "Genetic Counseling" New York: Raven Press, 1977.
18. Klein HG, Aledort LM, Bouma BN, Hoyer LW, Zimmerman TS, DeMets DL: A cooperative study for the detection of the carrier state of classic hemophilia. N Engl J Med 296:959, 1977.
19. Francke U, Felsenstein J, Gartler SM, Migeon BR, Dancis J, Seegmiller JE, Bakay B, Nyhan WL: The occurrence of new mutants in the X-linked recessive Lesch-Nyhan disease. Am J Hum Genet 28:123, 1976.
20. Morton NE, Lalouel JM: Genetic epidemiology of Lesch-Nyhan disease. Am J Hum Genet 29:304, 1977.

21. Swift M, Cohen J, Pinkham R: A maximum-likelihood method for estimating the disease predisposition of heterozygotes. Am J Hum Genet 26:304, 1974.
22. Corey LA, Nance WE, Berg K: A new tool in birth defects research: The MZ half-sib model and its extension to grandchildren of identical twins. In Summitt RL, Bergsma D (eds): "Cell Surface Factors, Immune Deficiencies, Twin Studies." New York: Alan R. Liss for The National Foundation—March of Dimes. BD:OAS XIU (6A): 193–200, 1978.

7
Patterns of Health Behavior

I.M. Rosenstock, PhD

INTRODUCTION

Responses of people to genetic counseling can be considered as a special case of a more general class of health behavior. Although there is not a substantial amount of knowledge regarding generic factors that influence responses to genetic counseling, there is a large body of information concerning the social-psychological determinants of health-related behavior undertaken in one's own behalf or in behalf of one's children. A summary of much of this literature has recently been published [1]. The applicability of this material to likely public responses to genetic screening programs also provides a framework for considering factors that may influence the kinds of responses counselees make to genetic counseling [2].

WHY PEOPLE USE HEALTH SERVICES

It will be helpful at the outset to distinguish among preventive health behavior, illness behavior, and sick-role behavior.

Preventive health behavior is defined as any activity undertaken by a person who believes himself to be healthy, for the purpose of preventing disease or of detecting disease in a presymptomatic stage.

Illness behavior is defined as any activity undertaken by a person who feels unwell, for the purpose of determining whether he or she is ill and for discovering a suitable remedy.

Sick-role behavior is defined as the activity undertaken by one who considers himself sick, for the purpose of regaining health.

Clearly, these three modes of behavior are continuous. Hardly anyone can be found who, upon intensive questioning, would report himself totally free of all symptoms; similarly, the edges between illness behavior and sick-role behavior are blurred. Nevertheless, the distinctions are useful because they refer to *modal mental* states that help to account for behavior.

139   © **1979 Alan R. Liss, Inc.**

Genetic Counseling and Preventive, Illness, or Sick-Role Behavior

Genetic counseling relates to preventive behavior, as in prospective counseling and genetic screening, and it relates to illness or sick-role behavior, as in retrospective, proband-oriented counseling. The major emphasis in this chapter will be on preventive behavior related to prospective counseling.

Conditions for Taking Health-Related Action

The health belief model. In recent years, a model has been developed to explain the conditions under which people take action to prevent, detect, and diagnose disease [1, 2].

Most of the relevant research has been done in connection with health conditions other than genetic conditions, although there has been one study on factors influencing the decision to participate in screening for the Tay-Sachs trait. Some of the findings on nongenetic conditions may be applicable to genetic screening or counseling programs, but more studies are needed of behavior specifically related to genetic problems.

The major variables in the model are drawn and adapted from general social-psychological theory, dealing with the subjective world underlying individual behavior and not with the objective world as observed by others. The model links current subjective states of the individual with current health behavior.

A truism in social psychology is that motivation is required first for perception and then for action. Thus, people who are unconcerned with a particular aspect of their health are not likely to be receptive to any material pertaining to that aspect. Even if, through accidental circumstances, they do perceive such material, they will fail to comprehend, accept, or use the information.

Such concerns or motivations are not only a necessary preconditon for action; motives also determine the particular ways in which the environment will be perceived. That a motivated person perceives selectively in accordance with his motives has been verified in many laboratory studies as well as in field settings [3].

Concepts pertinent to health behavior grow out of such evidence. Specifically, there are three classes of explanatory variables: 1) the general state of health motivation or health concern exhibited by the individual; 2) the psychological state of readiness to take specific actions; and 3) the state of belief that a particular course will be beneficial in relation to the psychological costs of taking that action.

Health motivation. Motivation may be defined as degrees of emotional arousal in individuals caused by some given class of stimuli — in this case, relating to health matters. Health motivation includes negative components (eg, avoidance of ill health or conditons that might put one at risk of suffering illness) and positive components (eg, striving for a sense of good health and well-being).

Readiness to act. Two principal dimensions define whether a state of readiness to act exists: 1) the degree to which an individual feels vulnerable or susceptible to a particular health condition and 2) the extent to which he feels that suffering from that condition would have personally undesirable consequences.

Perceived susceptibility. This refers to the subjective fear of contracting a condition or of possessing a particular transmissible trait. Individuals vary widely in their acceptance of personal susceptibility to a conditon. At one extreme is the individual who denies any possibility of his contracting or transmitting a given condition, or of possessing a particular trait. A more moderate case is the person who may admit to the statistical possibility of its occurrence, but to whom this possibility has little personal reality. At the other extreme is the person who feels in real danger of contracting or transmitting a given condition or of possessing a particular trait.

Perceived severity. Convictions concerning the seriousness of a given health problem may also vary from person to person. The degree of perceived severity may be judged both by the degree of anxiety aroused by the thought of a disease, and also by the personal consequences an individual believes a given disease will have.

A person may, of course, see a health problem objectively in terms of its medical or clinical features, but the perceived seriousness of a condition may, for a given individual, include broader and more complex implications, such as the effects of the problem on self-image, job, family life, and social relations. Thus a person may not believe that tuberculosis or the sickle cell trait are medically serious, but may nevertheless believe that either condition would be serious if it created important psychological or other tensions within himself or his family. There is probably some "optimal" level of perceived seriousness for producing a readiness to act. Too little or too much perceived seriousness can produce a response that is inappropriate to the actual situation.

Perceived Benefits of Taking Action, and Barriers to Taking Action

The acceptance of one's susceptibility to a disease or trait provides a force leading to action, but not necessarily the particular direction that action is likely to take. This is because the direction of action is influenced also by beliefs regarding the relative effectiveness of alternative courses of action. An action is more likely to be regarded positively if it promises to reduce one's perceived susceptibility to an illness or its severity. Again, the persons's subjective belief about the availability and effectiveness of various courses of action, and not objective facts about the effectiveness of action, determines what course will be taken. Beliefs in this area are undoubtedly influenced by the norms and pressures of one's social group.

Even when a given action is seen as likely to reduce the threat of disease, it may also have high psychological costs, including inconvenience, expense, unpleasantness, pain, or embarrassment. These negative consequences of health action can arouse internal conflicts. Several resolutions of these conflicts are possible. If the benefits of action are perceived as great and the costs or negative aspects are seen as relatively minor, the action in question is likely to be taken. Action is likely to be rejected when negative aspects are seen as outweighing perceived benefits. Where both are seen as great, the conflict will obviously be more difficult to resolve.

What does the individual do if there are no acceptable alternatives for resolving his conflicts? Experimental evidence suggests that one of two responses occurs. First, the person may attempt to insulate himself psychologically from the conflict by denying the threat or by directing his energies into activities that do not really reduce the threat; vacillation between choices is an example. Second, a marked increase in fear or anxiety may be aroused. If the conflict becomes intense enough, an individual can be rendered incapable of thinking consistently and behaving constructively about the problem. Even if he is subsequently offered a more effective means of handling the situation, he may not accept it, simply because he can no longer think rationally about it.

Cues to action. The variables that measure perceived susceptibility and severity and the variables that define perceived benefits and costs of taking action generally have been validated by research. However, one additional variable, which has not yet been subjected to careful study, is necessary to complete the model: A cue or trigger to trip off appropriate action is needed. The levels of motivation provide the energy or force to act; the perception of benefits in relation to subjective barriers determines a preferred direction of action. The combination of these can reach considerable levels of intensity without resulting in overt action unless some triggering event or catalyst sets the process in motion. In the health area, such events or cues may be internal (eg, perceptions of bodily states) or external (eg, interpersonal interactions, impact of data from the communications media or, of course, genetic counseling).

The intensity of the cue required to trigger behavior presumably varies with the level of readiness. With relatively low motivation and poor psychological readiness, intense stimuli would be needed to produce a response. On the other hand, with higher levels of readiness, even slight stimuli may suffice.

Evidence from a Tay-Sachs screening program. A large number of major investigations have been undertaken to test this model of health belief [1]. For the most part, they have provided support for its validity in helping to explain individuals' responses to preventive and screening programs and degrees of compliance with medical regimens.

The applicability of the model to genetic screening is confirmed by a recent study that analyzed factors influencing members of an identified Jewish population, in the Baltimore–Washington area, to participate in screening for the Tay-Sachs trait [4]. The education of the target community began 6 to 8 weeks before initiation of mass testing. Multiple educational approaches were used to saturate the communities with accurate and clear information. These included the press, TV, radio, letters from rabbis, fliers from community organizations, medical presentations to the community, telephone calls from trained volunteers, brochures from physicians, and other special mailings. Lists of the target population were available, so it could be ascertained that all members of the target group – Ashkenazi Jewish couples of childbearing age – were exposed to at least some of these educational activities.

As applied to the Tay-Sachs situation, the tested variables were defined as follows: 1) Health motivation included two components: (a) a positive response indicating a desire to have (additional) children and (b) a set of generalized items about typical health behavior, such as the frequency with which the person thinks about his own health and whether he generally goes to the physician if he feels sick. 2) Perceived susceptibility included the person's belief about whether he could carry the Tay-Sachs gene and transmit it to his progeny. 3) Perceived severity was interpreted as the potential impact on an individual of learning that he was a carrier, especially with regard to future family planning. 4) Perceived benefits were defined in terms of a subjective evaluation of how much good it would do the potential carrier to be screened for the trait. Did he really need to know or want to know his carrier status? 5) Barriers to action (costs) were not measured in this study. They would include, however, economic and convenience factors, as well as threats we currently know very little about, such as the impact on an individual of learning that he is a carrier of some recessive trait. How would it affect his self-image, his perception of his health and of his well-being? Would it affect his marriage? How would it influence future reproductive attitudes?

In all, nearly 7,000 adults, estimated to be 10% of the total eligible population of childbearing age, were screened during the first year of the study. Subjects were drawn from lists of synagogue membership and names in predominantly Jewish neighborhoods. All adults who appeared for screening were asked to complete a brief questionnaire before going through the screening process; 500 of these were selected at random to be the participant sample. In addition, 500 questionnaires were mailed to a random sample of nonparticipants who had been invited in for screening but had not attended; the response rate in this sample was 82%. It should be noted that both respondents and nonrespondents were presumed to have received broadcast and individual information on Tay-Sachs disease and screening. Comparisons were made between the 500 participants and the 412 randomly selected nonparticipants who had responded to the mailed questionnaire.

The participants were significantly younger than the nonparticipants, had fewer children, were less likely to have completed their families, and were slightly better educated. Regarding the health belief variables, the participants differed sharply in the first component of health motivation – desire to have children. Of those who expressed the desire to have more children, 82% participated in the screening program, while less than 19% who did not desire future children participated. There was no significant difference in participation according to the second motivational measure, general health behavior. The perceived susceptibility measure was highly significantly correlated with participation in the screening program. Perceived severity was negatively associated with participation.

When the three significant variables were combined, it became apparent that, while each of the three was associated with participation, the combination of perceived susceptibility and the desire to have more children interacted statistically, producing a much better prediction of participation that the sum of the two. Perceived severity, on the other hand, had an independent explanatory role. For persons who desire additional children, a moderate level of perceived susceptibility and low perceived severity best explains participation. Among those who are not motivated to have additional children, high perceived susceptibility and low perceived severity best explain participation. If we disregard motivation entirely, the combination of high perceived susceptibility and low perceived severity best accounts for participation.

Among those who planned to have more children, more nonparticipants indicated that their future family planning would be affected if either husband or wife were carriers. Possibly many of these nonparticipants may have been deterred from having more children because of misconceptions about their risk of Tay-Sachs disease appearing in a child, or about the availability of antenatal diagnosis for Tay-Sachs disease.

The impact of learning that one member of a married couple was a carrier had very different effects on participants and nonparticipants. Participants were much less likely than nonparticipants to alter their plans. More of the participants had learned that carrier status in just one member of a couple posed no dangers. However, in response to the question on the impact if both parents were found to be carriers, while participants were again less likely to change their reproductive plans, they reported they would reduce the number of intended children or they would use "other" approaches. In nearly every case where the "other" category was reported, participants went on to explain that they would elect to use antenatal tests for their planned pregnancies. Very few of the nonparticipants indicated awareness but indicated that they would not have additional children if they were found to be carriers.

Since more participants than nonparticipants learned about amniocentesis, screening conferred three potential benefits on participants: Testing could eliminate the possibility that both parents were carriers; if both were carriers, amniocentesis could assure that the fetus was unaffected; or if the fetus were affected, they could elect to abort it. While nearly all the respondents, both participants and nonparticipants, held attitudes favoring abortion in the event that a fetus had Tay-Sachs disease, the nonparticipants could not have seen as much benefit in screening, since they did not seem to have learned about amniocentesis.

Barriers to screening were minimized in this study by offering the test at low cost, to a relatively affluent group, at convenient times and locations. Such financial and situational factors could, however, prove to be important for other target groups.

One final consideration should be emphsized. It is believed that in this project, perceived severity associated with the Tay-Sachs trait reached such high levels in some persons that it caused them to avoid participation in the program. It has always been believed that what is needed for appropriate behavior is an "optimal" balance of perception of health motive, vulnerability, severity, and the psychological benefit—cost ratio; where the balance among these is either quite "low" or quite "high", professionally recommended behavior will not be followed. The validity of this assertion, however, can be tested only in future studies, using more sensistive measures for health behavior determinants than the measures used to date.

Relationship between the health belief model and demographic factors. Research on utilization of health services shows that demographic factors can help to distinguish high from low utilizers. Generally speaking, variables in the health belief model are distributed unevenly in the population, high scores on the belief variables tending to be more prevalent among whites, among females, among persons of relatively high socioeconomic status, and among the relatively young [1]. One might conclude that it is not the person's socioeconomic status, race, sex and age that determine aciton, but his motives and beliefs. However, well-designed research has shown that the seeking of periodic Papanicolaou smears for cancer of the cervix in women is determined both by beliefs and demographic characteristics. Even when beliefs are discounted, such action is more probable among whites, among persons of higher socioeconomic status, and among the relatively young [5]. Apparently, health beliefs and sociologic characteristics, though closely related, make independent contributions to behavior.

Health habits. There is, of course, a class of behavior determined by yet more complex variables, namely habitual behaviors and life-styles. Patterns of behavior that are developed in early life most likely are not motivated by the kinds of conscious health concerns that guide adult behavior. During the socialization process, children learn to adopt many health-related habits and practices that will permanently influence their adult behavior; for example, brushing teeth, nutritional practices, or visits to the physician and dentist. These habits in turn are probably determined by the habits, or the knowledge and belief the parents or guardians received from their parents. The implication of this process for improving people's use of health services is considered below.

Compliance with medical advice. Although genetic counselors generally attempt to be nondirective in their counseling, undoubtedly clients often receive strong nonverbal signals from counselors that suggest that one course of action is preferable to some other. Assuming that these signals are seen to be recommending a course of action, studies of patient compliance with prescribed regimens are relevant to client response to genetic counseling.

Kirscht et al have shown that the occurrence of symptoms is highly predictive of whether individuals will seek care. However, when allowance is made for symptom-occurrence, health belief variables account for much of the remaining variation in behavior [6].

Where a professional diagnosis of illness has already been made, the concept of susceptibility means perceived *resusceptibility* to the illness, or belief that the diagnosis is correct.

Of the four available reports examining subjective susceptibility and taking of medications [1], three have concentrated on rheumatic fever as the disease model. Heinzelmann demonstrated that adherence to regular taking of penicillin by college students with a history of rheumatic fever was related to subjective estimates of the likelihood of having another attack [7]. Similarly, Elling et al found significant association between a mother's belief in the possibility that her child would get rheumatic fever again and compliance both in administering the penicillin and in clinic attendance [8].

The only negative report, by Gordis et al [9] found only 58% of the compliers, as opposed to 73% of the noncompliers, believed that their child could get another attack of rheumatic fever. The authors speculated, however, that these results reflect an awareness on the part of the respondents that since their children were poor compliers, they were more susceptible, and that these results may not necessarily bear on the influence of perception of susceptibility on compliance status.

Finally, Becker et al [10] observed that mothers who felt the child was resusceptible to a present acute illness, otitis media, would more often give medication properly and keep clinic appointments.

Although Gordis could show no connection between the mother's "degree of worry about the child's health" and compliance, Becker found higher rates of compliance for mothers who felt their child was "easily susceptible to disease", "often ill," and "illness was a substantial threat to children in general." Only one study has looked at belief in the diagnosis; here, a score was constructed combining the mother's extent of agreement with the physician's decision and her opinion of how sure the doctor was that the child had an ear infection. This "degree of certainty score" successfully predicted compliance with the penicillin therapy.

The relationship of perceived severity to patient compliance with prescribed therapies is quite similar to that for perceived vulnerability. Heinzelmann [7] found that the patient's view of the seriousness of rheumatic fever, whether in an absolute sense or in comparison with other diseases, was predictive of compliance with prescribed penicillin prophylaxis. When Gordis et al [9] questioned mothers about their estimates of the severity of another attack of rheumatic fever, more compliers (44%) than noncompliers (25%) thought the impact on their children would be serious. In research conducted in several private pediatric practices, Charney et al [11] concluded that a mother's perception of severity of the disease (both streptococcal pharyngitis and otitis media) was significantly related to likelihood of giving the medication. Becker et al [10] and Francis et al [12] reported similar associations for perceived seriousness (in terms of both organic severity and interference with the mother's activities) and compliance with both prescribed therapy and appointment-keeping. An additional study also reported that parents' estimates of severity of the child's condition is positively related to compliance in obtaining follow-up care for a wide range of school-discovered illnesses and health problems [14].

1) Perception of benefits is also related to patient compliance with therapy. Both Elling [8] and Heinzelmann [7] reported positive association between belief in the ability of penicillin to prevent recurrence of rheumatic fever and adherence to the regimen. Becker [10] found that "belief in efficacy of clinic medications" predicted faithful administration of the penicillin, and that "belief in doctors' ability to cure illnesses" was related to keeping clinic appointments. Only Gordis et al [9] found no association between belief in the power of the drug to prevent another attack and compliance.

In studies of related sick-role behaviors Donabedian [13] identified "doubt about the recommended procedures" as a reason for elderly patients not following the physicians' instructions regarding their chronic illnesses, and Gabrielson [14] showed that faith in the effectiveness of professional care correlated with parents' compliance in obtaining follow-up care for their school-age children.

2) Perceived "costs" or barriers have been measured in a number of ways, and several variables have been dependable predictors of noncompliance. Fear of pain or discomfort, and of the monetary expense associated with obtaining dental care, is inversely associated with compliance, as are such "negative" aspects of prescribed regimens as: cost; extent to which new patterns of behavior must be adopted (especially if the patient is experiencing work, family, or other social problems); complexity; duration; and side-effects.

PROBLEMS IN IMPROVING PEOPLE'S USE OF HEALTH SERVICES

How should health-related behavior be modified? Although a multiplicity of factors influencing attitude and behavior have been considered in the behavioral sciences, they have yet to be applied systematically and experimentally to the solution of problems in patient behavior, let alone in response to genetic counseling.

Educational Diagnosis and Strategies

Whereas the health beliefs described earlier have been demonstrated to be modifiable [1], there is no a priori reason that interventions directed at any one dimension will, in the long run, prove more effective than attempts to alter another dimension. Health education programs might therefore legitimately focus on any one or any combination of health-behavior determinants. However, clues to the selection of appropriate health education strategies can be derived from examination of perceptions about specific health problems and from surveys of health beliefs held by various at-risk populations.

Studies have shown, for example, that although most persons regard cancer as extremely serious and without much possibility of beneficial intervention, other conditions, such as dental decay, seem to be perceived as highly prevalent, frequently very expensive to prevent or control, but not very serious [15]. It would seem, therefore, that an educational program in the area of behavior related to cancer should, on the average, attempt to reduce fear and to persuade people (where it may legitimately be done) that effective methods of prevention or control are available. On the other hand, a program whose objective is prevention of dental caries might better be directed toward *increasing* fear or concern, and toward suggesting relatively convenient and inexpensive methods for reduction of caries. Similarly, in connection with health problems of emerging importance, such as the genetic diseases, the public's knowledge and beliefs seem to be so inadequate that educational activities designed to engage *every* component of the health beliefs appear to be required. As has been shown, even after genetic counseling or directed educational activity, many clients are quite confused or incorrect in their opinions about the burden or severity of a disease should it occur, about risks of transmitting it, and about techniques available to prevent it [16].

Educators in health should also take into account the different belief levels toward a given condition that exist in different population subgroups. For example, it has been shown that health beliefs relative to tuberculosis vary significantly with educational level, social class, and ethnic group. One may therefore need to increase perceived susceptibility in one group, perceived severity in another, and belief in benefits in a third. These findings suggest, in turn, the value of collecting data about a particular population's health beliefs and motives as well as individual variations, for planning mass media or other health education efforts.

Children's health beliefs. While, in the short run, programs requiring voluntary participation must be attacked on a disease-by-disease basis with special campaigns devoted to each, in the long run this would appear to be a rather inefficient (and possibly ineffective) method. It is inefficient because it requires the target audience to acquire a unique set of facts and beliefs concerning each condition. It may be ineffective because it may involve attempts to transmit knowledge and motivation that cannot be adequately communicated in a brief pamphlet or through a series of short television, radio, or telephone announcements. Moreover, it is apparent that influencing life-styles is much more difficult than inducing people to maintain appropriate health behaviors in the first place.

It therefore seems essential to begin a multigenerational effort to introduce relevant health-related curricula into the education system of each age group, in order to enhance subsequent receptiveness of consumers to the potential benefits of voluntary health action. Few systematic efforts have been made to develop curricula specifically designed to stimulate the acquisition of desired health beliefs. Yet, it is interesting that the use of emotional appeals has successfully modified the health behavior of children [1]. Many opportunities exist in preschool, primary, and secondary education to influence children both to develop desirable health habits and to acquire desired health beliefs. Such curricula, beginning with instruction in human biology, including genetics, could build on theories of the natural causation of disease and germ theory, and could deal with the topics of susceptibility to various diseases, the personal and social consequences of unchecked disease, and the approaches to prevention, early detection, and control of disease. Thus, much can be done by educators to lay the foundations for later minimizing adult psychological barriers to accepting recommended and beneficial health services.

SPECIAL EDUCATIONAL PROBLEMS IN GENETIC COUNSELING

Promoting Health Motivation

How might the findings about health beliefs help to predict responses to genetic counseling? The same variables that explain health behavior and responses to symptoms may be useful in explaining why counselees respond as they do. Minimally, counselees must: 1) be motivated in a manner that makes them receptive to information about genetics; 2) be persuaded that they possess a genetic factor or factors that may produce a diseased child (susceptibility); 3) believe that the possession of genetic factors may have significant implication for themselves or their progeny (severity); 4) be convinced that methods exist for preventing or controlling the effects of genetic disease (benefits); and 5) believe that the economic or psychological barriers associated with taking these actions are not excessive (barriers).

There is little systematic information on the state of public awareness about genetics, but knowledge is probably low. Relevant research has found that the counselor's message is not equally well understood by all counselees; that many deny the seriousness of the disease or the possession of a harmful gene; that there is considerable variation in ability to grasp the meaning of odds; and that many fail to accept effective methods of intervention [4, 16].

The problem of the perception of odds is a most complex one, even for physicians. A recent national study of physicians' knowledge and attitudes concerning genetic screening revealed that physicians varied widely, both within specialties and between specialties, in their subjective assessment of the risk for genetic conditions *even when the objective odds had been specified for them* [17]. That is, physicians varied widely in whether they interpreted a probability of 1 in 4 as "high," "medium," or "low". In the earlier reported study of Tay-Sachs screening, less than 13% of the study group correctly recalled the actual odds of 1 in 30 for possessing the carrier state for the Tay-Sachs gene [4]. It is not clear what counselees understood by terms such as 1 in 4 (risk of two carrier parents having an affected child) or 1 in 3,600 (incidence of Tay-Sachs disease children born to the Ashkenazi population). It is questionable whether accurate knowledge of mathematical probability has a direct relationship to perceived susceptibiliy. Perhaps it is sufficient for an individual to believe there is *some* probability that his child will be affected, rather than to know that the actual chances are 1 in 3,600 or 1 in 4. Clearly, research is needed on the relationship between objective understanding of numerical odds and subjective perception of susceptibility, since each influences response to counseling. Similarly, it is necessary to ask what level of perceived severity is enough – but not too much – to instigate appropriate action. Clearly, if a counselee believes no possible harmful consequences exist for his progeny, he will not be receptive to counseling. On the other hand, even if he believes the consequences to be serious, he may deny the seriousness or behave in other maladaptive ways.

It has also been shown that people vary widely in their knowledge of diagnostic procedures such as amniocentesis and may, as a consequence, fail to take appropriate action [4].

At present, the public is not sophisticated about the concept of odds, about the meaning of genetic disease, or about methods of prevention or management. It is the responsibility of the genetic counselor to provide such knowledge and stimulate needed beliefs.

The Meaning of Perceived Severity in Genetic Disease

There is anecdotal evidence that perception of severity is profoundly different for genetic problems than for other diseases. In the infectious disease model, most people have come to regard disease as caused by a foreign invader to be despised and destroyed or contained. Mass media have reinforced this view by picturing bacteria and viruses as ugly, nasty little things. Even in the chronic degenerative diseases, it seems likely that most people believe their problems are due to the occurrence of something external to themselves, which then upsets the internal balance.

In genetics, however, the disease threat cannot be regarded as external; it is not an invasion, it is part and parcel of ourselves. As a cartoon character once said "we have met the enemy and they is us." We need to know about how the self-image is affected by the information that our own genes — our own persons — may produce disease in our children. Our educational system should make the public more sophisticated regarding heredity. Until then, parents may either fail to appreciate that they may be at risk of transmitting serious disease or, at the other extreme, exhibit excessive guilt over possessing "bad" or harmful genes. Concerning perceived impact of genetic disease on families or on the affected child, a national study of physicians [17] showed that fewer than half the respondents believed that cessation of treatment for all genetic disorders would have an extremely serious impact on affected children and their families. Is there reason to believe that the general public would have more sophisticated views than practicing physicians? We may be faced with a paradoxical task: First, of increasing fear or concern in our clients in order to attract their attention, and then spending considerable effort to reduce their fears in order to achieve an adaptive response.

Prenatal Diagnoses and Alternate Reproductive Options

Acceptance of carrier screening tests, newborn screening tests, and amniocentesis appears to be increasing, both among physicians and among selected subgroups in the population [17]. Nevertheless, it seems fair to conclude that neither the public nor the medical profession as a whole are yet ready to accept screening on a broad scale [17]. As genetic screening programs become more widely disseminated, they will, as a matter of course, come to be more accepted. If health curricula for the lay public can be improved, acceptance may increase still more readily.

Possible reproductive alternatives may be limited for a great many people. Most North American Jews appear to have no ethnic or religious antipathies to abortion in the case of prenatally diagnosed Tay-Sachs disease, but abortion or birth control for preventing other inherited diseases such as cystic fibrosis or the hemoglobinopathies are not likely to be widely accepted options in the foreseeable future.

When amniocentesis for such conditions does become available, the situation may change. To have children, at present, most families with such problems must risk having natural children, use artificial insemination, or adopt children. None of these alternatives may be acceptable. Some may go ahead and have children, taking the 3 in 4 probability that they will not have an affected child, and risking the 1 in 4 chance of an affected child along with uncertainty about the severity of disease or the life expectancy of the affected child.

Perceived Costs

For women who perceive bearing and rearing children as their only real chance for achieving something worthwhile in life, childlessness may be too high a price to pay for the assurance that genetically affected children will not be born. At the other extreme, for the middle-class family that can guarantee freedom from a genetic disease at the cost of, say, $500 per pregnancy, the cost may not seem high. The point is that the client's interpretation of costs has to be understood in terms of his or her personal circumstances, life-style, values and needs, and these will frequently be different — sometimes vastly different — from those of the counselor.

Education of the Public and the Profession

The previous material concerning client knowledge and client beliefs suggests that it is necessary for the genetic counselor to impart both comprehensible information and practical options that will fit the value systems of the client. Certainly, information concerning susceptibility, severity, benefits, and costs would seem to be required, although we have not yet determined precisely what information is needed in each of these areas.

For patient education to be successful on a large scale, it would seem necessary 1) to modify formal medical, public health, and allied health care curricula in in order to produce health care practitioners oriented toward prevention as well as treatment, and 2) to ensure that practitioners are also oriented toward the "whole person," his psychology, and the importance of preparing him for personal responsibility in health maintenance and disease control. Current medical education places little emphasis on the necessity for adequate patient education, and few medical schools provide any exposure to information related to counseling for genetic or other diseases; to the conditions under which patients will follow advice; or to methods for communicating with clients. Moreover, few medical schools provide interviewing skills for finding out what the patient knows, believes, or is concerned about. Thus, an important role to be shared by behavioral scientists and health educators alike is that of bringing into the education of health workers a greater emphasis on psychosocial factors that influence health behavior.

Counselors and other providers of health care must appreciate that 1) behavior is motivated 2) ingrained health beliefs predetermine a client's responses; 3) all persons possess these beliefs and motives to different degrees; and 4) factual information, while necessary, is often not sufficient to stimulate needed beliefs. In addition, health practitioners should be encouraged to accept responsibility for patient or client education and to view such activity as important. I therefore recommend that information concerning the role of health beliefs and how they may be modified become part of the curricula of all health care training programs.

Many patients who are highly knowledgable about the illness and its medication, nonetheless do not carry out the prescribed regimen. Various studies of health beliefs cited earlier have shown that, of the people who do not follow a health recommendation, some are unmotivated; some lack belief in their vulnerability to, or in the degree of severity of, the condition; and still others fail to see benefits in proposed actions or ways of overcoming barriers to such actions.

These individual differences suggest that no single educational prescription can be suitable for all. To devise a unique educational strategy for different individuals or groups requires knowing what health belief components require bolstering. I suggest that, for purposes of educational diagnosis, a brief, standardized set of questions employing model variables be administered to each patient, perhaps as a regular part of the history-taking process. Answers to these questions should aid the counselor in identifying the dimensions of the problem in each case. Thus, by knowing which model components are below a level deemed necessary for informed decision-making, the health worker can tailor interventions to suit the particular needs of each individual.

CONCLUSIONS

The description of the health belief model and its component beliefs may serve as a point of departure for more effective counseling, but knowing what beliefs clients lack does not ensure a specific strategy for providing what is neeeded. The counselor may know what a person lacks or needs, yet not know how to give it to him. Successful genetic counseling is both a skill and an art. While ongoing research may provide increases in information concerning educational methods, the experience and intuitive skills of the practitioner will probably always exceed the ability of technology to define or replace these skills. Personal aptitudes in human interactions will always be required: Individual differences in the personalities and values of clients will always necessitate individualized efforts and entail high levels of interpersonal skills on the part of counselors.

In the final analysis, the particular relationship between counselor and client defines the difference between effective and ineffective counseling. Greater knowledge of human behavior and better training of health professionals in the behavioral sciences, in interviewing skills, and in personal sensitivity, can greatly enhance the success of the counseling relationship.

ANNOTATED REFERENCES

1. Becker MH: "The Health Belief Model and Personal Health Behavior." Thorofare, New Jersey: C.S. Slack, 1974.

   This 150-page monograph describes the origins of the health belief model, a scheme for explaining 1) health related behavior taken in the absence of symptoms; 2) behavior taken in the presence of symptoms; and 3) behavior undertaken by people defined as ill. Potential applications to related areas are described. Efforts to modify health beliefs are discussed. Each chapter contains a detailed review of relevant literature.

2. Committee for the Study of Inborn Errors of Metabolism: "Genetic Screening: Programs, Principles, and Research." Washington, DC: National Academy of Sciences, 1975.

   This final report of the Committee for the Study of Inborn Errors of Metabolism concerns programs, principles and research relevant to genetic screening. Part I: a set of recommendations. Part II: prospects of screening. Part III: history of screening for phenylketonuria in the U.S.; Part IV: experiences with screening for a variety of genetically determined diseases. Part V: review of principles of health behavior affecting public attitudes toward screening and summary of a national study of the knowledge and attitudes of physicians with respect to genetic screening. Part VI: discussion of legal, ethical, and economic principles of screening, plus suggestions for future research. Part VII: procedural guidelines for planning new screening programs: Part VIII, various appendices.

3. Bruner J, Goodman C: Value and need as organizing factors in perception. J Abnorm Soc Psychol 42:37, 1947.

4. Becker MH, Kaback MM, Rosenstock IM, Ruth MV: Some influences on public participation in a genetic screening program. J Community Health 1:3–14, 1975.

To study the applicability of the health belief model in explaining voluntary cooperation in mass genetic testing, stratified random samples of 500 participants and 500 non participants were drawn from an identified at-risk population for Tay-Sachs disease. Participants were relatively younger and better educated, reported higher levels of perceived susceptibility to being a carrier, and stated more often that the impact of learning of being a carrier would be low. Participants were also more likely than nonparticipants to indicate they would not alter plans for future progeny.

5. Kegeles SS, Kirscht JP, Haefner DP, Rosenstock IM: Survey of beliefs about cancer detection and taking Papanicolaou tests. Publ Health Rept 80:815, 1965.

6. Kirscht JP, Becker MH, Eveland JD: Psychosocial factors as predictors of medical behavior. Med Care (in press).

7. Heinselmann F: Factors in prophylaxis behavior in treating rheumatic fever: An exploratory study. J Health Hum Behav 3:73, 1962.

8. Elling R, Whittemore R, Green M: Patient participation in a pediatric program. J Health Hum Behav 1:183, 1960.

9. Gordis L, Markowitz M, Lilienfeld AM: Why patients don't follow medical advice: A study of children on long-term antistreptococcal prophylaxis. J Pediatr 75:957, 1969.

10. Becker MH, Drachman RH, Kirscht JP: A new approach to explaining sick-role behavior in low-income populations. Am J Publ Health: 64:205, 1974.

11. Charney E, Bynum R, Eldredge D, Frank D, MacWhinney JB, McNabb N, Scheiner A, Sumpter EA, Iker H: How well do patients take oral penicillin? A collaborative study in private practice. J Pediatr 40:188, 1967.

12. Francis V, Korsch BM, Morris MJ: Gaps in doctor-patient communication: Patients' response to medical advice. N Engl J Med 280:535, 1969.

13. Donabedian A, Rosenfeld L: Follow-up study of chronically ill patients discharged from hospital. J Chron Dis 17:847, 1964.

14. Gabrielson IW, Levin LS, Ellison MD: Factors affecting school health follow-up. Am J Publ Health 57:48, 1967.

15. Kirscht JP, Haefner DP, Kegeles SS, Rosenstock IM: A national study of health beliefs. J Health Hum Behav 7:248, 1966.

16. Leonard CO, Chase GA, Childs B: Genetic counseling: A consumer's view. N Engl J Med 287:433, 1972.

17. Rosenstock IM, Childs B, Simopoulos AP: Genetic screening: a study of the knowledge and attitudes of physicians. Washington, D.C.: National Academy of Sciences, 1975.

8

Reproductive Attitudes and the Genetic Counselee

Paula E. Hollerbach, PhD

INTRODUCTION

One cannot predict the actions and decisions of individuals receiving genetic counseling without considering the social forces impinging on those individuals. In order to understand why so many individuals distort, ignore, or forget information they receive in counseling, one must understand 1) the stigmatization that childless couples experience; 2) the cultural pressures against bearing an "only" child; 3) the effect of sex preferences on fertility; and 4) the motivations for childbearing. These social forces strongly influence the personal and social meaning attached to genetic transmission of disease and the impact, on the individual and the family of bearing an affected child.

Extensive psychosocial and demographic literature exists on the reproductive attitudes of the general population [1–3], but there is regrettably little on the attitudes of genetic counselees [4, 5]. In this chapter I will review the fertility norms and reproductive attitudes characterizing the general population in the United States, since genetic counselees are subject to the same cultural influences and constraints. Second, I will discuss the reproductive attitudes of the genetic counseling population and explain how these attitudes are influenced by the threat that counselees may fail to fulfill fertility norms, and hence be regarded as deviants.

CULTURAL NORMS REGARDING APPROPRIATE FERTILITY BEHAVIOR

Sociologists define "norms" as standards of conduct that guide the actions of individuals. People are motivated to conform to norms to satisfy a variety of motives: to be right, to have predictable social interaction, and to maintain social approval [6]. Norms are typically learned through socialization, and a variety of formal and informal rewards and punishments are used to motivate compliance.

Demographers have long assumed that there are norms influencing fertility.

Only recently, however, have such norms been investigated to establish whether they control fertility or even exist. Some of the proposed norms include:

1. Societies prescribe the context or civil status in which childbearing should take place [7]. In the US this context is legal marriage. Married couples are expected to be childbearers, and they are assumed to be economically and emotionally prepared to care for children. It is tacitly accepted that children enhance the marital relationship.

2. Societies favor the reproduction of at least a minimum number of children within this context [7]. In the US the two-child family is the minimum accepted norm, and it is currently the most popular family size, although tolerance exists for up to four children. Informal negative sanctions are exerted on "deviant" couples who remain childless or have only one child, and comparable sanctions apply to those who exceed the accepted family size.

3. Not only are married couples expected to have children, they are expected to *want* them [3]. Voluntarily childless couples are deemed to be more deviant than the infertile; they are stereotyped, stigmatized, and subjected to informal sanctions, for they have *deliberately* violated the norm, and they pose a serious threat to generally accepted family values.

4. Preferences exist regarding sex composition of children [8]. Male and female children fulfill different functions within the family and provide different rewards. In the United States there are preferences for male children, especially as first-born children, and for balanced sex composition (having at least one child of each sex).

The Marital Context

In the United States, reproduction within marriage has higher status than that outside marriage, and children of formalized unions have greater legal protection than those born of informal unions [7]. Pregnancies are particularly stigmatized when the marital status of the parents violates cultural norms [9, 10]. Such situations include unmarried women who conceive by a man they cannot or do not wish to marry; women contemplating divorce; single or previously married women who are self-supporting or receive alimony or other support; and women who conceive after forcible rape. Analogous situations can exist for men.

The association between abortion and marital status indicates the existence of these norms. Legalized abortion has become a major factor in the unprecedented decline in illegitimate births in the United States [11, 12]. In 1975, for example, approximately 74% of the women receiving abortions were unmarried, and legal abortion ratios for unmarried women were invariably higher than those for married women [13].

Reproduction may be socially embarrassing for the unmarried or the newly married, but after a respectable interval (at least nine months), if the couple is economically secure, reproduction is expected. From 1970 to 1974, the median interval between marriage and the first birth was 1.7 years [14]. Virtually all people who ever bear children begin within the first 5 years of marriage [3]. Childless wives experience considerable pressure to become mothers after 1 year of marriage; pressure peaks during the third and fourth years and then declines [3].

In a 1972 Gallup poll, a sample of white Americans was asked, "Assuming that a couple can have a baby at about the time they want it, what in your opinion is a desirable length of time after marriage for the first baby to be born?" [15]. The average answer was 2.4 years, and the average birth interval between subsequent births was 2.1 years. Respondents agreed more closely on the desired age difference between offspring than they did on how soon reproduction should commence. College-educated respondents tended to select longer first-birth intervals (2.7 years) than did the grade school-educated respondents (2.0 years).

Recent evidence suggests that well-educated respondents may now accept an even longer interval before the birth of the first child [16–17]. Concern about overpopulation, increased freedom for women, desire for continuous growth and freedom, and ambivalence about the benefits of childbearing are cited as reasons for this change in attitude. Data on fertility in the United States, which has declined consistently since 1957, confirm that American women are marrying later and starting childbearing at older ages [18–20].

Although couples are postponing marriage and childbearing, the belief persists that children enhance a marital relationship. In a 1973 Gallup poll, 85% of the white Americans interviewed replied that, speaking for themselves, they thought married life was happier when there were children. Only 8% of the men and 6% of the women thought marriage was happier without children, and the remainder replied that they did not know [15]. Younger people of both sexes were somewhat more apt to think that marriage was happier without children. Moreover, the college-educated were more prone to reply "do not know" than were those with less education. This was especially true among college-educated women, whom Blake categorized as more "on the fence" than other groups: "not willing to affirm the virtues of childlessness, but not as ready as other women to extol the advantages of having children." Yet even among these college-educated women, 79% felt that children made a marriage happier, and 16% replied that they did not know [15; see also 17, 21].

In 1972 another poll asked: "A typical married couple goes through a number of stages in the family cycle from marriage to when the last child leaves home. Which of the following stages do you think is the happiest?" [15]. More than 40% of the men and 50% of the women thought that the happiest stage of marriage was "when the babies are being born and children are very young." This period of childbearing was the favorite among respondents of all ages and of all religions, although it did appear that less-educated women were much more likely to value the period of active reproduction as the happiest time. These couples were also asked to cite "the next happiest time." Again, clear preference was given to the childbearing and childrearing stages of life [15].

Despite the assumption that children enhance a marriage, no empirical support exists for this view. In fact, intensive longitudinal studies of couples at different points in the family life cycle have shown that marital satisfaction is highest prior to childbearing and in the later post-childrearing years [22], and that the first birth triggers a crisis in the marital relationship, resulting in post-partum decline in marital satisfaction and/or sexual satisfaction [22–24]. Feldman's research on middle- class and upper-middle-class respondents concluded that couples had positive feelings about their parental roles — ie, feelings of warmth toward children, of competence regarding their childrearing ability, and of being needed. However, this parental satisfaction differed markedly from their assessment of marital satisfaction [22]. A study of lower-class white women also indicated that parental satisfaction and marital satisfaction were not necessarily correlated. These women often found it easier and more gratifying to relate affectionately to their children than to their husbands, who often treated them with indifference [25].

The discrepancy between attitudes and empirical research may result because those responding to the Gallup poll interpret the "happiest stage of the family cycle" as the happiest stage with children rather than with spouse; or respondents choosing the happiest stage for the "typical" couple may select the stages that are culturally defined as the happiest, defining "typical" as the norm.

Norms Regarding Reproductive Goals

The second fertility norm posits that societies favor the birth of a minimum number of children within the appropriate marital context. A consistent preference for the two- to four-child family in the United States can be noted in surveys dating back to the 1930s, with relatively few respondents regarding fewer than two or more than four children as the "ideal," and relatively few "expecting" to have fewer than two, or more than four [26].

Population surveys conducted periodically by the U.S. Bureau of the Census have recorded a consistent drop in the average number of lifetime births expected by married women, during the seven-year interval since the first fertility expectations survey was conducted in 1967. Overall, wives aged 18–39 years in 1975 expected 2.5 births in their lifetime, down from 2.8 in 1971 and 3.1 in 1967 [14].

These changes in mean birth expectations signified an impressive shift in the proportion of wives favoring the two-child family (from 29.3% in 1967 to 44.1% in 1975), and a slight increase in the proportion expecting to remain childless (from 3.1% in 1967 to 4.6% in 1975) or expecting one birth (from 6.2% in 1967 to 10.6% in 1975) [14].

The two-child family was favored more by young wives, 18 to 24 years of age, and by wives not residing on farms. Mean expected births were lower for the better-educated; for women in the labor force; and for white wives, who expected a total of 2.5 births in 1975 in comparison to 3.0 births expected by black wives and 2.8 births by Spanish-origin wives. These racial, ethnic, and educational differences were less distinct among the younger wives [14, 27, 28]. In general, fertility expectations declined with increasing family income, although again this effect was less pronounced among the younger wives and did not always occur in the very highest and very lowest income groups [28; see also 15, 29].

Limited data are available on the characteristics of wives who expected to remain childless or to have one child. Younger wives favored these options. In 1974, 16.4% of the white wives and 25.9% of the black wives aged 18 to 24 years expected no births or one birth [28].

The two-child family has not only gained in popularity but is viewed as the minimum that a couple should have. Between two-thirds and four-fifths of Americans polled define a childless or one-child family as "too small." There is a less precise upper limit to family size, without as sharp a break as that between one and two children at the lower end. Three and four children are tolerated, especially by women, but five- and six-child families are typically defined as "too large" [15, 16, 30].

Stereotypes of Different Family Sizes

To reinforce compliance with norms regarding family size, informal negative sanctions are applied to couples who are deviant because they have remained childless or have had only one child, and to those who have exceeded the acceptable family size.

For instance, married couples expected to receive and actually do receive social pressure, especially from their parents, to have at least two children [16, 30–33]. After two children, pressure begins to limit family size, taking the form of hints, rhetorical or direct questions, advice, or signs of approval or disapproval [16, 30].

In addition, there are several derogatory stereotypes of the "typical" childless couple, of the only child, and of couples with very large families. It is impossible to test the validity of most of these stereotypes. Veevers has suggested, however, that validity is not important if the stereotypes are *believed* to be true and therefore serve both as sanctions in themselves and as a basis for further sanctions [3].

The childless couple. Various historical materials record that, in ancient societies, infertility was often looked upon as a curse — as a mark of divine displeasure or as an indication of sinful behavior in a previous incarnation [34–36]. Barrenness in a woman was grounds for divorce in some societies; in others, it reflected on the virility of the male and the adequacy of the female and affected societal attitudes toward these people. Producing a minimum number of children was viewed as the woman's moral and economic duty in marriage; those who deviated from this norm were criticized and often ostracized [7]. According to Thompson, these religious and legal dicta have since been supplanted by the assumed existence of maternal instincts to procreate and to nurture. The belief still persists that the nature and role of woman can be realized only through mother-hood [37].

Although the roles of husband and wife have changed, it would seem that attitudes toward the childless couple have remained constant for centuries. Veevers reported that in Canada voluntarily childless wives all thought they were somewhat stigmatized by their unpopular decision to forego parenthood. They felt they were negatively stereotyped as being abnormal, selfish, immoral, irresponsible, immature, unhappy, unfulfilled, and nonfeminine [31; see also 30, 38].

The stigmatization felt by the childless is not imaginary. Sara Kiesler of the University of Kansas asked approximately 900 middle-class wives to evaluate photographs of women whose number of children, age, and employment varied. They rated the childless women (especially the 38- and 48-year old childless women) with the lowest percentage of positive adjectives and the least anticipated liking. Better-educated, younger women, and those with lower parity or lower fertility intentions were less likely to view the childless woman negatively. Nearly 40% of the respondents claimed, however, that there were no good reasons for being childless. The remaining 60% checked a variety of different reasons, especially emotional ones.

One cannot appreciate the stereotypes depicting the childless couple without considering the social significance of parenthood. Veevers has presented a typology delineating the dominant cultural definitions of parenthood and the nature of parents in our society, compared with the perceived meanings of childlessness and the nature of the childless [36]. As noted in Table I, the social meanings of parent-hood and nonparenthood revolve around the central themes of morality, responsibility, naturalness, sex, marriage, and mental health. Minor themes and stereotyped traits of the childless which are less frequently suggested include: unconventional, fearful of pregnancy, pessimistic, career-oriented, ambitious, irreligious, irresponsible, lonely, inordinately fond of pets, materialistic, sensuous, afraid, and insecure.

The possibility of genetic problems is not included in this schema, nor is it ever considered by respondents as a characteristic of the childless, though sexual incompetence, frigidity, and sterility are mentioned. There are no studies indicating what proportion of couples remain childless for genetic reasons. One study of 862 childless couples in 1939 concluded that eugenic motives were only a negligible consideration [39].

Many, but not all people, probably subscribe in varying degrees to Veevers' definitions and characterize childless couples negatively [36]. Maternal instinct is assumed to be stronger than the male reproductive drive, and parenthood is thought to be more essential to female adult status than to male, so the relation-ship between childlessness and these character stigmatizations will be more pronounced for wives than for husbands [36].

The only-child family. Negative stereotypes also exist regarding parents who have a single child. The cultural pressures to bear a second child derive from

TABLE I. The Social Meanings of Parenthood and Nonparenthood: A Delineation of Ideal Types.

Dimension	Definition of parenthood	Definition of nonparenthood
Morality	Desire for parenthood is a *religious obligation;* being a parent is being *moral.*	Lack of desire for parenthood is a *flouting of religious authority;* not being a parent is being *immoral.*
Responsibility	Desire for parenthood is a *civic obligation;* being a parent is being *responsible.*	Lack of desire for parenthood is *avoidance of responsibility;* not being a parent is being *irresponsible.*
Naturalness	Desire for parenthood is *instinctive;* being a parent is *natural.*	Lack of desire for parenthood and/or not being a parent is *unnatural.*
Sexual Identity and Sexual Competence	Desire for parenthood is *acceptance of gender role;* being a mother is *proof of femininity* and of *sexual competence* as a woman; being a father is *proof of masculinity* and of *sexual competence* as a man.	Lack of desire for parenthood is *rejection of gender role;* not being a mother indicates *lack of feminity* and *sexual incompetence* as a woman; not being a father indicates *lack* of *masculinity* and *sexual incompetence* as a man.
Marriage	Desire for parenthood is the *meaning of marriage;* being a parent *improves marital adjustment* and *prevents divorce.*	Lack of desire for parenthood *destroys the meaning of marriage;* not being a parent *hinders marital adjustment and increases divorce proneness.*
Normalcy and "Mental Health"	Desire for parenthood is a sign of *normal mental health;* being a parent contributes to social *maturity* and *personality stability.*	Lack of desire for parenthood is a sign of *abnormal mental health;* not being a parent is associated with *immaturity* and *emotional maladjustment.*

Source: Veevers JE: The social meanings of parenthood. Psychiatry 36:291, 1973 [36]. Reprinted by special permission of the William Alanson White Psychiatric Foundation, Inc. Copyright held by the Foundation.

cultural beliefs concerning the negative personality and social characteristics of "only" children [37, 38]. For instance, Thompson reported that the only child (of either sex) was rated consistently more negatively than the male or female child with two siblings [37]. The only child was generally perceived as "maladjusted and socially inadequate, self-centered and self-willed, attention-seeking and dependent on others, temperamental and anxious, generally unhappy and unlikeable, and yet somewhat more autonomous than a child with two siblings" [37, pp. 95–96]. When subjects were asked to suggest other attributes, synonyms of the above terms were offered, but no neutral or positive attributes. Moreover, when questioned directly, subjects found it difficult to explain the basis for their choice of negative traits and exclusion of positive ones.

Opinion polls suggest that the negative attributes and consequences of bearing an only child are widely accepted. Most Americans agree that "people would say your child would be spoiled" [30], or that "being an only child is a disadvantage" [15, 40]. Respondents who are themselves only children are less likely to consider the only child disadvantaged than are those who had siblings. Even among the singletons, however, 60% of the male and 70% of the female respondents in one 1972 Gallup poll agreed that the only child was at a disadvantage [15]. Similarly, in a study of 300 married white women in Buffalo, Terhune found that liking of their own family size was lowest among those who were only children. Nearly half of the only children reported that they liked their family size "not at all." From these data, Terhune surmised that only children missed the emotional gratification of having siblings with whom to share experiences and confidences [41].

Unfavorable attitudes toward the one-child family influence fertility decisions. In the 1941 Indianapolis fertility study, the majority of wives reported that they were "influenced very much" in their decision to have a second child by the belief that the only child is "handicapped" [42]. Even today, although a number of advantages are associated with an only child (parental attention to the child, ability to provide materially for the child, fewer economic concerns, and general opportunities and freedom), the *perceived* costs seem to outweigh the advantages. Such costs include spoiling the child, lack of companionship for the child, lack of social benefits from siblings (such as learning to get along with others), and lack of development of responsibility in the child [41]. Thus, many parents feel it is necessary to have a second child in order to "save" the first and provide a play-mate and friend.

Contrary to these perceived consequences, data on the actual consequences of family size suggest that only children, like other first-born children, actually share a number of advantages relative to later-borns, in terms of higher I.Q. perform-ance, verbal ability, academic achievement, and leadership ability [37, 41, 43–46]. Purported to be dependent and to lack sociability, the only child tends to be more independent, socially outgoing and popular, and high in self-esteem [41].

Only a few aspects of the stereotype cannot be refuted. The only child's alleged tendency to be aggressive and domineering does receive slight support; and there is a tendency for only children to be more frequently neurotic or alcoholic, per-haps as a result of excessive parental pressures or unrealistic expectations for achievement and independence in some families [37, 41].

Other traits attributed to only children, such as egotism and conceit, have not been well measured; some traits, such as craving for attention, have not been measured at all. On balance, however, a largely positive characterization of the only child has emerged, contrary to popular notions. "The only child, it seems is more maligned than maladjusted" [41, p. 80].

In accounting for this discrepancy between research findings and perceptions of the only child, Terhune has suggested the following explanations: 1) Views on the only child are merely perpetuated myths. 2) Without siblings for companionship, children are more likely to interact with adults, thus lending credence to the parents' beliefs that the only child craves attention. 3) Parents of only children tend to expect more of them, therefore an inability to meet these high expectations is seen as a deficit. 4) Positive traits of the only child can be perceived negatively, perhaps through jealously or envy: for example, self-esteem can be seen as conceit; social popularity, as attention-seeking. 5) As the child matures, bad traits can become sublimated into more socially acceptable behavior – eg, attention-seeking may evolve into ambition and/or gregariousness. 6) Researchers have failed to examine the variables relevant to spoiling [41].

Wanting Children

Not only are couples expected to bear two children (but not more than four), they are expected to *want* them. It is for this reason that voluntarily childless couples are deemed to be more deviant than the infertile, for they have deliberately violated expected norms of fertility behavior. In contrast, childless couples who desire to bear children but are unable to do so because of infertility are more pitied than condemned [3].

Although demographers have long assumed that people want children, only recently have attempts been made to understand the reasons why people want or do not want children – that is, their motivations for and against childbearing [1, 32, 47–55]. Among a variety of suggested schemata, a theory developed by Hoffman and Hoffman postulated that fertility desires are determined by 1) the value of children, 2) alternative sources of the value, 3) costs (what must be lost or sacrificed to obtain a value), 4) barriers, and 5) facilitators (the factors that make it more difficult or easy to realize a particular value by having children). In their research, nine basic values of having children emerged [54, 55].

Adult status and social identity. Parenthood, more than any other role, establishes both men and women as truly mature, stable, and acceptable members of the community. This is especially true for women, for whom motherhood is defined as the most important role, the most satisfying activity, and the culmination of socialization. For some women, particularly less-educated women, few alternative roles may be acceptable; even among women who assume other roles, these are defined typically as being complementary or supplementary to the central role of motherhood.

Women tend to view "woman's role" as a more important reason for having children than prestige, religion, and marital happiness [56]. Hoffman and Hoffman conjectured that the achievement of adult status and identity for women was most salient with the birth of the first child, although subsequent births could reconfirm this status at crucial points in the life cycle, as when the youngest child entered school [54]. Among college students sampled by Kirchner and Locasso, high role-fulfillment motivation was associated with larger family size desires in both sexes [49].

Expansion of the self. Under this category are four distinct motivations for parenthood. Having children may satisfy a need for "immortality" – ie, the assurance that one's characteristics will be preserved in another life. Moreover, having children, especially males, allows for continuation of the family name and lineage. Men tend to express this motivation for childbearing more than women [48, 54], and urban lower-class and rural agricultural respondents show stronger orientation toward continuity of family name than do those from the urban middle class [48]. Children also help to expand parental self-images by providing ties to the larger society and ties from the past to the future, in that parents transmit to their children much of what they have received from their own parents. Finally, children can evoke new dimensions of the personality, such as feelings of being needed and desires to protect another human being [54].

Morality. Childbearing is often viewed as a moral act involving self-sacrifice for the sake of another person, for community welfare, religious tradition, or for norms supporting deferred gratification. Children may be necessary for the performance of religious functions, or they may be viewed as tokens of "Heaven's favor." Having children may help to perpetuate or increase the power of one's group, tribe, religion, nation, or caste [57], or provide the opportunity to be altruistic. For instance, men interviewed by Rainwater wanted large families because they wished to avoid a selfish identity [38]. Being a parent can help a man or woman feel virtuous and can provide a sense of self-worth [22]. Finally, children can bring stability and structure to a parent's life and thus provide a means to escape or avoid impulsiveness and too much freedom [54].

Primary group ties and affiliation. The affiliative value of children is of great importance in large and mobile societies. "Avoidance of loneliness" and companionship are frequent reasons for having children, especially many children, in the United States and elsewhere [38, 48]. I have already discussed the belief that children improve a marriage and have noted that some women, especially lower-class women or those in more segregated marital relationships, may derive much affiliation from their children, thereby compensating for a lack of closeness with their husbands [25]. Affiliation may also be a motive for parenthood among middle-class wives whose husbands' careers prevent them from fully satisfying their wives' needs [54]. Children may be valued as a source of affection for unmarried parents as well. It seems generally established that wives, especially in urban locations, emphasize companionship and the affectionate relationship with their children more than husbands do.

Stimulation, novelty, and fun. Children appear to add an element of unpredict-ability and excitement to the home. Watching them grow, develop, and change may be especially satisfying. Having children and playing with them can also be fun, allowing parents the joy of reliving their own youth. Pleasure from growth and development of children was cited most frequently as an advantage of having children by middle- and lower-class urban whites in a Hawaiian sample [48].

Creativity, accomplishment, and competence. Parents may gain a sense of creativity and accomplishment not only from physically producing a child but from meeting the challenges of childrearing [49]. Successful rearing of a child can be viewed as evidence of parental competence. Such feelings are expressed by respondents in all social classes, and by blacks as well as by whites [54].

Power, influence, and effectance. Although little research exists on this topic, parenthood may increase the power of the parent, especially the mother, by pro-viding an opportunity to teach, control, and exert influence over a dependent individual according to valued ideals and attributes [54].

Social comparison and competition. Children can also provide prestige and competitive advantages to parents. Having a large number of children (at least up to four) may be seen as an indication of one's fecundity, sexuality, and marital love. Other achievements of a woman, such as a career, may be enhanced if she also has a large number of children (the "Wonder Woman" model). On the other hand, competition with others may encourage parents to concentrate on producing a high-quality child rather than a large quantity of children [54]. Fawcett and his colleagues noted that "pride in children's accomplishments" and "children to carry out the parents' hopes and aspirations" were important psychological benefits for rural East-Asian respondents, who were frustrated by their own life situations and wished for better circumstances for their children. Husbands were also more likely than wives to stress the benefits of pride in children's accom-plishments [48].

Economic utility. The last and most frequently investigated motivation for parenthood is economic utility. Economic utility may be short-term (ability to contribute to the family income when young, provide tax deductions, assist in household chores, or care for other children) or long-term (provide old-age sup-port, carry on a family business, or inherit family property and money). Thus the utility of children can be realized through receiving or contributing to family income.

In developing countries, especially among rural agricultural respondents, children are valued primarily because of their economic utility. This is somewhat less so in the urban lower-class and is least salient in the urban middle-class [48]. The economic value of children declines with increased industrialization and urbanization, replacement of subsistence farming by wage-earning, greater pressure to educate children, and an increase in the educational level of parents [54]. In the United States, the average cost of childrearing increases in absolute terms as income increases, although the proportional cost declines [57]. It is generally believed that the economic utility of children in the United States is very low, and economic concerns are frequently cited as reasons for limiting family size rather than increasing it [25, 51]. Whether rural American families are more likely to consider children as economic assets than are their urban counterparts has not been studied.

Sex Preferences

Few researchers investigating motives for childbearing have included questions relating to desired sex. One six-country study, however, asked respondents their reasons for wanting girls and wanting boys [48]. The reasons given showed strong similarities across countries, presumably reflecting certain universals in sex-role prescriptions. Girls were wanted for their qualities while they were still children and living with their parents; that is, as companions for the mother and for their positive personality or behavioral qualities. In contrast, boys were wanted for reasons applying more to their adult state – eg, continuity of the family name and economic security for the parents.

In the United States there are two primary sex preferences: for males, especially as first-born children, and for sex balance – ie, having at least one child of each sex. These preferences reinforce the concept of a two-child family as the minimum acceptable family size, and they influence fertility intentions and behavior. Typically, couples with few or no sons [58–61] or those whose children are all of the same sex [58, 60–63] intend or expect to have more additional children than do other couples. Many people prefer a majority of boys among their offspring [64–66] or as a first-born or only child [61, 64, 65, 67]. Williamson, reviewing many cross-cultural studies, found a preference for male children in virtually all cultures [8].

Sex preferences also affect fertility, although the exact relationship may be undergoing change. During the 1950s and 1960s, couples whose first few children were of the same sex [60, 62, 68, 69] or those whose children were predominantly female [59, 63, 68] tended to have another child more quickly or to have larger completed families than did other couples.

In the United States, although sex preferences have not changed, these preferences may have lost strength in determining fertility intentions and behavior, as fertility norms have declined from the three- to four-child family of the 1950s to two children in the 1970s [58, 60, 61, 68, 70].

In the 1955 Growth of American Families Study (GAF), at second, third, and fourth parities, a progressively higher proportion of couples whose children were all of the same sex expected to have more children than the couples who had both boys and girls [60]. Longitudinal data from the Princeton Fertility Study, between 1957 and 1967, indicated that a third, a fourth, and even a fifth birth were more likely to occur if the preceding births were of the same sex; this was particularly true in cases of all-girl families [68].

The 1965 and 1970 National Fertility Studies (NFS) continued to show a modest influence of sex preferences on fertility desires or intentions among second-parity couples [58, 61]. Unlike the 1955 GAF and the Princeton Fertility Study, however, the 1965 NFS showed that sex of previous children did *not* distinguish third-parity couples who wanted no more children (80% of the group) [58]; no data were given for third-parity couples in the 1970 NFS [61].

Since 1970, the presumed effect of sex preferences on fertility intentions and actual fertility has declined. A 1971 probability sample of urban white wives indicated that couples with children of the same sex were only slightly more likely than couples with a boy and a girl to want a third child (the difference was only 3.1%). The addition of the wife's age as a control did not affect the relationship. Analyses of mean intended family size among wives at the third and higher parities yielded similar results [70].

A recent study in Great Britain also showed that the probability for an added birth to women of second parity was not related to son preference and only slightly to a preference for one child of each sex [58]; couples who did not achieve their sex preferences had no more children than couples whose preferences were fulfilled. Unfortunately, no recent comparable fertility tabulations are available for the United States.

The role of sex preferences is difficult to separate from other determinants of fertility. United States surveys during the 1950s and 1960s (when norms favored the three- to four-child family) demonstrated a modest effect of sex preferences on fertility intentions and on actual fertility. Smaller United States and British studies from the early 1970s (when norms favored the two-child family) suggested that sex preferences were less likely to influence birth plans. Although sex preferences have not changed, and parents may be disappointed that their desires are not fulfilled, other factors today seem to mitigate against having a third child. Further longitudinal data are required to corroborate whether the effect of sex preferences has in fact changed and whether it is related to shifts in the number of expected children [70].

Summary

Thus, the typical young American, although marrying somewhat later than previous cohorts, expects to marry and bear at least two children, hopefully a boy and a girl. Consciously or unconsciously, these children are conceived to provide affection, creativity, fun, adult status, role fulfillment, enhancement of the marital relationship, and various other intrinsic satisfactions; they are expected to represent what is best in their parents, yet be able to achieve and attain more than their parents.

THE GENETIC COUNSELEE AS DEVIANT

Screening programs, genetic counseling, or the birth of a defective child constitute, for many individuals, the first realization or confirmation that they carry a genetic problem that sets them apart from other people and may prevent them from achieving fertility norms. A person's expectations, self-conceptions, and self-esteem can be shattered on learning that he or she possesses a stigma, a deeply discrediting attribute, which may disqualify the individual from full social acceptance. Goffman terms stigmas "discredited" when the stigma is known, evident, or obvious, and he terms them "discreditable" when the stigma is not known by others or immediately perceivable [71]. For those individuals or couples who are carriers, the stigma is discreditable. Their children, if affected by genetic disease, have a discredited stigma. Some stigmas can change from discreditable to discredited, as when symptoms of Huntington Disease appear in a person at risk, or when information about carrier status is disclosed to a potential spouse. Other individuals, such as siblings of an affected child, who are normal but stigmatized because of their close association with a stigmatized individual, possess yet a third type of stigma, termed by Goffman a "courtesy stigma" [71, 72].

Having a genetic disorder is particularly stigmatizing because it involuntarily deprives the individual of a socially valued role under circumstances that reflect unfavorably upon his *capacity* for the role. The lost role of husband, wife, or parent, may be one that the individual had previously attained or desired. The moment of failure finds the person feeling that he or she was suitable for the role in question [73]. One of Fletcher's respondents aptly describes this situation:
"I am just crushed and disappointed. I had so hoped to give my husband a healthy baby, and now I know that I will not. You spend all your life looking at pictures of pretty babies and their mothers and growing up thinking that will be you. It is pretty gruesome when you are the one who is different" [74, p. 319].

THE DISCREDITABLE STIGMA

Disclosure of a genetic disorder can be made before the birth of an affected child, through genetic counseling of families who have had an affected member, or through screening programs to detect clinically normal carriers of conditions such as Tay-Sachs disease and sickle cell anemia. With few exceptions, carrier status does not carry with it any observable differences, as does the actual disease state; thus disclosure of this status is a discreditable stigma.

Identification as a parent at risk, however, involves more than knowledge of one's medical or genetic status. It may entail potential social and psychological problems, because of the social implications of carrier status [75]. Aside from a loss of privacy per se [76], disclosure may affect feelings of self-worth and competence and hinder the establishment or maintenance of social relationships [75], because it defines the individual as less capable or incapable of fulfilling expected fertility norms.

The extent of stigmatization depends greatly upon the probability that the discreditable stigma will become a discredited stigma. This, in turn, depends partly on the timing of disclosure of carrier status, with respect to the individual's reproductive career [75] and on the options open to the individual for preventing the disorder [77]. Other things being equal, when prenatal diagnosis of the condition is possible, disclosure of carrier status will be less stigmatizing than when freedom of mate selection or fertility is restricted. In the former situation, the discreditable stigma is prevented from becoming discrediting through the use of prenatal diagnosis and selective abortion, provided this is an acceptable choice for the individual. By this means, the counselee can still fulfill marital and reproductive norms, so the self can be redefined with little loss of credibility.

The Marital Context: Premarital vs Marital Counseling

If screening or genetic counseling is conducted prior to marriage, disclosure of a genetic disorder may change the person's desire to marry and restrict his freedom of mate selection. Since married individuals are expected to bear children, the threat of a severely or even mildly disabling disorder will cast doubt on one's parental capacity and thereby reduce an individual's desirability as a mate [75]. This doubt is not mitigated by the fact that *both* parents must be carriers for most genetic risks to materialize.

Available data indicate that premarital genetic counseling is currently the exception. Genetic counselors report that only 7% of their counselees seek premarital consultation. In the majority of these cases, the individuals know they are related, and are concerned about the possible consequences of their common ancestry [78]. There are no systematic data on the mating patterns of those individuals who receive premarital counseling for a genetic problem that may appear later in themselves, as in the case of Huntington Disease.

The Orchomenos study. Important data on the consequences of premarital counseling are available, however, for asymptomatic carriers of sickle cell anemia, in the peasant farming community of Orchomenos, Greece [77, 79]. Stamatoyannopoulos studied this major nonblack sickle cell population, in which 23% of the population were carriers and were well acquainted with sickle cell disease. From 1966 to 1969, 2,300 families were screened and counseled individually. In 1973, a total of 354 couples were reinterviewed to assess the effects of the screening program, including about 150 who had married after both partners had been screened.

The goal of the screening program was the premarital exchange of genetic information in the hope of avoiding matings that would lead to births of children with sickle cell disease. This goal was achieved. All of the 354 couples interviewed reported that, sometime during the arrangement for marriage, the parents or future spouses had revealed to one another their sickle cell status and had discussed the possibility that children with sickle cell anemia could result from the mating. Two-thirds of the marriages were arranged by the parents.

However, families with carrier children lost their freedom in the pursuit of marital arrangements. Because few carriers talked freely about their status, the courting couple lived in anxiety up to the moment that the hemoglobin status of the prospective spouse was revealed. This anxiety arose because social stigmatization occurred subsequent to the collapse of engagements. Almost one-fourth of all families, independent of carrier status, considered that having the sickle cell trait meant restriction of freedom and the risk of social stigmatization. All parents with carrier children taught them to avoid a carrier mate. In addition, however, *normal* children were advised by 10% of carrier parents and 20% of normal parents to avoid marrying a carrier. In both situations, this reaction could be attributed to the social embarrassment of the carrier state. Interviews of the smaller sample of married couples where both spouses had been premaritally screened indicated that the majority of noncarriers had not avoided a carrier spouse because they knew there was no risk of sickle cell anemia in the offspring.

The carriers, however, did not consistently exercise caution in mate selection. One-quarter reported that they had concealed their carrier status from the spouse, and one-quarter stated that hemoglobin status had been unimportant in spouse selection — they were ready to accept the risks. Only one-half of the carrier spouses had conscientiously avoided marrying a carrier and had inquired premaritally about the carrier status of the future spouse; among these, 20% stated that they had broken a marital engagement when they learned that the future spouse was also a carrier.

Although the screening program in Orchomenos encouraged the inhabitants to prevent sickle cell anemia by premarital consultation about the prospective couple's genotype, Stamatoyannopoulos concluded that the program failed to accomplish its goals concerning mate choice [77]. He estimated that, if matings had been completely random, the expected number of marriages between two carriers during the study period would have been 4.5. In fact, four such couples married in Orchomenos, all of whom had been tested and counseled premaritally. In two cases, one of the spouses had concealed the carrier status, and in the other two, the couples had married despite complete understanding of the risks.

Although the screening program benefited noncarriers by easing their anxiety, the program produced extensive stigmatization of carriers. It reduced their freedom of mate selection and the freedom of those noncarriers who mistakenly believed that a sickle cell carrier was a less desirable mate. Furthermore, it may not have reduced the incidence of sickle cell disease in this population.

This study of an isolated Greek community cannot be generalized without careful reservations. Nonetheless, there is no study of any community showing that genetic screening and counseling can be effective in altering marriage pairings or reproductive goals.

The Baltimore—Washington program. Fortunately, there are situations in which prenatal diagnosis of the condition is possible. Carrier detection programs for such disorders can be directed primarily to young married couples. In this situation, carrier disclosure need not impose limitations on mate selection or the reproductive goals of those who accept prenatal diagnosis and approve of selective abortion in case of a positive diagnosis. An example of this program is the Baltimore—Washington carrier detection program for Tay-Sachs disease in the Ashkenazi Jewish population, conducted by Kaback et al [80]. Among the nearly 7,000 individuals tested, 94% were married, 5% were engaged, and only 1% were single. Approximately 70% of the married individuals were tested as couples.

The program has so far identified 11 couples at risk for bearing a Tay-Sachs fetus among the nearly 7,000 individuals tested. None of these couples had previously borne a Tay-Sachs child. Five pregnancies have since occurred in this group; all were subjected to prenatal diagnosis, and one was aborted following positive diagnosis of Tay-Sachs [80]. Thus the program appears to be achieving its goal of disease prevention.

Three factors may account for the varying success of the Orchomenos and Baltimore—Washington screening programs. First, the educational levels of the two populations differed. The educational level among the Jewish population in the American screening program was very high [81]. Nearly 75% of those tested had completed college, and 43% had had some postgraduate education [80]. In contrast, Orchomenos is a peasant farming community, and its inhabitants were poorly educated. Also, the Greek program offered only negative alternatives, involving restriction of freedom to select mates or to reproduce. The Tay-Sachs screening program was conducted postmaritally. It offered positive alternatives and a guarantee of unaffected children through prenatal diagnosis and abortion of affected fetuses, which was acceptable to this target population [77]. Finally, it is likely that the extent of restriction of mate-selection and the extent of stigmatization produced was greater in a small community like Orchomenos than it was in a larger urban society [77]. Thus the characteristics of the populations, the options of the two screening programs, and the locales of screening would all seem important in explaining the difference in success of the two programs.

At present there is no information regarding the effects of carrier detection on established marriages. A long-term study of the impact and possible stigmatization resulting from carrier testing on the individual, couple, family, and community is being undertaken by Kaback and his associates in the Baltimore—Washington program, but this study will require continuing follow-up over a prolonged period. It is likely, however, that the stigmatization produced by disorders that are amenable to prenatal diagnosis, and therefore positive control, will be less severe than that produced by disorders such as sickle cell anemia, where the options available are much more restrictive in nature.

Effects on Norms Regarding Reproductive Goals

If screening or counseling is conducted prior to marriage, it may change an identified carrier's desire for children or produce guilt if marriage is to another carrier and a child with the disorder is born [77]. At present, there are few data for assessing the impact of known carrier status on reproductive plans. It is still too early, for instance, to assess the effect of counseling on the reproductive decisions of married carriers in Orchomenos.

On the basis of research discussed in Part I, it is assumed that pressure to bear children will be exerted on those couples who refrain from childbearing because of a known genetic disorder associated with a high risk factor or severity. Individuals who decide to remain childless or to limit their childbearing to one normal child will be stigmatized and negatively stereotyped, because they seemingly do not *want* to reproduce, or have reproduced a supposedly disadvantaged only child. Veevers' research suggests that childless counselees will be questioned freely, even by casual acquaintances, about the reasons for their deviant status. They will be subjected to the heaviest pressure to reproduce during the third and fourth years of marriage [3]. This pressure will be strong if couples choose not to reveal the underlying genetic rationale for their childlessness.

The life cycle stage of the genetic counselee is thus a strong factor influencing reproductive intentions. Counselees may feel the heaviest pressure (or the strongest desire) to reproduce after 3 years of marriage, or approximately 3 years after the birth of a normal child. Self-referred genetic counselees may be more prone to seek counseling at these times. The birth of an affected child and the severity of the disorder will probably modify the response of counselees considerably.

Those who explain their childlessness or one-child families on genetic grounds may escape some of the negative stereotyping and social pressure experienced by the voluntarily childless couples. In fact, genetic counselees may be considered *more* responsible, self-sacrificing, unselfish, mature, and stable because they have decided to forego childbearing. Although genetic counselees may have weaker social pressure directed at them to reproduce, they and the barren are likely to be "more open to despair in that they do accept the dominant value belief system, and are unable to fulfill what they themselves acknowledge to be legitimate expectations" [3, p. 585]. Moreover, in reducing stigmatization due to non-normative childbearing, the couple must reveal a different stigma: their genetic problem. The couple, like the barren, will then be defined as unfortunate and become an object for sympathy or pity rather than condemnation [3].

Of course not all couples seeking genetic counseling want additional children. Some may come hoping for a genetic rationale to refrain from childbearing that will convince their parents and others who urge them to reproduce. These couples hope that genetic information will soften the stereotypes of the non-childbearing or one-child families; redefine the couple as responsible, self-sacrificing, and mature; and ease the social pressure on them to bear children. Other couples may have already had their desired number of children but want information on genetic risks for their children's children.

THE DISCREDITED STIGMA: THE BIRTH OF AN AFFECTED CHILD

The birth of an affected child is the most traumatic way in which to learn of a disorder, precisely because the self cannot be completely redefined along defensible lines. If the child survives, the evidence of one's inadequacy is glaringly present, both to oneself and to others.

Fletcher eloquently describes this moment:

"The experience of learning that your child is defective immediately after birth can still be categorized among the most painful and stigmatizing experiences of modern people. It is as if the parents' *raison d'etre* were called into question before an imagined parental bar of justice and an ontological blow dealt to their hopes of continuing their identities" [82, p. 24].

As noted in Table II, many factors may influence the impact of a disorder on a family [74, 75, 83–94]; the listing is not exhaustive, and in many cases the research is outdated, poorly designed, limited in sample size, or in need of corroboration.

Studying the response of parents to the birth of an affected child is one way to understand the psychological meaning of stigmatization. A general sequence of response characterizes many parents. The literature relating to genetic disorders, chronic illness, and physical handicaps suggests the following immediate and long-term psychological responses.

Immediate Reactions

All agree that the initial experience of parents, and possibly of the health profession as well, is shock, disbelief, denial, and rejection based upon disappointed hope [95–97]. Solnit and Stark have defined the parents' experience as loss of the hoped-for and expected baby occurring simultaneously with the birth of the feared, threatening, and anger-provoking child [98]. Parents may be so shocked initially upon hearing the diagnosis and learning of its hereditary transmission that they repress the information. Several counseling sessions may be required for them to accept fully the fact that they have a child with an inherited defect [99].

This initial phase of disorganization is followed by stages of increasing awareness of the loss; acceptance of the implications of that loss; and attempts to reintegrate family functioning, to work through one's feelings, and prepare for problems of medical management. A variety of affective responses characterize this

TABLE II. Factors Affecting the Impact of a Disorder on Family Functioning*

A. Factors Pertaining to the Disorder Itself
  1. Severity of the disorder in terms of visibility, salience, or certainty of the disorder, and hence so acceptability and associated stigma–value.
  2. Extent of physical vs. mental disability.
  3. Nature of the disorder, genetic or nongenetic: if genetic, the objective and perceived risk of recu rence within the immediate family and within the larger kin group; if genetic, whether responsib for the disorder is unknown or can be attributed to one or both spouses.
  4. Potential harm to unaffected family members as a function of the disorder.
  5. Manageability of the disorder: Degree, type, and length of care required; degree of social disrupt to normal routines.
  6. Prognosis: Implications for reduced length of life and independence of functioning.
  7. Degree of control over health of future progeny: Existence of prenatal testing to diagnose the disorder.
B. Factors Relating to the Patient
  1. Age and sex of the patient.
  2. Relationship of affected family member and the number of members affected.
  3. Personality of the patient.
  4. Manner in which the patient perceives the disorder and the response mechanisms employed.
  5. Patient attitudes toward medical care and caretaking competence prior to the disorder.
C. Factors Relating to the Family and Close Relatives
  1. Family dynamics prior to the disorder: Existence of close, supportive, and satisfying relationshi stability of the group; and communication among members.
  2. Flexibility between and within roles; ability to diversify caretaking roles and vary approaches to problem-solving.
  3. Knowledge of others with similar problems and previous personal experience with the disorder.
  4. Personality of family members (eg, achievement orientation, internal–external locus of control, ability to cope with stress) and response mechanisms employed.
  5. Family's attitude toward the affected person.
  6. Health and needs of other family members.
  7. Ability to obtain family goals through nonaffected members.
  8. Manner in which the family learns of the disorder and the structure of the counseling or screeni program.
  9. Manner in which the family perceives the disorder, which may be related to various social and cultural factors (eg, life cycle stage, ethnic group, social status and economic resources available religion, and religiosity).
D. Factors Relating to the Society
  1. Attitudes toward abnormality.
  2. Normative fertility levels.
  3. Cultural emphasis on achievement vs. ascription.
  4. Community resources available for the treatment and rehabilitation of the disorder and integrat of patients into economic and social life of the community.
  5. Resources available to provide social support for the family.

*See references 74, 75, 83–94, especially 93.

stage: feelings of sorrow, depression, guilt, anxiety, helplessness, and anger. This grief reaction, followed by a long period of mourning for the loss of a normal child and the particular loss of the healthy limb, capability, or gene, has been noted by many specialists in the field [83, 96, 97, 100–102].

Parents employ a variety of defense mechanisms to safeguard them from despair, especially for life-threatening disorders. As noted by McCollum, Schwartz, and others, the most frequently observed defenses are denial, repression, isolation of affect, and avoidance [103–106]. These emotions and reactions are often accompanied by physical exhaustion, nightmares, psychosomatic illnesses, rejection of normal sexual relations, social isolation from others, and reliving of past mourning experiences [99, 107].

The final stage, sometimes referred to as mature adaptation, effective response, or acceptance, is the objective of counseling [82, 95, 97]. Few families achieve mature adaptation directly [108]. Lasting maladaptive reactions, such as those suggested by McCollum and Schwartz, are more common: chronic sorrow, anger, guilt, and anxiety [104, 105]. These situations seem particularly likely to occur in the aftermath of genetic disorders, especially those least socially acceptable – ie, genetic or chromosomal anomalies that impair mental functioning or create cosmetic deformities or crippling handicaps [75, 83, 85, 86, 109].

Long-Term Reactions

Sorrow. The central emotion aroused by a disorder is sorrow. As noted by McCollum and Schwartz, it is doubtful whether sorrow can be greatly assuaged by professional intervention [105]. Based on his counseling experience, Olshansky concluded that most parents who have a retarded child, for instance, suffer chronic sorrow throughout their lives, regardless of whether the child is kept at home or is institutionalized [84]. Although the parent–child relationship is not completely devoid of satisfaction, "the permanent day-by-day dependence of the child, the interminable frustrations resulting from the child's relative changelessness, the unaesthetic quality of mental defectiveness, the deep symbolism buried in the process of giving birth to a defective child, all these join together to produce the parent's chronic sorrow"[84, p. 192]. Olshansky urged that this sorrow be accepted by the individual and by the professional worker as a *natural* response to a tragic fate, rather than a *neurotic* response. However, based on psychiatric assessment of parents of 13 cyanotic congenital heart disease children, Rozansky and Linde concluded that parents commonly denied their repeated episodes of grief, especially parents of older children [106].

Anger. Whereas it is doubtful that sorrow can be greatly assuaged, anger can often be ameliorated. A variety of outlets may be chosen. Rejection of the child is sometimes manifest in the form of overprotectiveness, at times alternating with withdrawal [106, 110]. The marital partner or extended kin may be chosen as targets for anger, especially in the case of genetically transmitted disease [99, 105].

Anger may be directed toward God, resulting in a weakening of religious faith, or toward health professionals, especially when a medical error or incorrect interpretation has been made [106]. Finally, anger may also be directed inward, resulting in an abrupt loss of self-esteem and acute depression [106]. For instance, in a study of 100 families affected by cystic fibrosis, depression was reported as extremely common among mothers of affected children. Approximately 79% of the mothers described themselves as "run down or depressed," and 42% were receiving antidepressant drug therapy [111].

It is to be hoped that counseling will enable parents to acknowledge their anger, recognize its displacement, and discharge it in a nondestructive manner, which will free them to look to other people as sources of emotional support. Possible channels include talking to the social worker, discharge (sports, vigorous cleaning), and aggressive social activity (such as fund-raising, support of medical research, or working for various causes) [105].

Guilt. Nurture and protection of the offspring are central to parenthood. Therefore, when a child is threatened, most parents experience a painful but transient process of self-examination and self-reproach [105]. If the disorder is genetic in nature, guilt feelings will be particularly strong. Fletcher has noted the unusual sense of guilt and shame associated with genetic disease and has termed it "cosmic guilt" [74]. Severe guilt feelings are common to mothers of hemophilic children [110], cystic fibrosis children [111], and cyanotic children [106]. Guilt is not as characteristic of the noncarrier parent.

In situations where responsibility cannot be assigned to one parent, each parent may perceive the other's feelings of guilt and inadequacies and may blame the other for producing the abnormal offspring. Numerous psychosexual conflicts and a gradual deterioration of intrafamily communication may ensue [99]. Finally, the child may eventually reproach the parents for the misery of his illness, thereby reinforcing their guilt.

Anxiety. McCollum and Schwartz have suggested five possible sources of apprehension and anxiety [105]. Loss of mastery over the parental role is stimulated by: a sense of helplessness, knowing that the child is endangered; realization that the outcome cannot be altered; fears of being unable to cope with the situation and losing self-control or fears that their defensive reactions are not normal; intense separation anxiety in anticipation of the child's death; and stimulation of anxiety about the parent's own death. Complaints of worry and anxiety are frequently expressed by parents, especially mothers [102].

Effects on Norms Regarding Reproductive Goals

The intensity of these psychological responses reflects the parents' reluctance to accept new self-concepts and their feared inability to achieve fertility norms. The birth of an affected child, especially when first-born, defines the parent to him or herself and to others as less capable of childbearing. Fertility expectations and sex preferences are threatened and may go unfulfilled. In fact, as the typical family size declines to two children, there may be an attendant increase in the desire that children be as perfect as possible. The impact of a genetic disorder in a situation of declining fertility may thus be more devastating to parents and kin than it would be if fertility were higher [75].

In addition, an affected child does not fulfill certain of the motivations for childbearing:

1. Adult status and social identity: The birth of an affected child does not define the parent as a mature, stable, and acceptable member of the community. The parent is defined as a failure with a newly stigmatized social identity.

2. Immortality: Producing an affected child confirms that one's worst rather than best characteristics will be reflected in another. The lineage is tarnished. In fact, if the child's prognosis is poor or future childbearing is doubtful, the lineage may not continue at all, to the consternation of parents and kin.

3. Stimulation, novelty, and fun: The child may not add an element of excitement or fun to the home and may provide little opportunity for parents to relive their youth. Indeed, watching the growth and development of the child may be a painful, rather than a pleasurable process.

4. Social comparison and competitive advantage: Depending upon the severity of the disorder, pride in children's accomplishments and the ability of the child to carry out the parents' hopes and dreams may be an impossibility. The attitudes of close relatives, friends, and neighbors will heighten the parents' sensitivity and affect their self-esteem. Sometimes to compensate for the failure of having an affected child, other children in the family will be expected to work harder and be more successful than their peers [91].

5. Economic utility: The child may be unable to contribute to security in the parents' old age. On the contrary, the economic burden of rearing an affected child may overwhelm the parents, and later, the siblings.

Despite these limitations, however, the birth of an affected child may successfully satisfy other motivations for childbearing. The desire to feel essential and protect another human being may be enhanced. A need for affiliation may be fulfilled. A handicapped child can satisfy altruistic motivations for parenthood, since parental self-sacrifice for the child will produce feelings of virtue and self-worth. A parent may gain a sense of creativity and accomplishment from meeting the challenges of rearing an affected child. And, finally, the birth of an affected child may signify to the parents a test of their religious faith.

The Marital Context of Fertility

The disclosure of carrier status may not only affect fertility desires and prevent the satisfaction of certain needs: if a genetic disorder is disclosed within an established family unit, the husband and wife may develop severe chronic dissatisfaction with each other as marriage partners and may possibly seek other mates [75, 80], especially in cases in which prenatal diagnosis of the condition is impossible or unacceptable.

Regrettably, available studies on this topic have used comparatively crude measures of marital stability, such as self-reports of marital deterioration or dissatisfaction (which are subject to deception and distortion) or the proportion of separations and divorces within a group. The studies are further handicapped by a lack of longitudinal, post-counseling measures of marital adjustment; by failure to control for parity and the presence of normal children in the home; by failure to note whether responsibility for the disorder is unknown or rests with one or both spouses; and by self-selection among counselees. Given these limitations, all findings cited below are tentative.

Many studies have concluded that, for the majority of counselees, diagnosis of a disorder or the presence of a child with a disorder had no adverse effect on the marital relationship; some couples reported that their marriages were strengthened by the need to cope with the difficulties of rearing a defective child [87, 102, 111]. These responses seem suspect, given the evidence cited previously – that in homes with normal children, marital satisfaction is highest prior to childbearing and in the later post-childrearing years [22]; and that the first birth triggers a crisis in marital relationships, resulting in postpartum declines in marital satisfaction and/ or sexual satisfaction [22–24]. The responses of counselees may reveal the need to deny the tenacity of cultural beliefs that children, even those with disorders, improve a marriage. It is also possible that during the time span between the birth of an affected child and the study interview, some adjustment in the marriage has already taken place. Fletcher's sample of counselees, for instance, reported that they had "learned to live" with their situation, although the effect of the disorder had not worn off [74].

Some couples, albeit a minority, report that the marital relationship deteriorated following the birth of the child. Marital deterioration was typically aggravated by sexual difficulties and lessened sexual activity caused by exhaustion or the fear of having another affected child [111–116]. Fear of pregnancy seemed greater among populations using inadequate contraceptive techniques [111]. For many couples, the anxiety could be relieved through the use of contraception or sterilization [114], but for others it remained [111].

Other potential sources of marital friction, aside from fatigue and fear of pregnancy, lay in the mother's preoccupation with the affected child and the father's subsequent feeling of abandonment, his inability to accept the child, or his difficulty in finding a meaningful role in the care of the child [87, 105].

Divorce

Reports on the number of separations and divorces among genetic counselees differ. Simple follow-up studies have generally concluded that the divorce rate among these couples is *not* significantly greater than that for the general population, other patients in the hospital, or members of the same age cohort [111, 117–119]. Among couples who subsequently divorced, only a minority categorically stated that having a defective child was the cause of their marital problems [118, 120].

Some situations, however, may lead to a higher divorce rate within the counseling population. Among those suggested are preexistence of marital tensions or psychological problems, attribution of genetic responsibility to one spouse, and unfulfilled fertility desires.

Although a genetic disorder can be an important factor, it was rarely the sole factor precipitating divorce. Preexisting tensions and problems were often cited by the divorced [87, 102, 111, 118, 120]. Second, it is *assumed* that marital discord can result from telling parents which one is responsible for the disorder. Some counselors believe it is better to diffuse feelings of responsibility, by simply informing the couple that the child has a genetic problem and that both parents contribute to the genetic composition of the child [121]. There is no empirical evidence, however, that this procedure reduces marital discord or stigmatization, and the practice does not seem widespread. Some counselors report that in such situations, the carrier parent is notified privately and given the option of remaining silent or informing the spouse. Most counselees prefer to inform the spouse and return together for further counseling.

Finally, it has been suggested that divorce is more frequent among couples with unfulfilled fertility desires than among those who have already completed their desired family size [75]. Sorenson recomputed data from 455 genetic counseling couples, originally compiled by Carter and his associates [117]. The data were arrayed so that a comparison could be made between those who reported that counseling had affected their reproductive expectations and those who said that it had not. The rate of divorce in the unaffected group (one divorce among 252 couples) was below the divorce rate of the couples whose reproductive expectations had changed following consultation (6 divorces among 169 couples), and below the expected divorce rate for that age group. Sorenson concluded that the disclosure of carrier status could result in a higher incidence of divorce, especially in situations in which individuals had not completed their reproductive careers or where procedures such as amniocentesis were not possible [75, 122].

As Sorenson recognized, these are admittedly limited data. Remaining married does not indicate a successful marriage or the level of satisfaction enjoyed by the partners. Moreover, from a demographic standpoint, comparisons of divorce data between genetic counselees and the general population, even when age is controlled, are insufficient. Since a high proportion of genetic counselees are middle- or upper-class, and since social status is negatively related to the divorce rate, one would expect a lower divorce rate among counselees than among the general population. One study noted that the educational level of counselees made a profound difference in the rate of divorce [111]. Aside from educational attainment, parity should also be controlled. Second, one cannot ascertain from the original Carter data [117] whether altered reproductive careers were actually the major factor contributing to a higher divorce rate. It is also possible that those couples who stated that they were deterred from reproduction perceived the severity of the disorder (and its concomitant family stress) as greater or perceived a higher risk factor (which may have heightened fear of pregnancy and adversely affected the sexual relationship). Thus, greater family stress or deterioration in the sexual relationship may be as responsible for marital dissatisfaction and divorce as frustrated desires for children.

Finally, sampling bias will affect the incidence of divorce. Genetic counselees who are self-referred may have lower divorce rates than those who are referred to counseling by physicians or those who avoid counseling. Thus the referral source of counselees, as well as the incidence of divorce among noncounseled couples, must be considered before the effect of genetic disorders on marital satisfaction and adjustment can be assessed accurately.

The problem of marital disruption can extend beyond the nuclear family when risks apply to many relatives and multiple siblings are affected. Fear and anxiety can spread through an entire kindred, distressing those who are not even at risk for the disorder. Parents and kin sometimes cease reproduction after diagnosis of a genetic disease is made, thereby promoting disintegration of marriages and disruption of family units [99, 105, 116]. In other situations, however, as in dominant disorders, diagnosis of the disease can cement family relationships through distorted bounds of genetic identification [123, 124]. One early study of a large family in which 32 of the 170 members were affected with hereditary hemorrhagic telangiectasia reported that the disorder had drawn the family together. Frequent family reunions and clannish attitudes emphasized the lasting traditions, values, and achievements of the family. It was the group consensus that family assets far outweighed the dangers of telangiectasia, and reproduction was therefore encouraged [124].

Redefining the Self

Following the birth of a defective child, a couple may adapt to their failure and redefine their self-conceptions along defensible lines. Goffman has described a variety of adaptations to failure, many of which are applicable to genetic counselees [73].

First, a person may gain a status different from the one he lost or failed to attain, but which provides him with at least a compensatory identity. In this regard, social workers or physicians should encourage parents to accept the affected child as a replacement for the normal one they failed to obtain. Families, such as the one afflicted with telangiectasia, can sometimes provide special support and recognition for the achievements of their members.

Second, the couple can be offered another chance to qualify for the role at which they failed. After the birth of a defective child, parents may feel a great urge to compensate by initiating another pregnancy [115]. Among couples who have already borne one or two normal children, thereby fulfilling fertility norms and expectations, the negative impact on self-image and the urge to reproduce will be weaker. However, in situations where an only child is affected, parents and kin may need to prove to themselves and to others that they are indeed capable of producing something better. The desire to produce at least one normal (and hopefully male) child can be very strong. Support for continued reproduction, to replace a lost or affected child, may come from the larger family unit as well, as was the case in the family affected with telangiectasia.

When the disorder involves high risk to future offspring and cannot be diagnosed prenatally, parents will feel depressed and trapped; maladaptive adjustments to their situation may ensue. In such situations, couples may cease reproduction or, if acceptable, may decide to adopt, to utilize artificial insemination, or to sublimate their parenting impulses in social activities (fostering, teaching, scouting, etc). When future fertility is deterred, individuals may attempt to absolve themselves of personal responsibility by placing the blame elsewhere — on spouse, kin, doctor, or God. In these cases, deterioration of the marriage or divorce can occur, followed by a new marriage partner and a redefined self.

CONCLUSION

Disclosure of a genetic disorder is always stigmatizing. However, if the disorder can be prevented through informed mate selection or through prenatal diagnosis and selective abortion, the individual's self-concept can be redefined along defensible lines. If these preventive steps are not available, the couple may revise their fertility desires and attempt to find alternate gratifications for the psychic needs that children would have satisfied: they may decide to adopt a child, to utilize artificial insemination, or to reproduce despite a known genetic risk. The birth of a normal child may be needed to redefine the self, to fulfill normative fertility behavior, or to enhance the marital relationship.

Factors associated with genetic disorders, such as perceived risk and severity of the disorder, are important considerations in fertility decisions. However, fertility must be understood not solely within a medical—genetic context but within a social context. It is probable that the influence of genetic counseling upon fertility depends greatly upon the life cycle stage and reproductive intentions of individuals prior to counseling. Genetic counseling can be of value to counselees who are undecided or have decided to stop childbearing in the absence of full information — ie, among those who are still motivated to bear children. Among those who are no longer motivated to bear children (on the basis of correct information about the disorder) or among those who are highly motivated to bear children, regardless of what information they receive, genetic counseling will have a weaker influence in shaping fertility behavior.

ACKNOWLEDGMENTS

Appreciation is expressed to Y. Edward Hsia and Ruth Silverberg for their editorial advice and guidance, to Paul Neurath of Queens College for his assistance in translating articles, and to James Sorenson of Boston University and Nancy Williamson of the Population Council for their provision of references and materials.

ANNOTATED REFERENCES

1. Pohlman E: "The Psychology of Birth Planning." Cambridge, Mass: Schenkman, 1969.
   An excellent synthesis of the research literature on the motives for wanting children, the psychological costs of childbearing and child-rearing, especially the effects of unwanted conceptions, and the psychological meanings and problems associated with contraceptive methods and abortion.
2. Back KW, Fawcett JT (eds): Population policy and the person: Congruence or conflict? J Soc Issues 30(4), 1974.
   A special issue devoted entirely to goals, effects, and implementation of population policies. Topics of special interest to counselors include evolution and parenting (Bardwick), psychological effects of family size, especially the only child (Thompson), measurement of fertility desires, and components of fertiliy decision-making (Hass).
3. Veevers JE: The violation of fertility mores: voluntary childlessness as deviant behaviour. In Boydell C, Grindstaff C, Whitehead P (eds): "Deviant Behaviour and Societal Reaction." Toronto: Holt, Rinehart & Winston, 1972, pp 571–592.
   An integration of theory and data pertaining to the norms of having children and wanting children, stigmatization and stereotypes associated with childlessness, and the efficacy of sanctions.
4. Hilton B, Callahan D, Harris M, Condliffe P, Berkley B (eds): "Ethical Issues in Human Genetics: Genetic Counseling and the Use of Genetic Knowledge." New York: Plenum Press, 1973.
   Proceedings of the Fogarty International Symposium No. 13. Four studies of particular relevance include a discussion on screening (Murray), privacy (Lubs), sociological and psychological factors in applied human genetics (Sorenson), and findings from J. Fletcher's study of decision-making among 25 couples who underwent amniocentesis, 3 of whom subsequently elected abortion.
5. Lipkin Jr M, Rowley PT (eds): "Genetic Responsibility: On Choosing Our Children's Genes." New York: Plenum Press, 1974.
   Proceedings of a symposium, "Genetics, Man and Society," presented at the 1972 meeting of the American Association for the Advancement of Science. Articles pertain to genetic counseling and screening, and include psychological and social considerations (Sorenson, Fletcher), procedures, and assessment of effects (Hsia).
6. Kiesler CA, Kiesler SB: "Conformity." Reading, Mass: Addison-Wesley, 1969.
7. Hass PH: Wanted and unwanted pregnancies: A fertility decision-making model. J Soc Issues 30:125, 1974.

8. Williamson NE: "Sons or Daughters? A Cross-Cultural Study of Parenthood Preferences." Beverly Hills: Sage, 1976.

9. David HP: Unwanted pregnancies: costs and alternatives, U.S. Commission on Population Growth and the American Future. In Westoff CF, Parke Jr R (eds): "Demographic and Social Aspects of Population Growth. Vol I of Commission Research Reports." (Stock No. 5258-0005). Washington DC: Government Printing Office, 1972, pp 439–466.

10. Lee NH: "The Search for an Abortionist." Chicago: University of Chicago Press, 1969.

11. Sklar J, Berkov B: Abortion, illegitimacy, and the American birth rate. Science 185:909, 1974.

12. Tietze C: Two years' experience with a liberal abortion law: Its impact on fertility trends in New York City. Fam Plann Perspect 5:36, 1973.

13. Center for Disease Control: Abortion Surveillance 1975. Atlanta: Center for Disease Control, 1977.

14. US Bureau of the Census: Fertility history and prospects of American women: June 1975. "Current Population Reports" (C3.186:P-20/288). Washington DC: US Government Printing Office, 1976.

15. Blake J: Can we believe recent data on birth expectations in the United States? Demography 11:25, 1974.

16. Kiesler SB: "Social Norms and Family Size." Report prepared for the Center for Population Research, National Institute of Child Health and Human Development, DHEW, 1976.

17. Peterson RA: Change in college students' attitude toward child-bearing from 1971 to 1973. J Pers Assess 39:225, 1975.

18. Glick PC: Some recent changes in American families. "Current Population Reports" (C56.218:P-23/52). Washington DC: US Government Printing Office, 1975.

19. Sklar J, Berkov B: The American birth rate: Evidences of a coming rise. Science 189:693, 1975.

20. Anonymous: US fertility continues to drop although birth rate shows slight rise. Popul Dynamics Q 3(2):7, 1975.

21. Rabin AI: Motivation for parenthood. J Projective Techniques Pers Assess 29:405, 1965.

22. Feldman H: The effects of children on the family. "Family Issues of Employed Women in Europe and America." Edited by A Michel. Lieden, The Netherlands. EF Brill, 1971.

23. Dyer ED: Parenthood as crisis: A re-study. Marriage and Family Living 25:196, 1963.

24. LeMasters EE: Parenthood as crisis. Marriage and Family Living 19:352, 1957.

25. Rainwater L: "And the Poor Get Children." Chicago: Quadrangle Books, 1960.

26. Blake J: Ideal family size among white Americans: A quarter of a century's evidence. Demography 3:154, 1966.

27. U.S. Bureau of the Census: Prospects for American fertility: June 1974. "Current Population Reports" (C56.218:P-20/269). Washington DC: US Government Printing Office, 1974.

28. U.S. Bureau of the Census: Fertility expectations of American women: June 1974. "Current Population Reports" (C56.218:P-20/277). Washington DC: US Government Printing Office, 1975.

29. Eagly AH, Anderson P: Sex role and attitudinal correlates of desired family size. J Appl Soc Psychol 4:151, 1974.

30. Griffith J: Social pressure on family size intentions. Fam Plann Perspect 5:237, 1973.

31. Veevers JE: Voluntary childless wives: an exploratory study. In Kammeyer KCW (ed): "Population Studies: Selected Essays and Research" 2nd ed. Chicago: Rand McNally, 1975, pp 323-332.

32. Flapan M: A paradigm for the analysis of childbearing motivations of married women prior to birth of the first child. Am J Orthopsychiatry 39:402, 1969.
33. Pohlman E: The child born after denial of abortion request. In Newman SH, Beck MB, Lewit S (eds): "Abortion, Obtained and Denied: Research Approaches." New York: The Population Council, 1971, pp 59–74.
34. Berkow SG: "Childlessness: A Study of Sterility, Its Cause and Treatment." New York: Lee Furman, 1937.
35. Davis K: Changing modes of marriage: Contemporary family types. In Becker H, Hill R (eds): "Marriage and the Family." Lexington, Mass: DC Heath, 1942.
36. Veevers JE: The social meanings of parenthood. Psychiatry 36:291, 1973.
37. Thompson VD: Family size: Implicit policies and assumed psychological outcomes. J Soc Issues 30:93, 1974.
38. Rainwater L: "Family Design: Marital Sexuality, Family Size, and Contraception." Chicago: Aldine, 1965.
39. Popenoe P: Eugenic motivation of childless marriages. Eugen Rev 21:102, 1936.
40. Cutts NE, Moseley N: "The Only Child: A Guide for Parents and Only Children of All Ages." New York: GP Putnam's Sons, 1954 .
41. Terhune KW: "A Review of the Actual and Expected Consequences of Family Size" (Report prepared for the Center for Population Research, National Institute of Child Health and Human Development, DHEW) (NIH Publication No. [NIH] 75-779). Washington DC: US Government Printing Office, 1975.
42. Solomon ES, Clare JE, Westoff CF: Fear of childlessness, desire to avoid an only child, and children's desires for siblings. Milbank Mem Fund Q 34:160, 1956 (1941 Indianapolis Study).
43. Clausen JA, Clausen SR: The effects of family size on parents and children. In Fawcett JT (ed): "Psychological Perspectives on Population." New York: Basic Books, 1973, pp 185–208.
44. Kramer R: A fresh look at the only child. New York Times Magazine, October 15, 1972, p 77.
45. Eysenck HJ, Cookson D: Personality in primary school children: 3 – Family background. Br J Educ Psychol 40:117, 1970.
46. Belmont L, Marolla FA: Birth order, family size, and intelligence. Science 182:1096, 1973.
47. Bogue DJ: What are the motives for and against birth control in various cultures? In Bogue DJ (ed): "Mass Communication and Motivation for Birth Control." Chicago: University of Chicago, Community and Family Study Center, 1967.
48. Fawcett JT, Arnold F, Bulatao RA, Buripakdi C, Chung BJ, Iritani T, Lee SJ, Wu T-S: "The Value of Children in Asia and the United States: Comparative Perspectives" (Paper No. 32). Honolulu: East-West Population Institute, 1974.
49. Kirchner EP, Locasso RM: Motivations to have children: Factors and correlates. Presented at the annual meeting of the Eastern Psychological Association, Philadelphia, April 1974. University Park, Penn: Pennsylvania State University, Institute for Research on Human Resources. Mimeo.
50. Rabin AI, Greene RJ: Assessing motivation for parenthood. J Psychol 69:39, 1968.
51. Terhune KW: Fertility values: Why people stop having children. Presented at the annual meeting of the American Psychological Association, August 1973. Philadelphia: Temple University, Institute for Survey Research. Mimeo.
52. Beach LR, Townes BD, Campbell FL, Keating GW: Developing and testing a decision aid for birth planning decisions. Organizational Behavior and Human Performance 15:99, 1976.

53. Wyatt F: Clinical notes on the motives of reproduction. J Soc Issues 23:29, 1967.
54. Hoffman LW, Hoffman ML: The value of children to parents. In Fawcett JT (ed): "Psychological Perspectives on Population." New York: Basic Books, 1973, pp 19–76.
55. Hoffman LW: A psychological perspective on the value of children to parents. In Fawcett JT (ed): "The Satisfaction and Costs of Children: Theories, Concepts, Methods." Honolulu: East-West Population Institute, 1972.
56. Stolka SM, Barnett LD: Education and religion as factors in women's attitudes motivating childbearing. J Marriage Fam 31:740, 1969.
57. Espenshade TJ: "The Cost of Children in Urban United States" (Population Monograph No. 14). Berkeley: University of California, Institute of International Studies, 1973.
58. Coombs LC: Preferences about sex of children. In Freedman R, Coombs LC (eds): "Cross-Cultural Comparisons: Data on Two Factors in Fertility Behaviour." New York: The Population Council, 1974.
59. Freedman R, Coombs LC: "Cross-Cultural Comparisons: Data on Two Factors in Fertility Behaviour." New York: The Population Council, 1974.
60. Freedman DS, Freedman R, Whelpton PK: Size of family and preference for children of each sex. Am J Sociol 66:141, 1960 (1955 GAF).
61. Westoff CF, Rindfuss RR: Sex preselection in the United States: Some implications. Science 184:633, 1974 (1970 NFS).
62. Westoff CF, Potter RG Jr, Sagi PC: "The Third Child." Princeton: Princeton University Press, 1963 (Princeton Fertility Study, Second Report).
63. Westoff CF, Potter RG Jr, Sagi PC, Mishler EG: "Family Growth in Metropolitan America." Princeton: Princeton University Press, 1961 (Princeton Fertility Study, First Report).
64. Markle GE: Sex ratio at birth: Values, variance, and some determinants. Demography 11:131, 1974.
65. Markle GE, Nam CB: Sex predetermination: Its impact on fertility. Soc Biol 18:73, 1971.
66. Whelpton PK, Campbell AA, Patterson J: "Fertility and Family Planning in the United States." Princeton: Princeton University Press, 1966 (1960 GAF).
67. Dinitz S, Dynes RR, Clarke AC: Preferences for male or female children: Traditional or affectional? Marriage and Family Living 16:128, 1954.
68. Bumpass LL, Westoff CF: "The Later Years of Childbearing." Princeton: Princeton University Press, 1970 (Princeton Fertility Study, Third Report).
69. Gray E, Morrison NM: Influence of combinations of sexes of children on family size. J Hered 65:169, 1974.
70. Cutright P, Belt S, Scanzoni J: Gender preferences, sex predetermination, and family size in the United States. Soc Biol 21:242, 1974.
71. Goffman E: "Stigma: Notes on the Management of Spoiled Identity." Englewood Cliffs, NJ: Prentice-Hall, 1963.
72. Birenbaum A: On managing a courtesy stigma. J Health Soc Behav 11:196, 1970.
73. Goffman E: On cooling the mark out: Some aspects of adaptation to failure. Psychiatry 15:451, 1952.
74. Fletcher J: Parents in genetic counseling: The moral shape of decision-making. In Hilton B, Callahan D, Harris M, Condliffe P, Berkley B (eds): "Ethical Issues in Human Genetics: Genetic Counseling and the Use of Genetic Knowledge." New York: Plenum Press, 1973, pp 301–327.
75. Sorenson JR: Some social and psychologic issues in genetic screening. In Bergsma D (ed): "Ethical, Social, and Legal Dimensions of Screening for Human Genetic Disease." Miami: Symposia Specialists for The National Foundation:March of Dimes, BD: OAS X(6):165, 1974.

76. Lubs HA: Privacy and genetic information. In Hilton B, Callahan D, Harris M, Condliffe P, Berkley B (eds): "Ethical Issues in Human Genetics: Genetic Counseling and the Use of Genetic Knowledge." New York: Plenum Press, 1973, pp 267–275.
77. Stamatoyannopoulos G: Problems of screening and counseling in the hemoglobinopathies. In Motulsky AG, Ebling FJG (eds): "Birth Defects: Proceedings of the Fourth International Conference, Vienna, 1973." Amsterdam: Excerpta Medica, 1974, pp 268–276.
78. Sorenson JR: "Applied Human Genetics Study: Final Report." Princeton: Princeton University, 1971.
79. Horn P: Newsline: When genetic counseling backfires. Psychol Today 9 (4):20, 1975.
80. Kaback MM, Becker MH, Ruth MV: Sociologic studies in human genetics: I. Compliance factors in a voluntary heterozygote screening program. In Bergsma D (ed): "Ethical, Social and Legal Dimensions of Screening for Human Genetic Disease. "Miami: Symposia Specialists for The National Foundation–March of Dimes, BD:OAS X(6):145, 1974.
81. Greeley AM: "Ethnicity, Denomination, and Inequality Disease." Miami: (Sage Research Papers in the Social Sciences). Beverly Hills: Sage, 1976.
82. Fletcher J: Attitudes toward defective newborns. Hastings Cent Stud 2:21, 1974.
83. Johns N: Family reactions to the birth of a child with congenital abnormality. Obstet Gynecol Surv 26:635, 1971.
84. Olshansky S: Chronic sorrow: A response to having a mentally defective child. Social Casework 43:190, 1962.
85. Cummings ST, Bayley HC, Rie HE: Effects of the child's deficiency on the mother: A study of mothers of mentally retarded, chronically ill and neurotic children. Am J Orthopsychiatry 36:595, 1966.
86. Harasymiw S: Prejudice toward minority groups and familiarity with disabilities: Their relationship to attitudes toward the disabled. Boston: Boston Univeristy, New England Special Education Instructional Material Center, 1971. Mimeo.
87. Hare EH, Laurence KM, Paynes H, Rawnsley K: Spina bifida cystica and family stress. Br Med J 2:757, 1966.
88. Heffrom WA, Bommelaere K, Masters R: Group discussions with the parents of leukemic children. Pediatrics 52:831, 1973.
89. Livsey CG: Physical illness and family dynamics. Adv Psychosom Med 8:237, 1972.
90. Mahoney SC: Observations concerning counseling with parents of mentally retarded children. Am J Ment Defic 63:81, 1958.
91. Morris D: The psychological management of handicapped children in the first year of life. In Howells JG (ed): "Modern Perspectives on Psycho-Obstetrics." New York: Brunner/Mazel, 1972, pp 449–469.
92. Olsen H: The impact of serious illness on the family system. Medicine 47:169, 1970.
93. Rusk HA, Novey J: The impact of chronic illness on families. Marriage and Family Living 19:193, 1957.
94. Zuk GH: The religious factor and the role of guilt in parental acceptance of the retarded child. Am J Ment Defic 64:139, 1959.
95. Garrard SD, Richmond JB: Psychological aspects of the management of chronic diseases and handicapping conditions in childhood. In Lief HI, Lief VF, Lief NR (eds): "The Psychological Basis of Medical Practice." New York: Harper & Row, 1963, pp 370–403.
96. Goodman L: Continuing treatment of parents with congenitally defective infants. Social Work 9:92, 1964.
97. Falek A: Five steps to better counseling. Genetic Counseling 16:100, 1975.
98. Solnit AJ, Stark MH: Mourning and the birth of a defective child. In "Psychoanalytic Study of the Child." Vol 16. New York: International Universities Press, 1961, pp 523–537.

99. Tips RL, Lynch HT: Genetic counseling in a team setting. In Bergsma D (ed): "Human Genetics." Baltimore: William & Wilkins for The National Foundation–March of Dimes. BD:OAS IV(6):110, 1968.

100. Bentovim A: Emotional disturbances of handicapped pre-school children and their families – Attitudes to the child. Br Med J 2:579, 1972.

101. Kennell JH, Klaus MH: Care of the mother of the high-risk infant. Clin Obstet Gynecol 14:928, 1971.

102. Walker JH, Thomas M, Russell IT: Spina bifida – and the parents. Dev Med Child Neurol 13:462, 1971.

103. Blumberg BD: Psychic sequelae of selective abortion. (MD Thesis, Yale, 1974).

104. Kaplan DM, Smith A, Grobstein R, Fischman SE: Family mediation of stress. Social Work 18:60, 1973.

105. McCollum AT, Schwartz AH: Social work and the mourning patient. Social Work 17:25, 1972.

106. Rozansky GI, Linde LM: Psychiatric study of parents of children with cyanotic congenital heart disease. Pediatrics 48:450, 1971.

107. Anonymous: Having a congenitally deformed baby. Lancet 1:1499, 1973.

108. Crocker AC, Cullinane MM: Families under stress: The diagnosis of Hurler's syndrome. Postgrad Med 51:223, 1972.

109. Tringo J: The hierarchy of preference toward disability groups. J Spec Educ 4:295, 1970.

110. Agle DP: Psychiatric studies of patients with hemophilia and related states. Arch Intern Med 114:76, 1964.

111. McCrae WM, Cull AM, Burton L, Dodge J: Cystic fibrosis: Parents' response to the genetic basis of the disease. Lancet 2:141, 1973.

112. Emery AEH, Watt MS, Clack ER: The effects of genetic counselling in Duchenne muscular dystrophy. Clin Genet 3:147, 1972.

113. Emery AEH, Watt MS, Clack ER: Social effects of genetic counselling. Br Med J 1:724, 1973.

114. Leonard CO, Chase GA, Childs B: Genetic counseling: A consumer's view. N Engl J Med 287:433, 1972.

115. Macintyre MN: Genetic risk, prenatal diagnosis, and selective abortion. In Walbert DF, Butler JD: "Abortion, Society, and the Law." Cleveland: Case Western Reserve University Press, 1973, pp 223–239.

116. Tips RL, Lynch HT: The impact of genetic counseling upon the family milieu. JAMA 184:183, 1963.

117. Carter CO, Roberts JAF, Evans KA, Buck AR: Genetic clinic: A follow-up. Lancet 1:281, 1971.

118. Carter CO, Evans K, Norman A: Cystic fibrosis: Genetic counseling follow-up. In Mangos JA, Talamo RC (eds): "Fundamental Problems of Cystic Fibrosis and Related Diseases." New York: Intercontinental, 1973, pp 99–102.

119. Freeston BM: An enquiry into the effect of a spina bifida child upon family life. Dev Med Child Neurol 13:456, 1971.

120. Reynolds B, Puck MH, Robinson A: Genetic counseling: An appraisal. Clin Genet 5:177, 1974.

121. Stevenson AC, Davison BC, Oakes MW: "Genetic Counseling." Philadelphia: JB Lippincott Co., 1970.

122. Sorenson JR: Genetic counseling: Some psychological considerations. In Lipkin M Jr, Rowley PT (eds): "Genetic Responsibility: On Choosing Our Children's Genes." New York: Plenum Press, 1974, pp 61–67.

123. Tips RL, Smith GS, Lynch HT, McNutt CW: The "whole family" concept in clinical genetics. Am J Dis Child 107:67, 1964.

124. Bird RM, Hammarsten JF, Marshall RA, Robinson RR: A family reunion: A study of hereditary hemorrhagic telangiectasia. N Engl J Med 257:105, 1957.

9

Parental Choice and Family Planning: The Acceptability, Use, and Sequelae of Four Methods

Paula E. Hollerbach, PhD

INTRODUCTION

Fertility intentions are determined by many factors — cultural norms, genetic and nongenetic considerations, as well as the availability and acceptability of methods to prevent or promote fertility [1–10]. During the last decade, with the advent of the pill, the intrauterine device (IUD), and simpler surgical sterilization, the contraceptive practices of Americans have changed remarkably. The less effective, coitus-dependent methods (diaphragm, condom, withdrawal, foam, rhythm, and douche) are being abandoned in favor of newer coitus-independent methods, which offer greater contraceptive protection [10].

These methods have been adopted by *all* subgroups of the population — all racial, age, educational, and religious groups. As of 1973, 68% of white and 81% of black users had adopted the pill, IUD, or sterilization. There were some racial differences in methods used, but among young wives of both races, the pill was especially popular, and among older wives, male and female sterilization were the most widely used methods [10]. The contraceptive practices of Roman Catholics have also shifted radically. In 1955, approximately two-thirds of Catholic wives were abiding by the Church's ban on artificial contraception, reporting that their most recent contraceptive method was rhythm or no method at all. By 1970, however, approximately two-thirds of Catholic wives had used a method *opposed* by the Church [9].

These shifts in contraceptive usage have been so remarkable that "It seems highly probable that by the end of the 1970s, almost all married couples at risk of unintended pregnancy will be using contraception, and almost all contraceptors will be protected by the most effective medical methods" [10, p. 57].

Genetic counselees may use various methods to prevent or terminate fertility. The postconception measures of prenatal diagnosis and selective abortion can permit reproduction while preventing some disorders; sterilization can be used to terminate fertility; and future generations may utilize sex-predetermination to select the sex of the fetus at the time of conception, and thereby avoid sex-linked genetic disorders. Finally, an alternative to natural conception is available through artificial insemination.

In this chapter, I will consider the attitudes of the American population in general and the attitudes of counselees in particular toward the use of these four modes to terminate, replace, or promote fertility. I will discuss their current or potential use in both populations, and, finally, I will consider the psychological sequelae and contraindications associated with these methods.

STERILIZATION

Approval and Prevalence of Sterilization

Probably the most dramatic change in recent US contraceptive practice has been the acceptance of and increased reliance on surgical sterilization. The National Survey of Family Growth (NFSG) recorded an acceleration in surgical sterilization for nonmedical reasons from 16.3% in 1970 to 23.5% in 1973. Both male and female operations increased; female procedures, slightly more than vasectomies. Among couples where the wife was between 35 and 44, sterilization was the most popular form of contraception — used by more than one-third of all current contraceptive users — but the proportions electing sterilization at younger ages also increased substantially [10]. This earlier sterilization seemed related to lower fertility expectations [7].

Among whites, equal proportions of males and females (12%) utilized sterilization in 1973, but among blacks, female sterilization (23.1%) far exceeded vasectomy (1.7%). This trend was related in part to greater misinformation among blacks regarding the consequences of vasectomy on sexual physiology [6, 7] and its association with genocide by black males [8]. However, use of other male contraceptive methods, such as the condom and withdrawal, was also much lower among black couples than among white couples [10]. Education was negatively related to the incidence of tubal ligations and positively related to vasectomies. Twice as many Protestant couples were sterilized than those who were Catholic or who were mixed Protestant—Catholic [7].

A number of factors may have accounted for the increased popularity of sterilization: disillusionment with contraceptive methods that are more obtrusive, unattractive, ineffective, or have unpleasant side-effects; desire to enjoy sexual relations unhampered by contraceptive vigilance and fear of pregnancy; shifts in fertility expectations to a smaller two-child family and therefore an earlier termination of childbearing; increased publicity about the operation; decline in misconceptions about the consequences of sterilization on sexual physiology; easing of medical, legal age, and parity restrictions; and development of simpler surgical techniques that reduce the expense, surgical trauma, and convalescence associated with the more traditional methods such as tubal ligation [6, 7].

Psychological Sequelae of Sterilization

Conclusions regarding the psychological sequelae of male and female sterilization must be drawn cautiously, owing to inadequacies in research design and measurement.

The psychological effects of voluntary tubal ligations and vasectomies performed primarily for contraceptive purposes are reviewed [11–15], excluding hysterectomies, which often are medically indicated operations. Regrettably, little research has been conducted on the sequelae of laparoscopic tubal sterilization, a method that is gaining popularity in the United States (see Tubal Ligation later in this chapter) as a less traumatic, less expensive, and more convenient form of sterilization [16].

Vasectomy. The research on psychological sequelae of vasectomy suggests that

> A normal sexually well-adjusted male will experience no significant psychological changes following elective sterilization if he understands what he can expect during and after the procedure and if he is given an opportunity to express his fears and have his questions answered in advance. . . . When psychological problems do occur postoperatively, they can usually be explained by preoperative attitudes and conditions [see 15, p. 33].

In her review of the research, Wortman has suggested a number of such preoperative conditions in which vasectomy may be contraindicated:

1. Young unmarried men with psychological problems.
2. Hypochondria in relation to other bodily functions.
3. Borderline impotency, homosexuality, doubts about masculinity.
4. A troubled marriage, including incompatibility with the wife.
5. Disagreement or coercion by the spouse.
6. Belief by either partner that vasectomy is a temporary measure that can be easily reversed.

For the vast majority of men, however, vasectomy is not accompanied by deterioration in physical health, sexual enjoyment, or other psychological problems. For instance, in the largest study so far, of more than 10,000 British males one or more years after vasectomy, only 0.2% indicated that their health had deteriorated [17].

Furthermore, vasectomy does not seem to affect sexual capabilities. In most studies, the majority of men and their wives reported either no change or improvement in the quality and enjoyment of sexual intercourse, or in marital harmony,

which they attributed to freedom from fear of pregnancy [18]. Studies in Great
Britain and the United States demonstrated that from 44% to 73% of the men who
had vasectomies reported increased enjoyment of sex; less than 3% reported a decline in sexual pleasure; only 0.5% to 1.2% reported a decrease in marital harmony [17, 19]. The majority of couples who cited problems and requested counseling typically had previous histories of marital, sexual, or psychological instability [14, 20].

A few longitudinal studies have compared the sexual behavior and psychological attitudes of couples in which the husband had a vasectomy with couples who
were using other contraceptive techniques [11, 21]. Rodgers and Ziegler found
rather negative attitudes after two years, but four years later, both the vasectomy
couples and the pill couples rated their marriages and frequency of intercourse
similarly [11]. Janke and Wiest concluded that the psychological adjustment of
the vasectomy group was superior to that of the control group, presumably due
to relief of anxiety regarding pregnancy [21]. Finally, Edward Pohlman of the
University of the Pacific, California, has conducted an intensive, three-year (1972–
1975) longitudinal study of 800 subjects. Preliminary analyses from this study
have shown no evidence of negative sequelae from vasectomy for the sample as
a whole.

General retrospective studies on the acceptability of vasectomy invariably
have reported that most vasectomized men (90–99%) and their wives (88–90%)
were favorably inclined toward the operation and would repeat the procedure
[6, 11]: Less than 10% reported that they would not repeat the operation because of changes in their life situation (marital dissolution, remarriage, infant or
child mortality), but they denied significant deleterious emotional or sexual
effects [11, 17].

Tubal ligation. Reports on the psychological sequelae of tubal ligation indicate an overall positive or at least neutral reaction to the procedure, although dissatisfaction is typically higher than in the vasectomy studies. Suggested contraindications to tubal ligation are similar to those listed for vasectomy. Conclusions regarding the psychological sequelae of tubal ligation must be drawn
cautiously, however, since the research designs have been flawed by methodological problems.

In reviewing 22 studies conducted between 1949 and 1969 of women who
had received tubal ligations for contraceptive *and* medical purposes, Schwyhart
and Kutner found that psychological measurements of female reaction to sterilization had been limited largely to self-reports of regret or dissatisfaction (ranging
from 1–18%), reduced libido or sexual adjustment (2–25%), and menstrual problems, which may be psychogenic (7–45%) [12].

Although not tested, it has been suggested by these authors that the most important contraindications to contraceptive tubal ligations are :

1. Unsatisfied maternal (parental) desire, perhaps because pregnancy is regarded as highly ego-supportive.
2. Presence of psychopathology.
3. Presence of high religiosity or family pressure which could produce guilt.
4. Marital instability, doubts about marital permanence, negative spouse attitudes toward the effects of sterilization, or manipulation by the spouse to have the operation.
5. Misconceptions regarding the effects of sterilization, reversibility, or alternative methods of birth control.
6. Poor sexual adjustment prior to sterilization.
7. Inability to accept recent or severe loss [see 12, p. 366].

Approval and use of female sterilization have continued to increase markedly since the latest study (1969) analyzed by Schwyhart and Kutner. Studies conducted today should indicate a much lower incidence of regret or dissatisfaction. For instance, a recent follow-up survey of a cross-section of 200 women undergoing laparoscopic tubal sterilization found that almost none of the women reported regret about the procedure; 97% said they would recommend it to a friend, and in fact, 90% had already done so [16]. Clearly, more recent and better-designed research on the topic is needed.

Prevalence and Psychological Sequelae of Sterilization Among the Genetic Counseling Population

In the series of studies analyzed by Schwyhart and Kutner, only three included sterilizations performed for genetic indications [22–24]. However, findings from these studies have regrettably limited significance: the three studies were conducted in the late 1950s and early 1960s; all three dealt with non-U.S. populations (Japanese, Danish and Swedish); follow-up time varied between ½–1½ years and 5–6 years post-sterilization. In the Swedish study, 11% of the sample was sterilized for genetic reasons; in the other two, the proportion with genetic indications was smaller. High proportions of the women studied had abnormal personalities, and many received sterilizations and abortions concomitantly. The proportion expressing regret over sterilization was 4% in the Danish study, 8.6% in the Japanese study, and 18% in the Swedish study [12].

The studies provide few data on the incidence of sterilization or the characteristics of genetic counselees who elect the procedure. Some genetic clinics do not recommend sterilization, and if consulted, actively discourage it for lower-risk conditions [25].

Sterilization, especially female sterilization, is more frequently elected by couples whose children's risk for a disorder is high or serious in nature, by those who have attained desired family size, and by non-Catholics [4, 25, 26, 28, 29]. A number of anecdotal examples suggest that a genetic carrier may feel personal responsibility to undergo sterilization, rather than a noncarrier spouse, arguing that the spouse might later remarry and want to have children, or that the person at fault should "pay for it" [27]. Sterilization is rarely elected following positive fetal diagnosis and selective abortion [4, 27, 30, 82]; couples who did often cited personal (nongenetic) reasons for their decision – the emotional strain they experienced and their inability or unwillingness to undergo amniocentesis again [4, 11, 27].

Relevance of Research to the Genetic Counseling Population

The attitudes and reactions of those undergoing sterilization for contraceptive purposes are not necessarily applicable to individuals seeking genetic counseling. Motivations for contraceptive sterilization typically include multiparity, socioeconomic considerations, emotional factors, and fear of pregnancy, combined with dissatisfaction and/or inability to establish another suitable birth control plan [31].

Counselees may fear pregnancy, and their choice of sterilization may certainly be motivated by socioeconomic considerations or emotional factors. However, sterilization may also be motivated by awareness that they are genetically "less fit" to bear children. Therefore, an unknown proportion of counselees will face sterilization with some ambivalence. Especially when prenatal diagnosis is impossible, risk factors are unacceptably high, or the family has previously failed to gain a normal child after amniocentesis, counselees may elect sterilization to free themselves from fears of future abnormal pregnancies. Yet they may still desire normal pregnancies.

Despite these limitations, many of the reviewed findings regarding sterilization seem applicable to the genetic counseling population. One would expect greater approval of sterilization, especially vasectomy, among whites than among blacks (although blacks are more likely to use sterilization); the well-educated; non-Catholics; those who have reached their desired family size, especially those who have already experienced an unwanted birth; and those who are correctly informed about the consequences of the procedures [7].

Data on genetic counselees corroborate that sterilization is utilized more by non-Catholics and by those who have completed their desired family size. In addition, genetic carriers, those at high risk and/or those who risk a serious disorder in progeny seem especially likely to seek sterilization.

General contraindications to sterilization for both sexes have been demonstrated: preexisting marital, psychological, or sexual problems of the couple; objection to the operation by a spouse; misunderstanding regarding the permanence and irreversibility of the measure; coercion by spouse, family, or doctor; and religious objections to the procedure.

In addition, specific attention of genetic counselors is drawn to the following contraindications:

1. Given the evidence on changing life situations, counselees whose carrier status is uncertain should be dissuaded from sterilization.

2. Counselees with unsatisfied parental desires, those unable to accept loss, those who have experienced recent severe grief (such as recent positive prenatal diagnosis and abortion), and those who desire sterilization concomitant with abortion are more likely to regret their sterilizations. Sterilization should not be combined with abortion in situations in which the couple has not reached desired family size. A three- to six-month waiting period between abortion and sterilization would seem advisable to allow patients time to separate any feelings of disappointment and guilt regarding the abortion from their decisions regarding childbearing. Obstetricians and genetic counselors should refrain from urging patients to combine both operations and should instead advise caution in making irreversible decisions [27].

Because genetic counselees may be at higher risk for negative psychological sequelae, they should receive special attention. At the same time, however, counselors should not lose sight of the fact that the permanence, convenience, and effectiveness of sterilization are its greatest assests and that the vast majority of men and women electing sterilization will experience no negative psychological or sexual problems but often report improvement in functioning because they no longer fear pregnancy.

In situations in which fear of pregnancy is great and decisions regarding future fertility seem firm, contraceptive sterilization is a plausible, effective, and desirable measure.

ARTIFICIAL INSEMINATION BY DONOR (AID)

Approval and Prevalence of Artificial Insemination

Artificial insemination with a donor's semen is used primarily when the husband is infertile. In a smaller number of cases, AID is used when the husband has known genetic defects or when both parents are recessive carriers of an anomaly and any children run a high risk of inheriting the disorder [32].

Guttmacher estimated in 1960 that AID produced 5,000 to 7,000 births annually in the United States [33]. By 1964 there may have been more than 250,000 AID children in the United States and possibly another 100,000 in the rest of the world [34].

A 1970 United States national poll found that no more than 26% of those polled approved of artificial insemination using donor semen, and only 55% approved of artificial insemination using the husband's semen (AIH) [37]. Surveyed college students were more liberal in their views [35, 36].

Factors associated with greater acceptance of AIH and AID were: 1) being previously well-informed about artificial insemination; 2) having previously discussed

AI; 3) being a member of a church group other than the Roman Catholic Church or not being affiliated with a religion; and 4) having a high grade-point average in college. Females were more accepting of AIH than males, whereas males were more likely to accept AID than females [36].

In terms of demographic characteristics, couples actually electing AID were very similar to this description. Finegold reported that couples in his practice requesting artificial insemination were typically above average in intelligence, mostly college graduates (who were more exposed to information on artificial insemination). Typically it was the husband who initiated the request [34]. AID was preferred over adoption equally for genetic, emotional, legal, and financial reasons. The majority of AID parents in one survey reported that artificial insemination allowed them a closer relationship to the infant. They were dissatisfied with adoption procedures, believed that genetic factors were under better control with AI, and believed that their children derived benefits from maternal heredity. Other desired influences included the experience of pregnancy, the concealment of of infertility, and faith in the donor-selection process [38].

The primary reasons for rejection of artificial insemination included preference for adoption, belief that AI was morally wrong or constituted legalized adultery, Church disapproval, fear of marital friction, genetic considerations, lack of desire for a child that was only partly one's own, and belief in fate [36, 49].

Psychological Sequelae of Artificial Insemination

With increased AID, issues regarding its ethical, legal, medical, and psychological consequences have arisen [34, 39–48], but research is sorely lacking [50].

Various psychological outcomes have been reported. The husband may develop feelings of inferiority, jealously of the unknown donor, or resentment toward the child. The mother may develop an unnatural attachment to the unknown donor or to the doctor, or she may be overly possessive of the child, on the grounds that the child is biologically hers. The child, serving as a continual reminder of the husband's infertility, may promote eventual rejection of the husband as inadequate. Finally, both parents may fear that the child will discover the source of his or her origin. This is of special concern with regard to genetically motivated artificial inseminations. The donor child may believe that he or she has the genetic disorder of the social father, and in cases of this type some gynecologists insist that the child be informed of the AI background [34].

Despite possible psychological problems described in the literature, many physicians performing AI have been extremely positive about the procedure and have noted few difficulties in their clinical experience. Their patients purportedly viewed AID as a therapeutic medical procedure. A high proportion of patients were satisfied with the outcome, and legal problems were very rare [33, 34, 46–48].

One of the few follow-up studies of families with children born by AI, in Israel, has confirmed the absence of special psychological problems with either the parents or the children [32]. It is not known how attitudes toward AID of genetic counselees who have experienced natural parenthood, albeit of abnormal offspring, compare with those of the infertile.

All authors agree that couples must be carefully screened and selected with regard to their general attitude, emotional stability and maturity, intelligence, marital stability, motives for desiring a child, and their honesty and ability to keep confidences. Some physicians refuse to initiate AI until the couple is interviewed by a qualified psychologist. A three-month interval is often allowed between the time of initial acceptance and the first insemination to assure that the decision for AI is not impulsive [32, 34].

Approval and Prevalence of AID Among the Genetic Counseling Population

Artificial insemination is infrequently selected in genetic counseling as an alternate method of reproduction. In one recent study, there were no instances in which children born after genetic counseling were conceived by artificial insemination either in the total sample of mothers (43 women) or in the sample of moderate- or high-risk mothers (7 women) [51]. In Carter's study, only two couples among the 455 people interviewed used AID to avoid recurrence of a severe recessive condition. Both were in the high-risk deterred group, and both did it on their own initiative. However, the low incidence of AI in this sample may have been related to the practices of the particular counseling center: "Since this procedure is unacceptable to most couples, we do not discuss it unless the couples ask about it" [52].

Other genetic counselors, such as Motulsky, suggest that genetic counselors should not hold preconceived notions about the course which counselees should take and that all alternatives— sterilization, AID, various birth control measures, and adoption — should be discussed [53]. One recent survey of nearly 500 genetic counselors indicated that, in fact, 79% of the counselors felt it was primarily *their* professional obligation to raise and discuss alternative forms of parenthood, including adoption and AID, and only 21% considered this normally to be the obligation of the counselee [54]. However, adoption and AID were grouped together in the question; separation of these alternatives might have indicated greater differences among counselors in their willingness to raise the two topics.

Today more counselees are willing to accept medical management of childbearing with amniocentesis and selective abortion. It seems plausible that counselee approval and medical management of pregnancy through AID will increase as well, especially given the recent decline in numbers of children available for adoption.

It is unlikely that AID will become widely accepted, in part because of legal restrictions, the lack of adequate public information about the procedure, and the reluctance of obstetrician-gynecologists to offer AID as a mode of fertility management. It is obvious that many couples who have utilized AID have been satisfied with it. Just as increased availability and knowledge of sterilization and abortion have produced attitude changes and increased reliance on these methods, one would expect similar changes in attitudes and use of AID. It would seem presumptuous for counselors deliberately to exclude discussion of AID from counseling sessions, thereby deciding for the parents which alternatives should be considered appropriate.

PRENATAL DIAGNOSIS AND SELECTIVE ABORTION

The Availability and Incidence of Selective Abortion

Whereas voluntary sterilization is a means of ending natural reproduction and artificial insemination is an alternative to natural reproduction, prenatal diagnosis and abortion can be used as a means of selective reproduction, enabling parents to participate actively in determining some aspects of the biological quality of their children [55].

Before 1967, all abortion laws in the United States could be classified as restrictive; abortion was prohibited, except to save a pregnant woman's life [56]. Soon after, 13 states adopted less restrictive abortion legislation, expanding the circumstances under which an abortion could be performed to include preservation of the mother's physical and mental health, prevention of the birth of a child with severe genetic or congenital defects, or termination of pregnancy in the case of incest or rape. Nonrestrictive conditions have theoretically existed in all 50 states since January 22, 1973, the date of the Supreme Court decision to remove legal controls [57].

The National Academy of Sciences estimated that between 1967 and 1974, more than 6,000 pregnancies have been monitored in the United Sates and Canada by means of amniocentesis, most of them for suspected chromosomal disorders related to advanced maternal age [57]. Milunsky's review of the US and Canadian experience indicated that of the 1,663 cases surveyed, 1,368 were for chromosomal disorders, and of these, 602 cases were tested because the woman was 35 years of age or older. After testing, 102 therapeutic abortions were performed, constituting 6.1% of the cases [59].

Data on the proportion of US abortions performed for fetal indications, including genetic and nongenetic factors, are difficult to obtain. In 1971, 0.8% of the abortions reported by indication to the Center for Disease Control (CDC) were performed for risk of fetal deformity [60]; in 1972, this proportion was 0.6% [61]. It should be noted, however, that reports to CDC *by indication* are extremely low, usually 5% to 10% of all abortion figures supplied, so that these data should be interpreted cautiously.

Jean Pakter (Director, Bureau of Maternity Services and Family Planning, New York City Department of Health) indicated that of the 81,200 abortions to New York City *residents* in 1973, only 59, or 0.1%, were reportedly performed for fetal indications. Figures from Scotland and Sweden similarly showed that the proportion of women electing abortion for fetal abnormalities was typically less than 4% [62, 63].

Increasing Approval of Abortion in the United States

Legal change toward nonrestrictive abortion has been accompanied by a decline in public opposition to abortion, as documented by U.S. opinion polls and surveys [2, 58, 64]. The extent of approval, however, still depends greatly upon the circumstances involved.

Table I illustrates trends in US public opinion from 1962 to 1975, regarding the legal or moral circumstances in which it should be "all right" or "legally possible" for a women to obtain an abortion [2, 58, 64]. Although the phrasing of questions sometimes differs, the data clearly demonstrate that during this period, the acceptability of various indications for abortion remained approximately the same, according to their relative rankings. Second, during the same time, there was a general increase in the proportion of individuals approving of legal abortion for all reasons, especially in the immediate aftermath of the 1973 Supreme Court decision. The court's action seemed to have a legitimating effect on public opinion [58]. Third, a clear majority of U.S. population supported legal abortion only in situations that were perceived to endanger the health of the mother or the fetus (when a pregnancy would seriously endanger the woman's health or life or there was was a strong possibility of deformity of the child) or in circumstances that violated cultural norms regarding the appropriate context of childbearing (when the pregnancy resulted from rape or incest). These three indications are usually referred to as "hard" reasons for abortion. From 1962 to 1975, approval of abortion in case of the probable deformity of the child increased from 52% to 80% of the adults polled [2, 58, 64]. Approval also increased when the hypothetical risk factor for deformity was raised from one-in-ten to one-in-five [68].

Attitudes toward selective abortion. As noted in Table II, differentials in approval of selective abortion have narrowed considerably, but approval was still greater among non-Catholics, the college-educated, and white populations [2, 58, 64, 70]. Religious commitment and high confidence in organized religion, especially among Catholics, accounted for differences in abortion attitudes to a much greater degree than did denominational identification [58, 69]. A positive relationship existed between educational attainment and approval of selective abortion. Opponents were primarily those with a grade school education, and even these individuals had noticeably shifted to a more liberal position since the 1973 Supreme Court ruling. Finally, although whites approved more of selective abortion than did blacks or other racial groups, blacks were more likely than whites to terminate pregnancies [73]. This statistic suggested that attitude differences may be

TABLE I. General Public Opinion Polls and Surveys: Summary of Proportions Approving Abortion or Legalization of Abortion in Specific Circumstances, United States, 1962–1975

Circumstances	\multicolumn{11}{c}{Year of Survey}

Circumstances	1962[a]	1965[a]	1965[a]	1966[a]	1967[a]	1970[a]	1970[b]	1972[c]	1973[cd]	1974[c]	1975[c]
Endangers woman's health	91%	71%		77%	86%	83%	90%	83%	91%	90%	88%
Endangers woman's life						91					
Pregnancy as result of rape	58	56			72	80	71	74	81	83	80
Pregnancy as result of incest					69						
Probable deformity of the child	52	55	55	54	62	69	69	74	82	83	80
Mother not married	18	18	18	18	28	38	32	40	47	48	46
Couple can't afford another child	13	21	21	18	25	34	25	46	52	52	50
Couple doesn't want more children	8	15			21		22	38	46	45	44
Sample Size	n.g.	5,516 wives	1,484	n.g.	3,278	2,401 women	5,623[e] wives	1,613	1,504	1,484	1,490

n.g. = not given

[a]Ref. 2, pp 175–225.

[b]Interviews with national probability sample of married women, 1970 National Fertility Study [64].

[c]Interviews with representative samples of adults, National Opinion Research Center [58].

[d]Survey made in March 1973, two months after the Supreme Court decision.

[e]"Other" responses omitted from percentage bases; percentages weighted; number of women varies slightly for each question due to omission of those giving "other" responses. The sample size given, 5,623 wives, represents the smallest number in that category used as a percentage base.

exaggerated, or that abortion became more acceptable as women approached or exceeded their desired family size [72, 73]. When educational levels were controlled, black—white differences in abortion attitudes typically persisted only among those with less than a high school education [58]. More blacks than whites had a Southern background and belonged to fundamentalist Protestant religions, and these characteristics were also associated with less favorable attitudes toward abortion [58, 71, 72].

Differences in attitudes toward selective abortion by marital status or sex of respondent were not that marked. Finally, age differences in approval of selective abortion were also comparatively small by 1975, contrary to earlier surveys [68].

Three major factors may account for the increasing approval of selective abortion among all subgroups of the population [66, 67]: 1) increasing medical feasibility to diagnose, predict, and intervene in the reproductive process; 2) changing attitudes — legal, public, and private — toward abortion in general and toward abortion for fetal indications in particular; and 3) the strong cultural value placed on mastery of our environment and the improvement of man through biological and social mechanisms [66]. Given these factors, Sorenson foresees the development of a societal attitude that if a congenital abnormality can be avoided, then it should be, and that those who fail to take advantage of these advances will be ostracized [49, 67].

Attitudes toward prenatal diagnosis and selective abortion among potential users. In contrast to the detailed survey data available on the attitudes of the general population, only a few studies have been conducted on the acceptability of prenatal diagnosis and selective abortion among potential users.

A study of parents of cystic fibrosis children noted that 40% of the 57 couples felt they would consider or definitely make use of prenatal diagnosis when it became possible for cystic fibrosis, followed by selective abortion, if necessary. The couples who would not elect the procedure often stated that, for themselves, termination of pregnancy on any grounds was unethical [74].

Another study of genetic couselees reported that, whereas attitudes toward abortion in general were not overwhelmingly approving, unfavorable attitudes became favorable when prenatal diagnosis was a possibility [28, 65]. Religion was not an important influence in the formation of attitudes toward abortion, prenatal diagnosis, or contraception in this group, although many of the unplanned pregnancies did occur among Catholics, and they were more opposed to the use of sterilization [28].

Higher rates of acceptance have been reported in more recently conducted U.S. studies. At the Yale-New Haven Genetic Counseling unit, among 17 low-risk counselees who wanted more children and could be helped by amniocentesis, 12 intended to use it [75]. Among parents attending two spina bifida clinics, approximately two-thirds of the respondents indicated that they would want prenatal

TABLE II. General Public Opinion Polls and Surveys: Summary of Proportions Approving Abortion or Legalization of Abortion To Prevent Birth of Probable Deformed Child, by Demographic Characteristics of the Respondents, United States, 1962–1975

Demographic characteristics	1962[a]	1965[a]	1965[a] Women	1965[a] Men	1967[a]	1970[a]	1970[b]	1972[c]	1973[cd]	1974[c]	1975[c]
Total	52%	55%	55%		62%	69%	69%	74%	82%	83%	80%
Religion											
Catholic	33	44	43	48	50	61	59	72	80	80	77
Protestant	56		55	57	64	72		80	85	85	84
Jewish			100	88	93	100		93	100	100	95
Other								72	79	88	86
None								91	92	96	95
All non-Catholic		62					74				
Education											
Grade School		41	41	40		53		59	74	76	72
1–3 yr h.s.		52	48	59				78	80	83	80
4 yr h.s.		58	58	63				81	88	86	85
1–3 yr college		64	66	69		76		89	91	90	90
4+ college		69						93	89	90	89
Race											
White		57				72	71	82	86	87	85
Black						60	60	60	71	72	69
Other						49					
All nonwhite	40										

Sex							
Men	54	62		80	84	84	81
Women	50	61		78	85	86	85
Marital Status							
Married			69	79	84	86	82
Separated			71				
Widowed			78 ⎱	71	83	84	86
Divorced			68 ⎰		87	85	85
Single			68	85			
Age							
<29			68	84	85	88	85
30–39			70 ⎱	71	88	86	83
40–49			70 ⎰		82	83	82
>50			n.g.				

n.g. = not given

aFrom [2].

bFrom [64].

cInterviews with representative samples of adults, National Opinion Research Center. "Not given" and "don't know" responses omitted from percentage bases. These previously unpublished figures were provided by William Ray Arney, Department of Sociology, Dartmouth College. The data were made available by the National Opinion Research Center through Project IMPRESS at Dartmouth.

dSurvey made in March 1973, two months after the Supreme Court decision.

diagnosis if they were to have more children [55]. A study of Duchenne muscular dystrophy families concluded that prenatal selection on the basis of sex alone was acceptable to the majority of these families as a hypothetical option. Yet "very few of the mothers and daughters had actually been tested to see if they were carriers, despite their stated interest" [55].

In the largest study yet conducted, a comparison was made of questionnaire responses from 500 randomly selected individuals who volunteered for Tay-Sachs screening and 412 (of 500) nonparticipants who had been mailed the same questionnaire [76]. Comparisons of the compliant and noncompliant subjects showed no significant differences in religious background, despite suggestions that orthodox Jews might be less likely to undergo testing [77]. Compliant and noncompliant subjects also did not differ in their attitudes toward abortion of Tay-Sachs fetuses.

Attitudes toward prenatal diagnosis and selective abortion among past users. Small-scale studies of couples who had undergone prenatal diagnosis showed varied willingness to undergo such procedures again, depending on the outcome of the first amniocentesis.

Among couples receiving negative diagnoses, nearly all remained extremely favorable to amniocentesis, would repeat it in future pregnancies, and would recommend the test to others [27, 78].

Women who had received positive diagnoses and had undergone selective abortion presented inconsistent findings regarding attitudes and actual behavior. The overwhelming majority of these counselees stated that they did not regret the past abortion and would repeat the procedure. This was especially true among women undergoing abortion because of exposure to rubella, where there was no threat to future pregnancies [79–81]. Verbal approval of amniocentesis and selective abortion was high among women with risk of genetic disorders [4, 27]. However, it was not clear what proportion of these women actually did repeat amniocentesis [30, 82]. Most, in fact, apparently did not. Reluctance to repeat the emotional trauma, ambivalent attitudes toward childbearing, or changed fertility intentions often superseded the original decisions [4, 27].

Research on counselees has been so limited, that it is not known whether these results can be generalized to a larger population of counselees or whether these findings characterize women whose amniocenteses were performed at particular centers. No major study has determined how many couples return for a second amniocentesis after selective abortion, revise their fertility desires downward, or continue to reproduce without monitoring their pregnancies.

Psychological Aspects of Prenatal Diagnosis and Selective Abortion

The attitudes of past users toward prenatal diagnosis and selective abortion cannot be comprehended fully unless one understands the psychological aspects of these procedures: the factors underlying decisions about amniocentesis; the emotional context of the waiting period; the psychological sequelae of selective abortion, the causes of depression and guilt that are typical responses to selective abortion; and the conditions under which such reactions become prolonged and more severe.

Decisions about amniocentesis. In explaining their reasons for seeking genetic counseling, parents most frequently mention parental responsibility to assure the health of their children and the security of their families. Fairness to the unborn child, to their living children, to themselves, and to society are interwoven for the majority of couples. Several parents, although not a majority, also mention the concept of a "right to a good mental life." Parents seeking genetic counseling because of advanced maternal age cite social and economic reasons, as do parents who already have had defective children.

Some specific concerns also relate to the amniocentesis procedure itself: the hazard of fetal injury or miscarriage; unknown aspects of the test; decisions about an abortion if results are positive; and the effect of that abortion on the security of a child at home who is affected by the same disorder [27, 78].

The primary moral problem faced by parents during the process is the abortion question. "Caught between a loyalty to the life of their child and a loyalty to the norm of a 'healthy' life (as expressed in children with no genetic defects) there was considerable suffering expressed" [27, p. 310].

The waiting period following amniocentesis. The three- to four-week period following amniocentesis before the report of results is one of considerable tension and anxiety for both parents [78]. Counselees frequently express the hope that future developments will allow for a shorter waiting period [4, 78]. Women who subsequently terminate their pregnancies also recalled a significantly higher incidence of "depression" and "guilt about the possibility of having an abnormal child" than did women who received negative diagnoses [4, 78]. Distortion of recall due to the abortion experience may account for this difference. A more plausible explanation would be Blumberg's observation that the women receiving negative test results were primarily facing low risks of having a defective fetus; in contrast, the majority of women who subsequently aborted were facing a risk of up to 50% in cases of male fetuses. The awareness of greater risk may have stimulated deeper feelings of depression and guilt among these women [4].

Depth studies also showed that the waiting period and its attendant anxiety exacerbated whatever marital or family problems existed before. These problems occurred more among younger than older couples [27].

Following the report of negative results, anxiety is typically abated for the remainder of the pregnancy. Thirty-one percent of the women in one nonaborted group claimed to be unconcerned, but nearly 20% of the patients still had doubts about the accuracy of the results after they were told the sex of the child and the existence of no demonstrable abnormalities [78]. Counselees attending other genetic centers, in which couples receive more counseling and communication, seemed more trusting of test results [27].

Psychological sequelae of selective abortion. The overall prevalence of severe psychological reactions following abortion for psychosocial grounds is quite low [4, 57, 86–91]. Information on the sequelae of selective abortion, however, is hampered by a shortage of research subjects; the proportion of women for whom pregnancy is terminated for fetal indications is small in most series, and fetal-indicated abortions have been omitted from some studies of psychiatric sequelae [92].

During the 1960s a few U.S. and European studies compared the psychological sequelae of women undergoing abortions for psychiatric, organic, or fetal indications, primarily rubella exposure [79–81, 93–94]. A few additional studies focused exclusively on small samples of women undergoing amniocentesis and selective abortion for genetic indications [4, 27, 65, 78, 95].

As noted in Table III, methodological and definitional problems have plagued much of the abortion research on psychological sequelae, including those studies relating to selective abortion [57]. In addition, the majority of subjects studied have been self-referred and middle- or upper-class, reflecting the characteristics of the majority of people receiving genetic counseling in the United States [96, 97]. This class selectivity is due to a variety of factors: knowledge of the availability of such services [98], beliefs regarding the propriety of reproductive control and intervention [10, 99], willingness to seek medical assistance [100], and knowledge about various genetic disorders, which is positively associated with education and income [50, 98].

Considered together, the data support the following trends on the psychological sequelae of selective abortion.

1. Mild and transient depression and regret in the period immediately following abortion was characteristic of the psychologically healthier women [79]. Moderate to severe depression was higher among the psychiatric group [79, 80, 93, 94].

2. Both the rubella and psychiatric groups evidenced guilt following abortion [79, 93].

3. Those aborting for organic disease or rubella were more likely to react unfavorably *immediately* afterwards than those aborted for psychiatric reasons [80]. Unfavorable reactions included mild and brief depression, regret, or uncertainty regarding the abortion [79–80, 93].

4. The diagnostic indications for abortion did not appear to be as important a determinant of long-term abortion response as the overall psychological balance of the patient. Those most likely to have major long-term regrets were those women whose pregnancies were terminated for psychiatric reasons rather than medical–eugenic reasons [81].

5. The incidence of depression seemed lower among women exposed to rubella than those at risk for genetic disorders. Fletcher reported that decisions to abort

TABLE III. Definitional and Methodological Problems Noted in Research on Selective Abortion Sequelae*

1. Failure to include preabortion psychological assessment of the woman and her partner for baseline comparative data.

2. Failure to distinguish differential effects of abortion by indication (cytogenetic, sex-linked disorders, age factor, rubella, etc); by method (saline or prostaglandin infusion, hysterotomy, abortion with and without accompanying sterilization); and by probability of recurrence (low-normal as in rubella, vs continuing risk).

3. Small samples studied and inattention given to possible interviewer bias or sampling bias in the return of questionnaires.

4. Wide variation in timing of follow-up interviews and inadequate comparisons of short-term vs long-term effects of abortion.

5. Variation in timing of studies and the legal and cultural acceptability of abortion. Adverse psychological reactions noted may be due to the abortion itself or to other factors, such as social embarrassment or hostility of medical personnel, which relate more to the legal or cultural status of abortion.

6. Absence of appropriate control groups. Although the absence of such controls may be attributed partly to inadequate research design, it also stems from problems in the definition of an appropriate control group. For instance, should counselees undergoing selective abortion be compared to other second-trimester patients undergoing abortion for nonfetal indications, or to those giving birth to an affected child, or to those undergoing prenatal diagnosis but not selective abortion? Moreover, should women be selected as controls on a random basis or matched on a one-to-one basis in accordance with certain characteristics of women in the abortion group, such as age, parity, marital status, socioeconomic status, and race? The question of the appropriate comparison group is rarely addressed.

7. Use of ambiguous terminology and problems of definition and comparability of such concepts as "depression," "guilt," "regret," or "uncertainty." It is difficult to assess the meaning of these terms, their duration and severity, and it is even more difficult to make comparisons among studies.

8. Lack of standardized instruments to measure the effect of an abortion. Numerous approaches have been utilized to assess the incidence or severity of guilt and depression: Patients' self-assessment through interviews or questionnaire responses, which may be subject to selective recall or distortion; psychiatric evaluation through interviews, clinical experience, or actual records on therapy or psychiatric hospitalizations; and use of more standardized measures such as the Minnesota Multiphasic Personality Inventory (MMPI) and Beck's Inventory Scores.

*Many of these points are discussed in reference 57.

following a positive diagnosis were uniformly followed by grief, self-condemnation, and guilt in his sample [27]. Blumberg reported that 84% of the women and 64% of the men reported depression as an immediate response to selective abortion. Psychological sequelae seemed most persistent among those who had repeatedly failed in their subsequent attempts to produce a healthy child. In contrast, success in obtaining a healthy child through a subsequent birth or adoption seemed to resolve lingering postabortion emotional difficulties [4].

Factors Affecting the Intensity and Duration of Depression

Thus it appears that women undergoing selective abortion experience depression more often and more severely than do women undergoing abortion on psychosocial grounds. A variety of factors may explain this difference. In the following discussion, the term "general abortion" refers to studies on abortion for psychosocial grounds. The term "selective abortion" refers to abortions performed for fetal indications.

Desire for pregnancy. First and foremost, selective abortion represents termination of a desired pregnancy and precludes the birth of a wanted child. In contrast, psychosocially indicated abortions usually terminate unwanted pregnancies.

A variety of general abortion studies have found that woman who desire to have a baby or are reluctant to have an abortion experience more guilt following the procedure [79, 89, 102, 103]. Although selective abortion is preferable to the birth of a defective child, presumably no couple undergoes amniocentesis with the hope that abortion may be required; probably few actually believe that an abortion will be necessary [27].

Responsibility for the fetal disorder and the abortion decision. Grief, depression, and a sense of self-condemnation are also common reactions following stillbirths and infant deaths, especially those involving malformations or wanted pregnancies [104–106]. However, it has been hypothesized that selective abortion engenders more serious depression than a stillbirth, because parents perceive their role not only in the origin of the fetal disorder but in the decision to abort the fetus [4, 107].

The major moral problem faced by counselees is the consideration of abortion, which has been described as a double approach–avoidance conflict. Continuation of the pregnancy is fostered by a desire for a child and possible antiabortion attitudes of the parents. At the same time, termination of a pregnancy is fostered by the social acceptability of preventing the birth of a defective child and the perceived physical, economic, and emotional burdens of bearing a defective child [4]. The decision to abort is accompanied by an unusual sense of shame and guilt associated with genetic carrier status (termed by Fletcher as "cosmic guilt"), the realization that the experiment to obtain a healthy child has failed, and the anticipation of future difficulties [4, 83–85].

Prior stress during pregnancy. As previously discussed, couples who know they are at risk for a genetic disorder will experience anxiety during the pregnancy both prior to and especially during the waiting period of amniocentesis [27]. Although the relationship between preabortion anxiety and postabortion sequelae has not been well investigated, general abortion patients who feel more guilt over abortion find the procedure more difficult and evidence greater fear of the procedure [89]. It is possible that the anxiety endemic to prenatal diagnosis itself may serve to increase the amount of discomfort during selective abortion and the negative sequelae.

The trauma of second-trimester abortion. Therapeutic abortion done by dilation and curettage or vacuum aspiration in the first trimester seem of minor emotional concern. When abortion is delayed until the second trimester, as is necessary in selective abortion, negative postabortion response increases. The saline-infusion or prostaglandin methods produce premature labor, a remainder that this was, in fact, a pregnancy [108]. With prostaglandins, labor tends to be shorter, but medical complications tend to be more serious. Vomiting and diarrhea still accompany the procedure, and the abortion itself is more physically traumatic [142].

Second-trimester abortion also results in the delivery of a well-formed, sexually differentiated fetus, which clearly creates considerable emotional stress for the patient [109]. Blumberg's quotations from selective abortion patients provide vivid and ample evidence of this stress [4].

Identification with the fetus. Second-trimester abortion is potentially more upsetting because it takes place after "quickening," the advent of fetal movement. With or without quickening, however, identification and emotional involvement with the fetus has already taken place. The longer the period of gestation, the more likely the fetus will be viewed as a "baby" rather than a "pregnancy," and the more likely abortion will be accompanied by increased feelings of depression, guilt, or other acute adverse psychological reactions of a mourning process [4, 27, 63, 108, 110–112].

It should be emphasized, however, that quickening is not a necessary condition in fostering identification with the fetus [4, 113]. Desire for pregnancy may be a more important factor. For instance, Senay and Wexler found that women who wanted their pregnancies did not inhibit the process of fantasy formation about the fetus (eg, sex, names, certain qualities or achievements desired) as did those with unwanted pregnancies [113].

To this point, we have discussed a variety of factors that are shared by the majority of selective abortion candidates: desire for pregnancy, responsibility for the fetal disorder and for the decision to abort, prior stress during pregnancy, the trauma of second-trimester abortion, and identification with the fetus.

In addition to these shared experiences, which promote negative sequelae, other characteristics of selective abortion candidates can increase or decrease the the sense of ambivalence with which they make their decisions to terminate or not to terminate a pregnancy. As noted previously, any situation that increases a couple's ambivalence or reluctance to abort will increase the sense of depression or guilt if abortion is elected. Some of the factors associated with abortion decisions for genetic risk are discussed below.

Mode of inheritance. From a genetic perspective, three subgroups compose the selective abortion group. Risks of recurrence can be Mendelian (dominant, recessive, or sex-linked), multifactorial, or age-related. In most studies these groups are too small to make comparisons permitting statistical analysis, but clinical data suggest some interesting hypotheses.

First, ambivalence regarding the abortion decision may be associated with the degree of uncertainty regarding fetal diagnosis. Although perceived severity of the disorder is of utmost importance in decision-making, there is some indication that couples undergoing amniocentesis for sex-linked disorders are less likely to elect abortion after diagnosis of an "affected" fetus by sex, because the risk of disorder is 50% rather than 100% [4, 59, 78]. Counselees at risk for sex-linked disorders who do elect abortion may deny the possibility that a normal male fetus might have been aborted [4].

Second, depression seems less severe in cases of nonrecurring disorders in which couples can anticipate another pregnancy under low-risk conditions. Conversely, the greater the risk factor, the greater the sense of personal responsibility for the fetal disorder and the more severe the postabortion depression. Although the intensity and duration of depression varies, the incidence of depression among genetic counselees is much higher than for rubella patients [79]. Depression among genetic counselees is also greater than that usually associated with elective abortion for psychosocial indications or with delivery of a stillborn, where future normal pregnancies can also be anticipated [57, 95].

Social support for the abortion decision from family and friends. Close, supportive family relationships result in far less postabortion distress than do situations of conflict [79, 80, 114]. However, genetic counselees are more likely to report conflict. Marital separations either prior to or subsequent to amniocentesis have been noted — separations that typically are instigated by husbands and viewed as an acting out of the anger, depression, and cosmic guilt surrounding the genetic circumstances of disorders. Seven of the 13 families interviewed by Blumberg also reported that "people misunderstood," were "cold" or "insensitive" [4].

Social support for the abortion decision from the medical community. Negative and hostile attitudes of hospital and counseling personnel also relate directly to the incidence of postabortion guilt, remorse, and depression experienced by abortion patients [91, 109, 115]. Staff members may find that their own standards of morality conflict with the actual roles they are expected to play. The tendency for the staff to identify with the fetus can create anger and resentment toward the abortion patient and resentment toward the doctor who performs the procedure but leaves the nurse to dispose of the products of conception [116].

One might expect, given increasing cultural approval for selective abortion in the United States, that a more supportive atmosphere for abortion would be perceived by genetic counseling patients, and that this might serve to reduce the incidence and severity of immediate guilt and depression. Depth interviews of genetic counselees, however, reveal that patients must frequently contend with conflicts with obstetrician-gynecologists prior to entering genetic counseling [27] and that their actions are sometimes viewed as morally unacceptable to the hospital staff where the procedures are performed. An objectively clinical stance by the genetic counselor or obstetrician is also interpreted by the patient as a rejection of the subjective qualities of the experience [4].

Coercion by family, friends, or the medical community. Just as social support reduces negative postabortion sequelae, coercion by parents, sexual partners, or physicians is related to greater distress. The evidence is considerable [79, 80, 103, 117–120].

Counseling centers and genetic counselors differ in their orientation toward counselees. The interpretation of risk factors and the perceived severity of disorders is sometimes made by the counselor rather than by the family. Individuals who are low on ego strength or who are more externally oriented will be more susceptible to the influence of the counselor [114].

Counselors also disagree on whether amniocentesis should be performed when the couple is ambivalent about abortion. Some caution that, because of the attendant risks and the desirability of avoiding impulsive abortion decisions, amniocentesis should be performed only if the patient and physician are prepared to interrupt the pregnancy, given a positive diagnosis [121–124]. Others argue that patients should not be compelled to agree to abortion prior to amniocentesis, "for this position works against the voluntarism inherent in present practice" [27, p. 325]. Golbus and his associates noted that even when a decision is made to continue the pregnancy, knowing the results of amniocentesis may enable couples to cope better following the birth of an affected child [78].

Religious or moral opposition. The attitudes of family, friends, and physicians all contribute to ambivalence regarding fetal testing, but of even greater importance are the counselees' own attitudes. Sorenson has suggested that the use of amniocentesis is more dependent upon moral prohibitions than is premarital or preconception genetic counseling, since amniocentesis will imply an acceptance of selective abortion in the event of a positive diagnosis.

Studies of general abortion patients as well as genetic counselees do not agree as to whether Catholics are more likely to experience ambivalence about abortion and, therefore, greater depression thereafter [4, 27, 89, 120]. Although increasing cultural acceptance of selective abortion may reduce this difference, it is probable that some groups, notably Catholics, will be less likely to undergo amniocentesis than others [66]. Just as Catholics have evinced greater autonomy with regard to contraceptive use, however, one might expect religious differentials in the use of amniocentesis to narrow over time. Among couples actively seeking amniocentesis, religious differences in acceptance of abortion are likely to be small.

Previous emotional health and experience with the disorder. Considerable evidence from studies of general abortion patients demonstrates that women who are psychologically healthy respond to abortion more easily than do those with previous psychiatric disorders [93, 117, 125–127].

Couples who have borne children with serious disorders, especially mental disorders, must cope with feelings of depression, cosmic guilt, chronic sorrow, and personality disorders following the birth of the child [27, 85, 128]. It is unknown what proportion of this group will elect prenatal diagnosis and selective abortion in planning future pregnancies. Among women having selective abortion, those who have previously borne affected children need not display higher levels of pre- and postabortion depression than general abortion patients. In fact, evidence suggests that previous experience with the disease facilitates the decision to abort and eases the psychological sequelae of abortion [4, 65].

Previous and subsequent experience with amniocentesis and selective abortion. Although previous experience with illness seems to ease psychological sequelae, multiple failures to obtain a healthy child may, by use of selective abortion, intensify depression. Some genetic counselors have noted clinically that a high proportion of their counselees return for subsequent amniocentesis. However, small-scale studies have shown that couples, especially wives who are "repeaters" with earlier abortions, bear vivid memories of their past failures and often view the present pregnancy as their final attempt. Those who later require another abortion suffer deep depressions and require special counseling and support [4, 27].

Need for Counseling

Some parents view amniocentesis as a miracle, enabling them to exercise some control over the health of future progeny and to bear children without fear. For others, however, who receive positive diagnoses, amniocentesis and selective abortion result in anguish, especially for the unfortunate couples who experience repeated failures in their attempts to produce a healthy child.

At present, earlier amniocentesis, reduction in the stressful waiting period, and abortion prior to quickening are not possible. Although psychological stress cannot currently be reduced through changes in the procedures employed, improvements can be made in counseling and the provision of emotional support during the periods surrounding both amniocentesis and selective abortion [4, 27, 87]. Most parents prefer to exercise moral autonomy in decision-making, relying on their own judgment rather than consulting others [27]. However, a sense of isolation and despair can be experienced by counselees subsequent to positive diagnosis and the decision to abort. Various approaches involving *voluntary* group and individual family counseling should be tried to see which is best in ameliorating these psychological sequelae. Research may indicate the usefulness of a variety of approaches, depending on the characteristics of the couples themselves [129].

FUTURE ALTERNATIVES: SEX PREDETERMINATION

Approval of Sex Predetermination

As discussed previously, counselees at risk for sex-linked disorders can utilize amniocentesis to determine the sex of the fetus during pregnancy. Such counselees appear to experience severe depression and guilt following selective abortion, perhaps because they perceive similar high risks in future pregnancies.

At present the only reliable means of sex determination is that involving amniocentesis. A variety of sex-predetermination methods have been suggested, however, that might enable couples to choose the sex of their children at the time of conception. Some researchers claim that their regimen regarding timing of coitus is relatively effective as a sex-predetermination method [130–131]. Although these natural insemination techniques have gained popularity in the mass media, contradictory findings exist regarding the type of insemination (artificial vs natural) and the human sex ratio at birth [132]. The inability to determine precisely the day of change on basal temperature charts and the inability to predict correctly the time of ovulation, which varies from month to month for each woman, increases the probability of error in coital-timing methods. Morever, the quality of pregnancy achieved with sperm aged in the female reproductive tract is often ignored [141]. There is no conclusive evidence on the influence of douching. Finally, sperm separation techniques are still primitive, and it is difficult to replicate findings, since many uncontrolled variables are associated with the procedures [133]. One method that does appear promising is the Ericsson method, which selects morphologically normal, primarily Y-bearing sperm of high motility. Ericsson's findings have been confirmed in four laboratories, although two others could not duplicate the results [141].

Of course, the development of sex-predetermination techniques will encourage their use not only by counselees but by the general public. However, sex preferences and the acceptability of various techniques would differ within the population, depending primarily upon the method required and whether it facilitated the birth of male or female.

When asked how they would feel about the ability to choose the sex of a child, 46.7% of wives sampled in a national survey indicated that they were against sex predetermination, 38.8% were in favor, and 14.6% were neutral. Women with all boys or all girls were slightly more in favor of such techniques (40.1% and 42.7%, respectively). Those with equal numbers of boys and girls were least in favor (32.7%). Westoff and Rindfuss have cautioned that it is difficult to assess attitudes before the actual introduction of the technology. They concluded, however, that, at a minimum, the data suggested the existence of cultural lag in the acceptability of such technology [134].

The characteristics of the technology, not considered in the 1970 National Fertility Study question, also determine acceptability. James Sorenson of Boston University reported that only 5% of U.S. doctors surveyed would perform amniocentesis for sex-preselection purposes. The relative complexity of amniocentesis; the necessity of having second-trimester abortions, which carry higher risks; and the perceived superficiality of sex determination as a rationale for pregnancy termination are major factors preventing its widespread adoption as a sex-preselection technique [135].

Reports of amniocentesis rarely mention sex determination as the sole indication for these procedures. However, from 1970 to 1973, among 170 amniocenteses performed by the Downstate Medical Center Laboratory (New York), prenatal determination of sex was done in four instances because of "crucial psychological conditions of the parents" [136].

It is also believed that separation methods requiring AI would be unpopular. As noted previously, little research exists on the acceptability of AI, especially with the husband as donor. Among a small sample of college students, who in general approved of sex predetermination, 17% replied that they would not use a method requiring artificial insemination, and an additional 33% were unsure [137].

Finally, acceptability of the technology and the demand for such measures would also differ within the population. It is expected that Catholics would be less in favor of artificial insemination or selective abortion as possible sex-predetermination methods. Yet those most knowledgeable about and accepting of sex-predetermination — the better-educated, those with egalitarian sex-role ideologies, Protestants, and those with no religious denomination — might also demonstrate less preference for male first-borns and lower demand for the technology [138]. On the other hand, since the better-educated are more likely to plan the number and timing of their births, sex-predetermination techniques might be in heavy demand to enable couples to plan a two-child family and ensure sex balance.

Perceived Social and Psychological Effects of Sex Predetermination

Despite the fact that no sex-preselection method is likely to be fully effective and widely used, researchers have attempted to forecast the effect of sex predetermination as if such methods were available and acceptable. Forecasts differ, some claiming that sex predetermination would result in smaller families, more males than females, a higher sex ratio, and dramatic social change [137]. Others claim that the effects would be short-lived and transitory; a surplus of males would encourage a reevaluation and rise in the status of women, a surplus of female births, and a corresponding rebalance in the sex ratio [134, 138, 139].

In areas where the one-child family is more prevalent (Scandinavia, Eastern Europe), the introduction of such technology might have more noticeable effects on sex ratios, marriage rates, and future fertility. Sex-control technology might also have a more radical impact on the sex ratios of developing nations, where there is greater cultural emphasis on having sons. Given the historical preference for male children, it is assumed that any method ensuring the production of sons would be more popular than one selecting for females.

Examining the situation from a psychosocial perspective, Pohlman has noted the psychological benefits of sex predetermination in terms of the parents' and child's adjustment. He suggested that the disappointment that some parents feel when a child is the "wrong" sex, and the negative effects such feelings can have on the child could be greatly alleviated. He further concluded, as have others, that in a culture that prefers sex balance, the possibility of sex predetermination could reduce birth rates somewhat, since it would make it unnecessary to continue reproducing in the hope of having a child of the desired sex [140]. It is possible, of course, that such predetermination techniques might encourage fertility for some couples because they would be assured of the results beforehand. Given current expectations of a two-child family among most Americans, however, this alternative seems unlikely.

Finally, just as couples undergoing amniocentesis noted that foreknowledge of the sex and health of the fetus served to strengthen the parent–child bond [65], knowing the sex of the fetus through sex predetermination may reinforce emotional attachment to the child, before and after birth, thereby benefiting both parents and children.

CONCLUSION

It seems unfortunate that much of the research in genetic counseling has focused on aspects of the disorders themselves, such as risk factors and severity of disease, in attempting to isolate the factors that will maximize information retention and "responsible childbearing." In contrast, comparatively little is known about the factors influencing parental choice of the alternatives of sterilization, artificial insemination, prenatal diagnosis, and selective abortion, or the potential acceptability of various sex-predetermination techniques. Even less is known about the psychological sequelae of these procedures, aside from the pioneering work on amniocentesis done by Blumberg, Fletcher, and Golbus. Some inferences can be drawn based on investigations of larger U.S. samples, but, clearly, research on counselees themselves is required because of the unique character of their situation.

This chapter has provided information on the general acceptance and prevalence of four modes of family planning, the characteristics of those most likely to elect these alternatives, the situations that may contraindicate choice of a procedure, the general psychological or social sequelae that can be anticipated following a procedure, and the factors that may serve to intensify or prolong negative reactions. More sophisticated research is required on these issues. The forthcoming results would not only facilitate the use of family planning among counselees, but also would help to ensure that they emerge from the counseling situation more emotionally intact.

ACKNOWLEDGMENTS

I would like to express my appreciation to many individuals who provided references and reprints of otherwise inaccessible materials: Rhonda Aizenberg, my research assistant, Jean van der Tak of the Population Reference Bureau, and the New York Committee to Combat Huntington Disease. Special thanks are also extended to William Arney of Dartmouth College for the tabulation and provision of unpublished NORC data on abortion attitudes, and to Christopher Tietze of the Population Council for his review of the manuscript.

ANNOTATED REFERENCES

1. US Commission on Population Growth and the American Future: "Demographic and Social Aspects of Poulation Growth. Vol I of Commission Research Reports," Westoff CF, Parke R Jr (Eds). (Stock No. 5258-00005). Washington, DC: US Government Printing Office, 1972.
One volume in a series of research reports on demographic and social aspects of US population growth presented to the Commission by independent scholars and research organizations. Chapters of special interest to genetic counselors focus on wanted and unwanted fertility in the US, demographic and social aspects of contraceptive sterilization, attitudes toward abortion, and genetic implications of population policies.

2. Moore-Čavar EC: "International Inventory of Information on Induced Abortion." New York: Columbia University, International Institute for the Study of Human Reproduction, 1974.
An excellent compendium of recent literature on religious, ethical, legal, medical, psychological, and demographic aspects of abortion, as well as acceptability, incidence, and prevalence of abortion. Includes tables synthesizing data from national and foreign sources.

3. Fawcett JT (ed): "Psychological Perspectives on Population." New York: Basic Books, 1973.
A comprehensive review of topics in the field of population psychology. Chapters of particular interest cover psychological studies in abortion, factors in the acceptance and use of oral contraceptives, psychological reactions to sterilization, and reviews of the literature pertaining to motivations for childbearing, family structure and fertility control, and the effects of family size on parents and children.

4. Blumberg BD: Psychic sequelae of selective abortion. (MD Thesis, Yale University, New Haven, Conn, 1974).
Although this volume is not easily accessible, it is one of the few studies conducted on the psychological sequelae of selective abortion among a sample of 13 couples who underwent amniocentesis and abortion. Material is presented in case history form, followed by a discussion of the factors that intensify depression. Also included is a comprehensive review of the general literature on psychological sequelae of abortion.

5. Hilton B, Callahan D, Harris M, Condliffe P, Berkley B (eds): "Ethical Issues in Human Genetics: Genetic Counseling and the Use of Genetic Knowledge." New York: Plenum Press, 1973.
Proceedings of the Fogarty International Symposium No. 13. Four studies of particular relevance include a discussion on screening (Murray), privacy (Lubs), sociological and psychological factors in applied human genetics (Sorenson), and findings from J. Fletcher's study of decision-making among 25 couples who underwent amniocentesis, three of whom subsequently elected abortion.

6. Presser HB, Bumpass LL: Demographic and social aspects of contraceptive sterilization in the United States: 1965–1970. In Westoff CF, Parke Jr R (Eds): US Commission on Population Growth and the American Future. "Demographic and Social Aspects of Population Growth. Vol. I of Commission Research Reports." (Stock No. 5258-00005). Washington, DC: US Government Printing Office, 1972, pp 505–568.
7. Bumpass LL, Presser HB: The increasing acceptance of sterilization and abortion. In Westoff CF (Ed): "Toward the End of Growth: Population in America." Englewood Cliffs, NJ: Prentice-Hall, 1973, pp 33–46.
8. Darity WA, Turner CB: Research findings related to sterilization: Attitudes of black Americans. Presented at the 51st annual meeting of the American Orthopsychiatric Association, San Francisco, April 8–12, 1974. (Amherst, University of Massachusetts, Department of Public Health. Mimeo.)
9. Westoff CF, Bumpass LL: The revolution in birth control practices of U.S. Roman Catholics. Science 179:41, 1973.
10. Westoff CF: Trends in contraceptive practice: 1965–1973. Fam Plann Perspect 8:54, 1976.
11. Rodgers DA, Ziegler FJ: Psychological reactions to surgical contraception. In Fawcett JT (Ed): "Psychological Perspectives on Population." New York: Basic Books, 1973, pp 306–326.
12. Schwyhart WR, Kutner SJ: A reanalysis of female reactions to contraceptive sterilization. J Nerv Ment Dis 156:354, 1973.
13. Westoff LA: Sterilization. New York Times Magazine, September 29, 1974, p 31.
14. Wolfers H: Psychological aspects of vasectomy. Br Med J 4:297, 1970.
15. Wortman J: Vasectomy – what are the problems? Population Reports (George Washington University Medical School) Series D, No 2:25, 1975.
16. Association for Voluntary Sterilization, Inc.: AVS News, December 1975, p. 1.
17. Simon Population Trust: "Vasectomy: Follow-up of a Thousand Cases." Cambridge, England: Simon Population Trust, 1969.
18. Freund M, Davis JE: A follow-up study of the effects of vasectomy on sexual behavior. J Sex Res 9:241, 1973.
19. Savage PM: Vasectomy and psychosexual damage. Health Serv Res 89:803, 1972.
20. Ferber AS, Tietze C, Lewit S: Men with vasectomies: A study of medical, sexual, and psychosocial changes. Psychosom Med 29:354, 1967.
21. Janke LD, Wiest WM: Psychosocial and medical effects of vasectomy in a sample of health plan subscribers. Psychiatry Med (In press).
22. Ekblad M: The prognosis after sterilization on social-psychiatric grounds: A follow-up study of 225 women. Acta Psychiatr Scand 37 (Suppl. 161): 32, 1961.
23. Jensen F, Lester J: Ten years of tubal sterilization by the Madlener method. Acta Obstet Gynecol Scand 36:324, 1957.
24. Koya Y, Muramatsu M, Agata S, Suzuki N: A survey of health and demographic aspects of reported female sterilizations in four health center of Shizuoka Prefecture, Japan. Milbank Mem Fund Q 33:369, 1955.
25. Carter CO: Comments on genetic counseling. In Crow JF, Neel JV (Eds): "Proceedings of the Third International Congress of Human Genetics." Baltimore: Johns Hopkins Press, 1966, pp 97–100.
26. Emery AEH, Watt MS, Clack ER: The effects of genetic counseling in Duchenne muscular dystrophy. Clin Genet 3:147, 1972.
27. Fletcher J: Parents in genetic counseling: The moral shape of decision-making. In Hilton B, Callahan D, Harris M, Condliffe P, Berkley B (Eds): "Ethical Issues in Human Genetics: Genetic Counseling and the Use of Genetic Knowledge." New York: Plenum Press, 1973, pp 301–327.

28. Leonard CO, Chase GA, Childs B: Genetic counseling: A consumers' view. N Engl J Med 287:433, 1972.
29. McCrae WM, Cull AM, Burton L, Dodge J: Cystic fibrosis: Parents' response to the genetic basis of the disease. Lancet 2:141, 1973.
30. Kaback MM: Discussion comment. In Hilton B, Callahan D, Harris M, Condliffe P, Berkley B (Eds): "Ethical Issues in Human Genetics: Genetic Counseling and the Use of Genetic Knowledge." New York: Plenum Press, 1973, pp 339–340.
31. Baudry F, Herzig N, Wiener A: Assessment of patients seeking tubal sterilization on psychosocial grounds. Obstet Gynecol 38:411, 1971.
32. Langer G, Lemberg E, Sharf M: Artificial insemination: A study of 156 successful cases. Int J Fertil 14:232, 1969.
33. Guttmacher AF: Role of artificial insemination in treatment of sterility. Obstet Gynecol Surv 15:767, 1960.
34. Finegold WJ: Artificial Insemination. Springfield, Ill, Charles C Thomas, 1964.
35. Greenberg JH: Social variables in acceptance or rejection of artificial insemination. Am Sociol Rev 16:86, 1951.
36. Vernon GM, Boadway JA: Attitudes toward artificial insemination and some variables associated therewith. Marriage and Family Living 21:43, 1959.
37. Francoeur RT: "Utopian Motherhood." Garden City, NY: Doubleday, 1970.
38. Ferris EJ, Garrison M: Emotional impacts of successful donor insemination. Obstet Gynecol 3:19, 1954.
39. Epstein CJ: Medical genetics: Recent advances with legal implications. Hastings Law J 21:35, 1969.
40. Knight B: Legal Aspects of Medical Practice. London, Churchill Livingstone, 1972.
41. Peyer HS: Untoward effects of artificial insemination. NY State J Med 65:1876, 1965.
42. Pollok M: Sex and its problems. 8. Artificial insemination. Practitioner 199:244, 1967.
43. Gerstel G: A psychoanalytic view of artificial donor insemination. Am J Psychother. 17:64, 1963.
44. Heiman M, Kleegman S: Insemination: A psychoanalytic and infertility study. Fertil Steril 17:117, 1966.
45. Levie LH: An inquiry into the psychological effects on parents of artificial insemination with donor semen. Eugen Rev 59:97, 1967.
46. Kleegman SJ: Therapeutic donor insemination. Conn Med 31:705, 1967.
47. Rubin B: Psychological aspects of human artificial insemination. Arch Gen Psychiatry 13:121, 1965.
48. Watters WW, Sousa-Poza J: Psychiatric aspects of artificial insemination (donor). Can Med Assoc J 95:106, 1966.
49. Sorenson JR: Some social and psychologic issues in genetic screening, In Bergsma D (Ed): "Ethical, Social and Legal Dimensions of Screening for Human Genetic Disease." Miami: Symposia Specialists for National Foundation—March of Dimes, BD:OAS X(6): 165–184, 1974.
50. Sorenson JR: "Social Aspects of Applied Human Genetics." (Social Science Frontier Paper). New York: Russell Sage Foundation, 1971.
51. Reynolds B, Puck MH, Robinson A: Genetic counseling: An appraisal. Clin Genet 5:177, 1974.
52. Carter CO, Roberts JAF, Evans KA, Buck AR: Genetic clinic: A follow-up. Lancet 1: 281, 1971.
53. Motulsky A: The significance of genetic disease. In Hilton B, Callahan D, Harris M, Condliffe P, Berkley B (Eds): "Ethical Issues in Human Genetics: Genetic Counseling and the Use of Genetic Knowledge." New York: Plenum Press, 1973, p 65.
54. Sorenson JR: Counselors: A self-portrait. Genetic Counseling 1:29, 1973.

55. Hsia YE: Strategies for the appraisal of genetic counseling. In Lubs HA, de la Cruz F (Eds): "Genetic Counseling." New York: Raven Press, 1967.

56. Kindregan CP: "Abortion, the Law, and Defective Children: A Legal–Medical Study." (Corpus Papers 5). Washington, DC: Corpus Books, 1969.

57. National Academy of Sciences: "Legalized Abortion and the Public Health." (Report of a Study by a Committee of the Institute of Medicine). Washington, DC: National Academy of Sciences, 1975.

58. Arney WR , Trescher WH: Trends in attitudes toward abortion, 1972–1975. Fam Plann Perspect 8:117, 1976.

59. Milunsky A: "The Prenatal Diagnosis of Hereditary Disorders." Springfield, Ill: Charles C Thomas, 1973.

60. Center for Disease Control: "Abortion Surveillance Report – Legal Abortions, United States, Annual Summary, 1971." (DHEW Publication No. [HSM] 73-8205). Atlanta: US Center for Disease Control, 1972.

61. Center for Disease Control: "Abortion Surveillance, Annual Summary 1972." (DHEW Publication No. [CDC] 74-8205). Atlanta: US Center for Disease Control, 1974.

62. MacGillivray I, Dennis KJ: Gynaecological aspects. In Horobin G (Ed): "Experience with Abortion: A Case Study of North-East Scotland." Cambridge: Cambridge University Press, 1973, pp 47–95.

63. Ottoson J-O: Legal abortion in Sweden: Thirty years' experience. J Biosoc Sci 3:173, 1971.

64. Jones EF, Westoff CF: Attitudes toward abortion in the United States in 1970 and the trends since 1965. In Westoff CF, Parker Jr R (Eds): US Commission on Population Growth and the American Future. "Demographic and Social Aspects of Population Growth. Vol. I of Comission Research Reports." (Stock No. 5258-00005). Washington, DC: US Government Printing Office, 1972, pp 569–578.

65. Fletcher J: The brink: The parent-child bond in the genetic revolution. Theological Studies 33:457, 1972.

66. Sorenson JR: Sociological and psychological factors in applied human genetics. In Hilton B, Callahan D, Harris M, Condliffe P, Berkley B (Eds): "Genetic Counseling and the Use of Genetic Knowledge." New York: Plenum Press, 1973, pp 283–300.

67. Sorenson JR: The rationalizing of reproduction and parenthood: Some societal develkopments. Presented at Conference on Decision-Making and the Defective Newborn, Skytop, Penn., May 1975, sponsored by New York University and the Foundation for Child Development, New York (proceedings to be published).

68. Peyton FW, Starry AR, Leidy TR: Women's attitudes concerning abortion. Obstet Gynecol 34:182, 1969.

69. Schneiderman LJ, Prichard L, Fuller S, Atkinson L: Birth control, sterilization and abortion. West J Med 120:174, 1974.

70. Westoff CF, Moore EC, Ryder NB: The structure of attitudes toward abortion. Milbank Mem Fund Q 47 (No. 1, Part 1): 11, 1969.

71. Ryder NB, Westoff CF: "Reproduction in the United States, 1965." Princeton: Princeton University Press, 1971. (1965 National Fertility Study).

72. Furstenberg FF Jr: Attitudes toward abortion among young blacks. Stud Fam Plann 3:66, 1972.

73. Center for Disease Control: "Abortion Surveillance, Annual Summary 1974" DHEW Publication No. [CDC] 76-8276). Atlanta, US Center for Disease Control, 1976.

74. Carter CO, Evans K, Norman A: Cystic fibrosis: Genetic counseling follow-up. In Mangos JA, Talamo RC (Eds): "Fundamental Problems of Cystic Fibrosis and Related Disease." New York: Intercontinental, 1973, pp 99–102.

75. Hsia YE, Silverberg RL: Response to genetic counseling: A follow-up survey. Pediatr Res 7:290 (Abstr) 1973.
76. Kaback MM, Becker MH, Ruth MV: Sociologic studies in human genetics: I. Compliance factors in a voluntary heterozygote screening program. In Bergsma D (Ed): "Ethical, Social and Legal Dimensions of Screening for Human Genetic Disease." Miami: Symposia Specialists for The National Foundation—March of Dimes, BD:OAS X(6): 145–163, 1974.
77. Chase GA: The background of couples who request genetic counselling. In Porter IH, Skalko RG (Eds): "Heredity and Society: Proceedings of a Symposium Sponsored by the Birth Defects Institute." New York: Academic Press, 1973, pp 143–155.
78. Golbus MS, Conte FA, Schneider EL, Epstein CJ: Intrauterine diagnosis of genetic defects: Results, problems, and follow-up of one hundred cases in a prenatal genetic detection center. Am J Obstet Gynecol 118:897, 1974.
79. Peck A, Marcus H: Psychiatric sequelae of therapeutic interruption of pregnancy. J Nerv Ment Dis 143:417, 1966.
80. Niswander KR, Patterson RJ: Psychologic reaction to therapeutic abortion. I. Subjective patient response. Obstet Gynecol 29:702, 1967.
81. McCoy DR: The emotional reaction of women to therapeutic abortion and sterilization. J Obstet Gynecol Brit Comm 75:1054, 1968
82. Fletcher J: Discussion comment. In Hilton B, Callahan D, Harris M, Condliffe P, Berkley B (Eds): "Ethical Issues in Human Genetics: Genetic Counseling and the Use of Genetic Knowledge." New York: Plenum Press, 1973, p 339.
83. Cohen P: The impact of the handicapped child on the family. Social Casework 43:137, 1962.
84. Langsley DG: Psychology of a doomed family. Am J Psychother 15:531, 1961.
85. Olshansky S: Chronic sorrow: A response to having a mentally defective child. Social Casework 43:190, 1962.
86. Callahan D: "Abortion: Law, Choice, and Morality." New York: Macmillan Co., 1970.
87. Illsley R, Hall MH: Psycho-social aspects of abortion: A review of issues and needed research. Presented at the Conference on Psychosocial Aspects of Induced Abortion, Prague, August 1973, Aberdeen, Scotland, MRC Medical Sociology Unit. Mimeo.
88. Simon NM, Senturia AG: Psychiatric sequelae of abortion, review of the literature, 1935–1964. Arch Gen Psychiatry 15:378, 1966.
89. Osofsky JD, Osofsky HJ: The psychological reaction of patients to legalized abortion. Am J Orthopsychiatry 42:48, 1972.
90. Osofsky HJ, Osofsky JD (Eds): "The Abortion Experience: Psychological and Medical Impact." Hagerstown, MD: Harper & Row, 1973.
91. Walter GS: Psychologic and emotional consequences of elective abortion: A review. Obstet Gynecol 36:482, 1970.
92. Malmfors K: Den abortsökande kvinnans problem (Problems of the woman seeking abortion). Svenska Läkartidn 48:2445, 1951.
93. Simon NM, Senturia AG, Rothman D: Psychiatric illness following therapeutic abortion. Am J Psychiatry 124:59, 1967.
94. McCance C, Olley PC, Edward V: Long-term psychiatric follow-up. In Horobin G (Ed): "Experience with Abortion: A Case Study of North-East Scotland." Cambridge: Cambridge University Press, 1973, pp 245–300.
95. Blumberg B, Golbus M: Psychological sequelae of abortion performed for a genetic indication. Am J Hum Genet 26:15a (Abstr) 1974.
96. Juberg R: Heredity counseling. Nurses Outlook 14:28, 1966.

97. Reed SC: Counseling in human genetics, Part III. Dight Institute, Bull No. 8. Minneapolis, University of Minnesota Press, 1953.
98. Feldman JJ: "The Dissemination of Health Information." Chicago: Aldine, 1966.
99. Westoff CF, Ryder NB: Recent trends in attitudes toward fertility control and the practice of contraception in the United States. In Behrman SJ, Corsa Jr L, Freedman R (Eds): "Fertility and Family Planning: A World View." Ann Arbor: University of Michigan Press, 1969, pp 388–412.
100. Mechanic D: "Medical Sociology: A Selective View." New York: Free Press, 1968.
101. Kretzchmar RM, Norris AS: Psychiatric implications of therapeutic abortion. Am J Obstet Gynecol 198:368, 1967.
102. Pare CMB, Raven H: Follow-up of patients referred for termination of pregnancy. Lancet 1:635, 1970.
103. Friedman CM, Greenspan R, Mittleman F: The decision-making process and the outcome of therapeutic abortion. Am J Psychiatry 131:1332, 1974.
104. Cullberg J: Mental reactions of women to perinatal death. In Morris N (Ed): "Psychosomatic Medicine in Obstetrics and Gynaecology: Third International Congress, London, 1971." Basel: S Karger, 1972, pp 326–329.
105. Kennell JH, Slyter H, Klaus MH: The mourning response of parents to the death of a newborn infant. N Engl J Med 283:344, 1970.
106. Walker JH, Thomas M, Russell IT: Spina bifida – and the parents. Dev Med Child Neurol 13:462, 1971.
107. Wilson D: Psychiatric implications in abortions. Va Med Mon 79:448, 1952.
108. Kaltreider NB: Psychological factors in mid-trimester abortion. Psychiatry Med 4:129, 1973.
109. Marder L: Psychiatric experience with a liberalized therapeutic abortion law. Am J Psychiatry 126:1230, 1970.
110. Bibring G, Dwyer TF, Huntington DS, Valenstein AF: A study of the psychological processes of pregnancy and of the earliest mother–child relationship. "Psychoanalytic Study of the Child." Vol 16. New York: International Universities Press, 1961, pp 9–72.
111. Bracken M, Kasl SV: Delay in seeking induced abortion: A review and theoretical analysis. Am J Obstet Gynecol 121:1008, 1975.
112. Szontágh FE: Psychic motives in the decision of women requesting induced legal abortion. "In Psychosomatic Medicine in Obstetrics and Gynaecology: Third International Congress, London, 1971." Basel: S Karger, 1972, pp 531–533.
113. Senay EC, Wexler S: Fantasies about the fetus in wanted and unwanted pregnancies. J Youth Adolescence 1:333, 1972.
114. Bracken MB, Hachamovitch M, Grossman G: The decision to abort and psychological sequelae. J Nerv Ment Dis 158:154, 1974.
115. Harper MW, Marcom BR, Wall VD: Abortion: Do attitudes of nursing personnel affect the patient's perception of care? Nurs Res 21:327, 1972.
116. Tourkow LP, Lidz RW, Marder L: Psychiatric considerations in fertility inhibition. In Hafez ESE, Evans TN (Eds): "Human Reproduction: Conception and Contraception." Hagerstown, MD: Harper & Row, 1973, pp 615–627.
117. Ekblad M: Induced abortion on psychiatric grounds: A follow-up study of 479 women. Acta Psychiatr Neurol Scand (Suppl. 99–102):3, 1955.
118. Ford CV, Atkinson RM, Bragonier JR: Therapeutic abortion: Who needs a psychiatrist? Obstet Gynecol 38:206, 1971.
119. Patt SL, Rappaport RG, Barglow P: Follow-up of therapeutic abortion. Arch Gen Psychiatry 20:408, 1969.

120. Smith EM: A follow-up study of women who request abortion. Am J Orthopsychiatry 43:574, 1973.

121. Fuchs F: Amniocentesis: Techniques and complications. In Harris M (Ed): "Early Diagnosis of Human Genetic Defects: Scientific and Ethical Considerations." (HEW Publication No. [NIH] 72–25). Washington, DC: US Government Printing Office, 1971, pp 11–16.

122. Littlefield JW: The pregnancy at risk for a genetic disorder. N Engl J Med 282:627, 1970.

123. Macintyre MN: Counseling in cases involving antenatal diagnosis. In Dorfman A (Ed): "Antenatal Diagnosis: Conference on Antenatal Diagnosis, University of Chicago, 1970." Chicago: University of Chicago Press, 1972, pp 63–67.

124. Nadler H: Risks in amniocentesis. in Harris M (Ed): "Early Diagnosis of Human Genetic Defects: Scientific and Ethical Considerations." (HEW Publication No. [NIH] 72-25). Washington, DC, US Government Printing Office, 1971, pp 129–137.

125. Ford CV, Castlelnuovo-Tedesco P, Long KD: Abortion: Is it a therapeutic procedure in psychiatry? JAMA 218:1173, 1971.

126. Jacobs D, Garcia C-R, Rickels K, Preucel RW: A prospective study on the psychological effects of therapeutic abortion. Compr Psychiatry 15:423, 1974.

127. Meyerowitz S, Satloff A, Romano J: Induced abortion for psychiatric indication. Am J Psychiatry 127:1153, 1971.

128. Cummings ST, Bayley HC, Rie HE: Effects of the child's deficiency on the mother: A study of mothers of mentally retarded, chronically ill and neurotic children. Am J Orthopsychiatry 36:595, 1966.

129. Bracken MB, Grossman G, Hachamovitch M, Sussman D, Schrieir D: Abortion counseling: An experimental study of three techniques. Am J Obstet Gynecol 117:10, 1973.

130. Shettles LB: Factors influencing sex ratios. Int J Gynecol Obstet 8:643, 1970.

131. Séguy B: Les méthodes de sélection naturelle et voluntaire des sexes (Methods of natural and voluntary selection of the sexes). J Gyne Obste Biol Reprod 4:145, 1975.

132. Guerrero R: Type and time of insemination within the menstrual cycle and the human sex ratio at birth. Stud Fam Plann 6:367, 1975.

133. Rinehart W: Sex preselection–not yet practical. "Population Reports" (George Washington Univ Medical School) Series I, No 2:21, 1975.

134. Westoff CF, Rindfuss RR: Sex preselection in the United States: Some implications. Science 184:633, 1974. (1970 National Fertility Study).

135. Etzioni A: Selecting the sex of one's children [Letter to the Editor]. Lancet 1:932, 1974.

136. Valenti C, Lungarotti MS: Responsibilities, limitations and prospects in genetic counseling. In Motulsky A, Ebling FJG (Eds): "Abstracts of Papers, Fourth International Conference on Birth Defects, Vienna, 1973." (International Congress Series No. 297). Amsterdam: Excerpta Medica, 1973, p 77.

137. Etzioni A: Sex control, science, and society. Science 161:1107, 1968.

138. Largey G: Sex control, sex preferences, and the future of the family. Soc Biol 19:379, 1972.

139. Walter SD: The transitional effect on the sex ratio at birth of a sex predetermination program. Soc Biol 21:340, 1974.

140. Pohlman E: Some effects of being able to control sex of offspring. Eugen Q 14:274, 1967.

141. Glass RH: Sex preselection: Is it a possibility? Contemp Obstet Gynecol 9:99, 1977.

142. Grimes DA, Schulz KF, Cates W Jr, Tyler CW Jr: Midtrimester abortion by intra-amniotic prostaglandin $F_2\alpha$: Safer than saline? Obstet Gynecol 49:612, 1977.

10

Decision-Making and Reproductive Choice

John Pearn, MD, PhD

INTRODUCTION

All decisions are based on complex value systems which estimate the consequences of alternative actions, each with its own set of risks and uncertainties.
In genetic counseling one helps parents, patients and clients to reach decisions by
the provision of information, and by support, discussion, and help with interpretation.

In common with decision making in general, decisions concerning future children require certain core information which includes factual data on alternative
options, outcomes, and risk. Decisions are subject to time restraints and must be
made on the basis of information available to the decision-maker at the time he
has to make his decision.

In the genetic context, decisions confronting parents are almost without exception decisions that have to be made under the threat of some potentially unfortunate outcome. That is, decisions are made under the shadow of varying
degrees of risk and do not simply entail the choosing of one of several relatively
neutral alternative paths.

An understanding of the dynamics of decision-making processes has evolved to
a point of considerable sophistication in the realms of logic, statistics, and psychology [1, 2]. Although the direct application of this knowledge to clinical situations
is in its infancy, an understanding of the influences inherent in, and bearing on
decision making is of great help in interpreting what happens in genetic counseling settings.

Doctors and counselors are constantly approached by individuals or parents
who are confronted with a genetic uncertainty of the type "Should I get married?,"
or "Should we have further children? " Such questions are inescapable if responsible individuals have knowledge of possible genetic disorders or hereditary risks
to their future children.

When individuals or parents become aware of real or imagined genetic implications within their family kindreds, such decision-requiring questions follow automatically. In practice, the most common clinical situations occur when parents discover that a child has a genetically determined condition – either obvious at birth or one that has become apparent subsequently during infancy or childhood – or alternatively when they themselves may have a disease believed to have genetic implications.

In such situations individuals or parents are forced to make one of three mutually exclusive decisions:

a) We shall not have further children.
b) We shall have further children.
c) We shall defer the decision.

In the parlance of students of decision making, these three possible decisions constitute all possible courses of action. Another apparent decision is to try for a future pregnancy and, if prenatal diagnosis reveals an affected fetus, to accept therapeutic abortion. In reality, this decision is a special case of 1) "We shall not have further children – unless these can be shown to be unaffected."

DELIBERATION AND VACILLATION

The first two of these possible decisions are definite and polar and are made by many parents without the benefit of formal genetic counsel. Many of these are made instinctually or impulsively, and may change with the passage of time.

The third option is, of course, a decision in itself – a decision to do nothing at the moment, or to defer a decision – is in fact a decision in itself [3].

This third possible decision occupies an important practical place in clinical experience for several reasons. First, parents who have reached this decision comprise the majority of those seeking counsel. One view of the fundamental role of genetic counseling (but not the only one) is to help couples reach a definitive polar decision about future reproduction. If counseling is to be realistic and effective, therefore, it might be hoped that a majority of the "deferred decision" parents would change, after counseling, to one of the two polar decisions.

Second, if parents do change their minds – say, from decision a) to decision b) – they usually pass through the intermediate decision stage in the process. It is this change from the decision to defer a choice that logically demands informed opinion. Therefore, it is likely that parents who have elected to defer the decision will be the ones to seek formal genetic advice.

Third, although the deferment of a polar decision is a decision in itself, it has escapist overtones, and it is known that this type of avoidance of a final decision may lead to conflict and anxiety [4].

Common experience and objective psychological testing [5, 6] reveal striking individual differences in both style and tempo of decision making behavior. Some people are more cautious or reflective; others are more impulsive. Although there is no specific data for decisions made in the genetic context, other evidence suggests that the time taken to reach decisions mirrors the personality trait of reflectivity; also, that the amount of time taken to reach a choice is not necessarily linked to the quality or optimality of the decision reached [7]. In the experimental situation at least, and probably in genetic counseling as well, the posession of facts concerning all possible outcomes of a gamble greatly reduces the period of vacillation and uncertainty before a definitive decision is made [8].

Sub-Themes of the Decision-Making Process

Decision-making under conditions of risk entails a consideration of two quite distinct and independent themes [9]. These are 1) The desirability of the outcome to the individual or individuals concerned, and 2) The perceived risk of a feature result (in this case, a Genetic Defect) eventuating.

In some instances these two themes may be mutually antagonistic, as occurs when a child is desperately desired but the perceived risks are very high. In other instances the desire for children may be low, but so may be the perceived risk. Each of these two influences can be thought of as having a hypothetical quantitative value – a "utility" score expressing the degree of desire for children, and a "risk" index comprising the perceived mathematical odds. As each of these can vary across a hypothetical continuum, it can be seen that the interplay between the two can vary along a broad spectrum.

It is the logical resolution of these two themes that forms the dynamics of decision-making in the context of human clinical genetics. This process is almost always subconscious on the part of parents or client; nevertheless, the same encompassing principle is that optimality of choice follows from the acceptance, albeit subconsciously, of an indifference point on the utility–risk continuum; if this point is exceeded, the parents will try for future children. If it is not reached, any future genetic gamble will not be accepted.

Decision-making is an everyday part of life, but few decisions assume greater dimensions for a couple than the decision to have children in the face of a genetic threat.

The process inherent in deciding whether to try for future children has a number of characteristic features not necessarily encountered in other life situations.

Compulsion. From the moment a genetic threat is known, the need for a decision is inescapable. There is no alternative to making a decision, even if the decision is to defer making a decision. The compulsory nature of the required decision often explains the stress, anxiety and apparent irrationality seen in members of such families.

Reality. For most patients, there is no doubt that the genetic threat is a real one – and for many, all too real, in spite of the long odds in many cases. The existence of a living proband within the kindred ensures that the topic is not of simply theoretical moment: if several members of a kindred are affected by a significant genetic condition, the perceived reality of the threat may be quite magnified, compared with an otherwise disinterested view.

On the other hand, in genetic screening for carriers of an inherited condition, or antenatal testing of older mothers for chromosomic abnormalities in the fetus, lack of familiarity with the condition in question may distort reality — for better or for worse.

Anticipation. Central to the willingness to commit oneself to a decision is the capacity to anticipate all the possible consequences. For parents who have already had an affected child, this may be relatively easy. Possible dangers here are wide differences in clinical expressivity in both autosomal dominant and polygenically determined conditions. Here it is essential to point out that if a genetic gamble is accepted, a subsequently affected child may be more — or less — severely affected than the propositus.

Responsibility. Most parents confronted with a genetic decision feel the responsibility very heavily. The result cannot be changed, and responsibility cannot be shifted to even the smallest degree. The genetic decision is of an unusual type in modern society, in that parents are both makers of the choice and acceptors of the consequences. From time to time, contemporary influences within society seek to minimize the options open to parents confronted with genetic decisions; it is essential from the point of view of medical ethics and from that of the individual dignity of man that such influences be resisted.

PROCREATIVE DRIVE

Decisions concerning the possibility of having future children depend in large part on the *intensity* of the desire for them. The intensity of this procreative drive can be thought of as the "utility" score mentioned above.

The desire for children, and in particular, for healthy children, is a basic human characteristic that is predetermined by cultural and personal influences [10]. This procreative drive is fixed in early childhood, and is determined by both individual experience in one's own family, and by more widespread cultural influences of the society in which that individual and family live. Being culturally determined, the intensity of the desire to have a child (or many children) will vary with time and place, depending on the socio-environmental norm of the individual seeking counsel. Racial and religious influences may also be important. In some societies, and in some families, there is a stigma attached to the state of childlessness; this in turn intensifies the "utility" value of having children and so modifies the dynamics of decision-making.

In the human species, the very strong motivation to have children may not be merely a true "basic drive" explicable by neurophysiological mechanisms.

It is probably a culturally determined phenomenon, controlled by a complex set of external environmental stimuli. Such factors producing the motivation to have children act from earliest childhood, and produce this motivational state long before any genetic risk can be appreciated. Most modern societies engender, as part of their culture, family goals which augment this motivation; in many instances the goal being a two-child family or larger.

The whole question of weighing a genetic gamble depends not only on the intensity of the procreative drive but also on a realistic assessment of alternatives. Adoption, artificial insemination, and prenatal diagnosis (with subsequent therapeutic abortion if appropriate) may be acceptable alternatives for some parents. In these instances, the desire for normal children may be satisfied with a lesser degree of risk. Of course, from the point of view of a given couple, the "utility value" of this substitute may be zero; or it may be so much less than that of the natural situation that the utility–risk resultant fails to exceed the neutral reference point, and the decision is made not to have children. Parents vary widely in such attitudes. To many, whether a future child in their family is biologically their own, or whether he is adopted is inconsequential. In this type of instance the "utility value" of the anticipated adopted child may be the same or almost the same as that of a natural biological child, and the risk of the future genetic condition infinitely less.

SUBJECTIVE INTERPRETATION OF ODDS

For the great majority of clients who seek genetic counsel, provided a diagnosis can be made, a more-or-less quantifiable mathematical risk can be calculated from the laws of genetic inheritance; this must be considered together with an assessment of penetrance and of the carrier state in appropriate cases.

The compilation of the mathematical risk may be simple, as in the case of cystic fibrosis, or it may require sophisticated mathematics such as the use of Bayesian techniques in complicated X-linked pedigrees. Even in instances in which there is uncertainty about the type of inheritance involved, it is usually possible to give some mathematical expression to the order of risk—that is to express the risk as odds, or as a percentage.

Although risk, odds, or probability can be expressed in absolute mathematical terms, this in itself has little relevance in the clinical context. It is universal experience that the same objective odds mean different things to different people and may mean different things to the same person at different times. It is clear from both everyday and clinical observation that people differ widely in their attitudes to word risk. What to one person is a high risk, is a low or acceptable risk to another.

It is this individual personal "feeling" about a fixed mathematical risk that is the significant factor in situations involving a genetic threat. It is this feeling that determines how parents or individuals will act. The counselor's own personal feeling about the odds he offers may not (and often does not) bear resemblance to his client's feeling, although each may be talking in the identical fixed mathematical terms. This phenomeneon has been called the "subjective interpretation of odds" [11]. The theme was formally recognized in 1926 by the logician and mathematician, Frank Ramsey, in his essay on "Truth and Probability." He spoke specifically about "degrees of belief" [12].

Acknowledgment of this phenomenon leads to two inescapable sequelae. First, it becomes illogical to adopt a judgmental approach to the behavior, in the genetic sense, of parents or individuals who seem to be rejecting a "low" genetic risk or accepting a "high" genetic gamble. Provided that a parent or client is sufficiently intelligent to understand the meaning of odds and risk figures, and does not suffer from a psychosis (itself often the diagnosis of the propositus — eg, Huntington chorea), an honest decision concerning future children is right for him, however inappropriate this may seem to the counselor or to society in general.

Second, it is very important that the genetic counselor be aware of the known subjective factors that can modify an otherwise objective interpretation of risk. Only in this way can the effects of such factors be reduced to a minimum; only in this way can the counselor interpret his own attitudes toward the genetic risks of patients who seek his advice; and only in this way can the occasional apparently "irresponsible" behavior (in the genetic sense) of his patients be understood.

These modifying factors are: 1) intelligence; 2) perceived general risk background; 3) presentation of risk figures; 4) the "risky shift" phenomenon; 5) anticipated risk odds; and 6) nature of outcome.

Intelligence

Intelligence is obviously very important in the interpretation of odds. A certain amount of intelligence is required to understand the mathematical symbols used to express risk; at the least, intelligence is required to appreciate relative orders of risk. A realistic interpretation of odds depends on how well subjects are able to use numbers in their actual perception of probabilistic events or in their perception of degrees of certainty and uncertainty [13].

Education and experience are also probably important in determining how an individual feels about a fixed mathematical risk. The *relative* influence of intelligence, education, and experience in determining the final subjective interpretation of a fixed mathematical risk is, however, unknown. Decision-making under conditions of risk is known to be illogical even in the case of trained math - ematicians confronted with gambling situations, at least in laboratory experiments [14].

Perceived General Risk Background

Whether a fixed mathematical risk is regarded as "high" or "low" depends very much on its value relative to that of the general risk background appropriate to the situation. For example, a risk of 1 in 100 for a specific individual might well be considered "high" if the risk to everyone else was 1 in 1,000,000. Alternatively, the same mathematical risk of 1 in 100 would probably be considered "low" if everyone else ran a risk of 1 in 10. (One often hears this type of comparison of risks in everyday conversation — eg, " 'so-and-so' is less risky than trying to cross the road!").

In the genetic context, the specific risk run by any individual or couple must be seen in the perspective of what they correctly or incorrectly believe to be the general risk. Many genetic counselors use as a working figure a general risk of approximately 1 in 50 to 1 in 30 that any living newborn infant will have a significant abnormality of one type or another; it is also common practice specifically to mention this general risk to couples seeking counsel concerning a particular problem.

This phenomenon of the general risk background has two implications for genetic counseling. First, the general risk should be added to the specifc genetic risk determined for a particular couple. Second, individuals and couples react differently when they view their own specific risk in the perspective of this general risk background; often, couples offered a specific risk of "intermediate" size (say, 1 in 10 to 1 in 20) seem to be comforted by the knowledge of a general risk of the approximate order of 1 in 30. It is probable in many instances that risks of this intermediate order are subjectively reduced to odds of less threatening levels, but individual differences occur and vary widely.

Some parents consider, correctly or incorrectly, that their own family trees are heavily burdened with genetic disease.

One has to be circumspect about introducing the concept of general risk. Perhaps 5% of women are already pregnant when they seek genetic counsel (a fact not necessarily revealed to the counselor), and most women are horrified to learn that the general risk of a significant congenital abnormality is so "high."

To summarize, the interpretation of a risk, when offered in genetic counseling, depends on its comparison with the sum of all other risks that could produce a similar outcome; namely, an abnormal child.

Presentation of Risk Figures

The manner in which risk figures are expressed is important, and have a significant influence on the patient's interpretation of the formal mathematical odds given to him. For example, a proffered risk of "1 in 4" is mathematically the same as a "3 to 1 chance against" the occurrence of a future result. Some genetic counselors use this type of approach to produce a legitimate directed interpretation of the risk. A proffered risk of "3 to 1 against", or "75%

probability of being unaffected" is an encouraging type of approach, and is sometimes used to reinforce manifest tendencies or attitudes that are already present. The alternative form of presentation of the risk, "1 in 4", or "25% probability of being affected" has implicit in it greater emphasis on the threat of an of an abnormal child.

The first form of presentation of fixed odds — that is, the optimistic or encouraging approach ("3 to 1 against" an affected child being born) — may be emphasized in two particular clinical situations. The first of these occurs when a woman is already pregnant, is seeking genetic advice, and there is no possibility of a therapeutic abortion, or of antenatal diagnosis. Personal research figures suggest that over 5% of women seeking counsel are pregnant. In this difficult situation, it is always kindest to express the odds in the least threatening form, if indeed specific odds are insisted upon. The second situation is when a couple so desperately want a living child of their own after having lost several affected children that they are going to go ahead in spite of an objectively high risk of recurrence that is involved. If it can be pointed out that they have a 3 to 1 chance (for example) of a normal child, then they obtain some reassurance and comfort in what is always a very worrisome period of waiting.

When to use this type of approach is arbitrary, and depends very much on the personal, ethical, and philosophical attitudes of the counselor, and the degree of responsibility he feels for his clients' decision.

The "Risky Shift" Phenomenon

It is well known from both personal and professional experience that the subjective interpretation of a risk is subject to shift; for example, odds previously regarded as high may subsequently assume less threatening proportions. One of the dynamic processes involved in this in known as the "risky shift". Research by experimental psychologists has revealed that prior discussion of a risk situation leads to an increasing willingness on the part of the average discussant to take greater risks [15–17]. It may well be that the very discussion of a risk can reduce its threat to an individual. In addition, group support is important to the way an individual interprets risk. The group may be a nuclear or extended family, friends, or a series of professional acquaintances such as clergy, and other doctors.

It is probable that the discussion (in considerable depth) that occurs during a genetic counseling interview also produces this "risky shift," although this has not yet been formally tested. It is probable that the ventilation of all aspects of a genetic problem that occurs ideally during any genetic counseling interview or series of interviews acts as a catalyst for further reflection in the privacy of the home. It might be hoped that a lot of subtopics relating to a genetic problem, previously taboo, might be frankly discussed that afterwards produces this "risky shift" influence in the clinical genetic sphere.

Anticipated Risk Odds

When parents or relatives consult a geneticist, they usually have some preconceived idea about the likelihood of disease recurrence. This prior belief may or may not be correct, but it serves as an unconscious reference point for the professionally supplied risk, and so modifies the patient's final subjective interpretation of the latter [11]. Although no accurate research figures are available, it is probable that the majority of patients leave the genetic counseling clinic furnished with risk figures smaller than those anticipated and feared prior to consultation, but many exceptions may occur.

Nature of the Outcome if Risk Eventuates

This is perhaps the most obvious factor influencing the subjective interpretation of odds. The theme has two important genetic overtones.

First, it implies that parents can assess specific genetic risks only if they are informed of the implications of all sequelae. This assessment is often most appropriately undertaken by their own general practitioner. In some exceptional cases (for example, when a woman is in late pregnancy) it would be totally inopportune to raise these issues. Again, when parents have obviously made an irreversible decision to have or not to have further children, it would not be appropriate to dwell on this point. These exceptions aside, the same risk may be interpreted quite differently by different parents who are informed of the full implications of a lost gamble. Parents are sometimes prepared to take higher risks if a child who is affected will die in infancy [18, 19].

Second, it implies that a specific, genetically determined disease can mean different things to different people. The subjective attitude toward the disease or lesion itself may be quite at variance with what informed medical opinon would regard as a realistic appraisal. Relatively minor limb or facial defects with cosmetic overtones are examples here. On the other hand, some patients regard with considerable equanimity genetic lesions that are of major medical significance. Thus, there is a two-stage process involved in the interpretation of risk in this context. First, the client or parent forms a very subjective personal view of the disease or lesion itself, and then he or she forms a subjective interpretation of the risks for that concept of the disease.

For parents seeking genetic advice, both the above themes are understood if they have had personal past experience of the specific genetic problems about which they are concerned. In test situations, past experience has been shown to lead to a more realistic assessment of mathematical odds [20]. Furthermore, even in the case of intelligent parents, it has been found that the individual learns to make optimal choices in a betting situation only after a number of such trials; decision-making under risk is known to be illogical, especially for random or single gambles [8]. This is probably applicable to the current genetic situation where family sizes tend to be small.

Even moderately informed opinion does not mean that people think similarly about genetic diseases. Figure 1 shows some results obtained from a survey involving approximately one hundred final year medical students. At the end of a course in medical genetics, the students were shown a series of color slides, projected on a six feet by six feet screen. These included a child with the fatal infantile form of spinal muscular atrophy; a grossly subnormal female with 47,XXX karyotype; a child with typical Down syndrome; and a child with primordial dwarfism (ie, normal-proportioned dwarfism).

The medical, clinical, and domestic overtones of each condition already well known to these graduating doctors, were reinforced. The students were then asked to assume they were personally contemplating a pregnancy, with each one of the above outcomes as a possibility. They were then asked to give the maximum risk they would accept before proceeding to have a baby under these circumstances. The results confirmed that even medically informed individuals view disease very differently.

THE COUNSELOR'S ROLE

Competence in decision-making is regarded as an important attribute of socialization in our culture. Few decisions are subject to such public scrutiny and judgmental comment as those taken in the face of a genetic risk. The counselor's role is to enable parents or clients to make such decisions, that have hereditary implications, in an informed and realistic way.

Irrespective of individual differences in style and approach among different genetic counselors, effective counseling follows a standard basic pattern (Fig. 2): the establishment of the diagnosis of the index case; the compliation of the kindred; the determination of the mode of inheritance involved; the calculation of recurrence; the presentation of such risks to the client or patient; the subjective interpretation of these risks by the client; and the final decision by the client concerning his reproductive choice.

The first four links of this seven-link chain make up the scientific components of genetic counseling. The counselor's role here is well defined and depends on his training and expertise in clinical medicine, formal genetic theory, and basic mathematics. Efforts in carrier detection may also be included here.

The next two steps of the counseling sequence do not involve scientific considerations primarily, but are the most important from the point of view of the outcome of the entire endeavor — ie, the final reproductive choice. Here, the art of counseling and the personal attitudes of the counselor are influential in shaping the client's decision-making process. The counselor's role here is not so well defined, and wide differences of opinion exist; it is essential, however, that the counselor have some knowledge of the relevant applied psychology rapidly accumulating in this field [11].

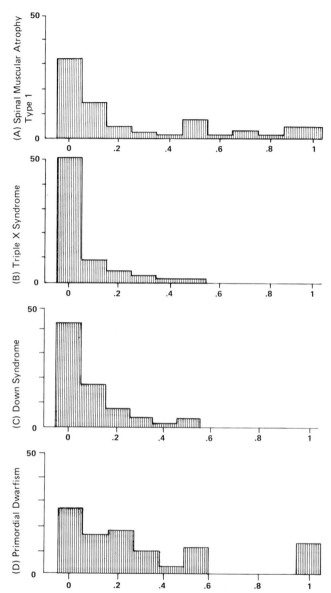

Fig. 1. This series of histograms shows the way in which 100 graduating doctors viewed the risk of different medical conditions. The abscissa shows the maximum acceptable risk for a theoretical pregnancy by self or spouse. The ordinate shows percent of subjects. (A) Spinal muscular atrophy Type I, a rapidly fatal paralyzing disease of infancy; autosomal recessive. 32% would not embark on a pregnancy if there were any risk of this disease, whereas 8% would accept odds of 1 in 2. (B) Triple X syndrome, associated with severe mental subnormality. No subject would accept a risk greater than 1 in 2 (0.5). (C) Down syndrome or mongolism. No subject would accept a higher risk than 1 in 2, but 3% would accept a risk of 1 in 2, in spite of the well-known consequences. (D) Primordial dwarfism. Here the distribution of risk opinion is much more evenly distributed, and 8% would be undeterred even if the outcome of having such a dwarfed child were 100% certain.

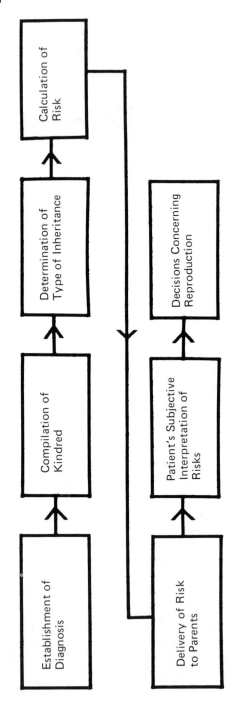

Fig. 2. This flowchart illustrates the seven-step basic sequence common to all genetic counseling situations. The first four of these steps comprise the scientific components of counseling; in almost all instances quantifiable risk odds can be given. Most counselors would agree on the objective mathematical risk appropriate to a specific case. By contrast, the last three steps of this sequential process are subject to wide variation, with wide divergence of attitudes and interpretations by both counselor and client.

A crucial responsibility in this phase of counseling is to ensure that the parents are making a truly informed decision. Experimental studies have shown that optimality of choice in any decision-making task under risk is significantly improved with increasing knowledge of the results of such a decision. Fuller knowledge of the consequences of a lost gamble affects motivational factors [7].

The final effector step, a decision concerning reproductive choice, cannot by its nature be made by the counselor. What is his role here? Because of the interplay of the many variables discussed earlier, an individual client's or couple's position will not necessarily coincide with the counselor's own view of the optimal reproductive decision. In spite of this, his role should be supportive, whether or not his own views concur with those finally reached by his patient. Many clients wish for active guidance from the counselor [21]. For others, risk-taking may be commonplace in their daily lives [22], and such individuals may not feel the stress of a specific genetic decision to the same degree. As the subjective interpretation of risk and the degree of procreative drive are so individual and personal, many believe that it is not the place of the counselor to express strongly his own point of view; rather, it would be more logical and certainly more humane to support the parents in whatever decision is ultimately reached. This presupposes that the client has become informed, in the fullest sense, of all the medical, social, domestic, and financial consequences of a lost genetic gamble.

Not all genetic counselors adopt this view; some feel a strong moral and professional obligation to dissuade parents from a positive reproductive choice when risks are high. Some feel that this approach denies that the counselor's own view are subjective, but this type of approach is neither inconsistent nor illogical, provided that the counselor himself is aware that his attitudes are subject to the same variables as those of his client.

SUMMARY

The appreciation of the dynamics of decision-making processes has reached considerable sophistication in the realms of logic, statistics, and psychology. Although the direct application of this knowledge to clinical situations is in its infancy, an understanding of such processes can be of great help to the genetic counselor.

In the context of genetic counseling, decisions leading to final reproductive choice depend on the degree to which primary procreative drive is modified by a perceived risk of genetically determined disease. The intensity of the procreative drive itself will have been reinforced both positively and negatively by many non-genetic factors, including family experience and pressures and sociological influences operating within the population of which the individual is a part.

Decisions about the biological conception of future children depend on the subjective manner in which a fixed, objective, mathematically precise risk is individually interpreted. Factors that, in turn, modify this subjective interpretation of risk or mathematical odds offered in genetic counseling include the parents' intelligence, the general risk background, the risky shift phenomenon, and the level of risk anticipated prior to formal counseling.

The counselor's presentation of the risk figures and his role and manner of informing the parent of the consequences of an eventuated risk are important in shaping the final manner in which a specific mathematical risk is interpreted.

Genetic counseling consists of a series of steps commencing with confirmation of the diagnosis in the propositus and ending with the client's decision concerning future reproduction. There are at least five intermediate links in this sequence, and the counselor's role in each of these impinges on and modifies final reproductive choice. An understanding of the counselor's relative influence at each of these steps enables more effective counsel to be delivered and often explains final reproductive decisions of the parents, which occasionally may seem inappropriate.

ANNOTATED REFERENCES

Decision-Making in the Medical Context

1. Edwards W, Tversky A (Eds): "Decision Making." Baltimore: Penguin Books, 1967.
   A comprehensive survey of decision-making with an extensive compendium of listed authors.
2. Lindley DV: "Making Decisions." London: Wiley–Interscience, 1971.
   A comprehensive text book covering all aspects of modern decision therory. Discusses numerical measures of uncertainty, the laws of probability, Bayes' theorem, and decision trees, all helpful reading for the genetic counselor.
3. Lifson MW: Decisions, decisions, decisions. Ann Biomed Engineer 1:285, 1973.
   An excellent, readable account of decision theory in the general health context. Clear exposition of the differences between decisions and conclusions; includes a description of maximized utility versus estimate of risk as the basic data input of the decision process.
4. Rangell L: The decision-making process. A contribution from psychoanalysis. Psycoanal Study Child 26:425, 1971.
   A discursive study of some theories about human decision-making. Includes a good section on motives and sequelae of decision-making in the medical context.
5. Janis I, Mann L: A conflict-theory approach to attitude change and decision-making. Greenwald AG, Brook TC, and Ostrow TM (Eds): "Psychological Foundations of Attitudes." New York: Academic Press, 1968.
   A reference account of some of the theories of decision-making, especially those developed to test conflict resolution.
6. Ekehammar B, Magnusson D: Decision time as a function of subjective confidence and amount of information. Percept Mot Skills 36:329, 1973.
   A short article confirming that subjective confidence in decision-making increases with increasing amounts of information about the decision task.

7. Mann L: Differences between reflective and implusive children in tempo and quality of decision making. Child Dev 44:274, 1973.
   An excellent study investigating the acquisition of decision-making expertise. Evidence is presented to show that the time taken to reach decisions is not necessarily linked to the quality or optimality of the decision.

8. Meyer DE: Differential effects of knowledge of results and monetary reward upon optimal choice behavior under risk. J Exp Psychol 75:520, 1967.
   A milestone study showing a quantitative relationship between optimality of choice in decision-making and the amount of relevant information available to the person prior to a gamble under risk.

9. Tversky A: Utility theory and additivity analysis of risky choices. J Exp Psychol 75:27, 1967.
   An excellent account of the processes of decision-making under risk. The utility theory of decision-making between risky alternatives can be described as the maximization of the patient's subjective expected utility.

Procreative Drive in the Genetic Context

10. Itkin W: Some relationships between intrafamily attitudes and preparental attitudes towards children. J Genet Psychol 80:221, 1952.
    An extensive survey of preparental attitudes toward the need for, and desirable features of, children. The survey has shown that, very largely, attitudes are influenced by the subjects' own parents.

Subjective Interpretation of Odds

11. Pearn JH: Patients subjective interpretation of risks offered in genetic counseling. J Med Genet 10:129, 1973.
    A review article discussing in depth the influences that modify the ways risk is interpreted by parents and individuals exposed to a genetic threat.

12. Ramsey FP: Truth and probability. In Braithwaite RB (Ed): "The Foundations of Mathematics amd other Logical Essays." London: Kegan Paul, Trench, Trubner Co. Ltd., 1931.
    One of the classics of the philosophy of the subjective interpretation of risk, and of mathematical odds. Ramsey wrote about the degrees of belief, its mathematical expression, and its implications for logical decision-making.

13. Howell WC: An evaluation of subjective probability in a visual discrimination task. J Exp Psychol 75:479. 1967.
    An important paper measuring directly the role of intelligence in assigning a mathematic expression of risk in a decision-making context.

14. Beach LR, Swensson RG: Instructions about randomness and run dependency in two-choice learning. J Exp Psychol 75:279, 1967.
    It is common experience that indivduals use a belief in run dependency in the process of decision-making, In spite of the mathematical fallacy of this procedure, in a real-life gambling situation its appeal is irresistibly seductive. This paper shows that formal education does not protect against its influence.

15. Rettig S: Group discussion and predicted ethical risk taking. J Person Soc Psychol 3:629, 1966.
    One of the earlier papers formalizing the concept of the "risky-shift" phenomenon.

16. Chandler S, Rabow J: Ethnicity and acquaintance as variables in risk-taking. J Soc Psychol 77:221, 1969.
   A valuable follow-up contribution ot the study and understanding of the "risky-shift" phenomenon. Shows the importance of discussion and group dynamics as an influence on the subjective interpretation of risk. It probably has direct relevance to genetic counseling where parents are inescapably subject to group influence, often the immediate family, in their choice and decisions concerning future children.

17. Horne WC: Group influence on ethical risk taking; the inadequacy of two hypotheses. J Soc Psychol 80:237, 1970.
   Follow-up studies on the dunamics of the "risky-shift" phenomenon. Although accepted as an established fact, the mechanisms of its action are ill-understood.

18. Murphy EA: The rationale of genetic counseling. J Pediatr 72:121, 1968.
   A milestone paper codifying the whole subject of the objective mathematical risk given in almost all instances of genetic couseling. This paper gives an excellent account of the different types of process by which recurrence risks can be assessed. The author describes modular, empirical, and particular types of data used in the formation of risk. A good doublet of papers is this one by Murphy followed by that of Pearn [11].

19. Carter CO, Roberts JAF, Evans KA, Buck AR: Genetic clinic. A follow-up. Lancet 1: 281, 1971.
   One of very few studies on the ways parents and clients act after receiving informed genetic opinion. This comprehensive study gives data on 455 couples seen at a second follow-up. In general, a risk of 1 in 10 (or greater) was interpreted as high enough to dissuade couples from trying for future children.

20. Beach LR, Phillips LD: Subjective probabilities inferred from estimates and bets. J Exp Psychol 75:354, 1967.
   This experimental study has shown that past experience and increased information concerning a gambling situation allows a more realistic interpretation of risk or odds.

21. Vertinsky IB, Thompson WA, Uyeno D: Measuring consumer desire for participation in clinical decision making. Health Ser Res (Summer): 121, 1974.
   A research article giving a helpful insight into the attitudes of patients to the respective doctor-patient roles in medical decision-making.

22. Moran E: Clinical and social aspects of risk-taking. Proc Roy Soc Med 63:1273, 1970.
   This paper discusses risk-taking in general, and many implications for genetic counseling can be inferred from it. In particular, the author illustrates how some patients are subject to a risk-taking milieu as part of their daily lives; ie, repeated high-risk taking is for some a micro-environmental norm.

11

Psychosocial Advocacy

Audrey T. McCollum,MS,ACSW, and Ruth L. Silverberg,MSSA,ACSW

INTRODUCTION: THE TASKS DEFINED

Genetic counseling is a potential crisis experience that may afford constructive benefits or lead to impaired self-esteem and disturbed interpersonal relationships. Many who request counseling have already been traumatized. They may,
for example, have been identified in a screening program as carriers of a deleterious
gene; they may have learned of an inherited disorder in the family; or they may
have borne a child afflicted with an illness known or suspected to be inherited.
The very decision to seek genetic information may have been painful and con-
flicted. For these reasons, the client is vulnerable from the outset.

The counseling experience confronts the client with psychological tasks that
must be accomplished if the process is to have a constructive outcome. The nature
and complexity of these tasks should be understood by those who undertake
genetic counseling. Either the geneticist or an appropriate colleague should
develop the depth and scope of insight that will enable him or her to serve as
advocate of the client's psychosocial needs.

In this chapter, we shall define these psychological tasks and delineate the
contribution of "psychosocial advocacy" through each stage of the counseling
process: evaluation and preparation of the client, presentation of genetic findings,
follow-up. Discussion of the professional identity of the advocate is found in
Chapter 13.

Assimilation of Genetic Information

The first psychological task confronting the client is the assimilation of the
genetic information presented. The health professional who listens attentively to
patients or their families soon learns that most persons have confused and inaccurate ideas about their bodily structures and functions that reflect the
complexity of the mental concept of the body — the "body image," composed
of the totality of an individual's ideas (realistic and imaginary), attitudes, and
emotions concerning the physical self.

239

Mental images are most readily formed of those bodily structures (eg, skin, eyes, mouth, rectum), products (eg, blood, urine), or processes (eg, heartbeat, elimination) that produce sensations or that can be directly observed. These images are influenced not only by perceptions but also by emotions such as pride, fear, or shame. They are molded by family, ethnic, and cultural attitudes, as well as by experiences of illness or injury. Those organs (eg, liver, spleen) or processes (eg, metabolism) that are not subjectively experienced, and are therefore only abstract, are extremely difficult to conceptualize.

Genetic information concerns structures and processes not subject to direct observation. Furthermore, its terminology is unfamiliar to the layman. Chromosomes and genes, dominant and recessive, autosomal and sex-linked, penetrance and expression, and statistical probabilities — such concepts are difficult for laymen to assimilate; difficult to understand and difficult to recall. They are all the more difficult for the client whose own body, whose own reproductive potential, or whose mate and children are implicated. When the information is painful and threatening, conceptual confusions tend to proliferate, since unbearable ideas are likely to be denied or forgotten and replaced with wish-fulfilling thoughts.

Physicians caring for families with serious inherited illnesses feel understandable urgency in attempting to prevent the birth of another affected child and may use genetic information to discourage a family from bearing children. However, no person can be coerced to assimilate unwanted information. We have observed instances in which many years have passed before parents of children with inherited disorders (eg, cystic fibrosis) could realistically consider the matter of genetic transmission.

Becoming informed is not an event, as it tends to be viewed in a medical center, where staff are busy and may dislike or dread imparting painful facts repeatedly. Rather, it is a continuing process. Disturbing information can be assimilated only gradually. Understanding can be enhanced with the guidance of professionals who accept the clients' pace and are available for repeated explanations and clarifications as needed.

Understanding and Coping With Associated Affect

Before the information can be fully assimilated, clients must also deal with the second task posed by genetic counseling. In those fortunate instances in which a genetic defect can be ruled out, reassurance and relief usually follow. When a disorder is identified, intense emotions are aroused which must be acknowledged, understood, and discharged in acceptable ways, at a tolerable pace.

The wish to reproduce varies according to an individual's position in his or her life cycle, interpersonal attachments, and various social and ethnic influences. This wish is an issue distinct from the potential for reproduction, which is an important component of one's body image. At least from puberty onward, the potential to have normal offspring constitutes a significant element in a person's view of himself or herself as a fully adequate male or female. Knowledge of a genetic defect violates this sense of sexual adequacy and impairs the sense of capacity for unhampered choice.

Furthermore, it may insult the individual's feeling of relatedness to the future. Motives for child-bearing are varied. (See Chapter 8.) One profoundly important motive arises from the wish to deny the limitations of human existence and to seek perpetuity. Although organ donations play a role, biological immortality is attained chiefly through reproduction. The denial of this possibility may gravely threaten an individual's sense of signifcance.

These violations of an individual's sense of adequacy and importance are likely to produce sadness and resentment. Guilt may arise, often having its source in irrational ideas about connections between cause and effect, as when the genetic "taint" is viewed as a consequence of evil thoughts, impulses, or deeds. Guilt may also be stimulated by the disclosure that an ill or dead child was afflicted with a disorder transmitted by one or both parents.

Anxiety may arise from the idea of being defective and undesirable as a mate. Should the client be pregnant, or be the mate of a pregnant woman, there may be grave concern about the normality of the fetus.

The intensities of these affects do not necessarily correspond to the realities of a problem. Rather, they are expressions of personality structure, existential position, hopes for the future, and the significance accorded the information in a client's fantasy life. Indeed, genetic information may produce genuine despair.

Unbearable feelings, like unwanted information, are warded off by a variety of psychic defenses. These are invoked because they are needed (as surely as a bandage is needed to protect a laceration). Aggressive attempts to penetrate these defenses are less than humane and usually are futile. However, sensitive and well-timed exploration of emotions at the threshold of consciousness can support the client in recognizing, understanding, and coming to terms with his or her own feelings.

Safeguarding Significant Relationships

In numerous ways, knowledge of a genetic defect, and the emotions associated with that knowledge, can burden meaningful relationships. For example, the guilt aroused when a child is found to have an inherited disorder may be expiated by an inappropriately indulgent and protective style of child-rearing, or can contribute to depressive withdrawal, depriving loved ones of needed attention and affection. If intolerable, the guilt may be projected outward as anger and blame, with the spouse as a likely target.

Anger may also be directed toward a parent who was a carrier, or toward siblings or offspring who escaped affliction. Heightened and diffuse irritability may damage friendships. Sometimes there is loss of religious faith or rejection of a God who appears so cruel and punitive.

Apprehension about further pregnancies can disrupt the sexual relationship even if a couple is fully informed about contraception. (Most adults can cite a few instances of contraceptive failure, supporting their fears.) The lowering of self-esteem, with a fantasy of being undesirable as a mate, can lead to withdrawal from either potential or actual sex partners.

Emotional responses to genetic information may only be slowly recognized. Similarly the impact upon significant relationships may become slowly apparent. For these reasons, follow-up to explore the affective and interpersonal responses to genetic information is as much a professional obligation as follow-up care after surgery.

Reproductive Planning

This is the fourth task imposed by genetic counseling. If genetic studies establish that a feared genetic trait is not present, the client is freed to make unfettered reproductive choices or to complete an existing pregnancy with reduced anxiety.

If a genetic defective is identified, complex issues concerning dating and choice of mate, sexual activity and contraception, and prenatal diagnosis and abortion, as well as the physical and psychological significance of the disease itself, will all need to be understood and resolved. There is no way to overstate the importance of these issues for most individuals, nor the difficulties of the psychological work required to resolve them.

The Psychosocial Advocate

In the four respects described above, genetic counseling can be a crisis experience. There are optimal situations for genetic counseling, such as a genetics service staffed by a skilled interdisciplinary team.

Laymen are, unfortunately, usually exposed to genetic information and mis-information through the mass media, from relatives and friends, in schools, and in community screening programs. Their physicians, after diagnosis of an in-herited disorder, are likely to include genetic information as well as advice about reproduction in discussing the illness with patient and family members. (The authors have known instances in which diagnosis, prognosis, and inheritance patterns of a fatal illness have been discussed in one single conference.)

Genetic information is frequently presented in a way that reflects the bias of the informant. For example, a group of guilt-laden parents of children with a serious inherited disease were told by their children's physician that society would someday make reproduction illegal for persons known to carry genetic defects. This declaration, profoundly distressing to the parents, was not unkindly intended. It reflected the physician's identification with the suffering of his patients, and his anger that such children should be born to suffer.

Adventitious, thoughtless, or wounding remarks occur in medical centers as well as in communities outside. In any setting, the likelihood that genetic counseling will be a constructive, need-fulfilling experience for the client is enhanced if a professional person qualified to serve as a client advocate collaborates with the physician or geneticist. (We recognize that there are instances in which no such professional person is available. In such cases, the genetic counselor would be well advised to make every effort to deepen his or her understanding of the psychosocial implications of imparting genetic information). The advocate should be trained to evaluate the clients' adaptive strengths and vulnerabilities, to understand their psychosocial characteristics and needs, to safeguard their right to self-determination, to offer personal and family counseling, or to effect appropriate referrals. He should understand the importance of privacy, protection from interruptions and auditory distractions, and ample time for conversation when sensitive information is discussed.

Genetic counseling should be a longitudinal process that begins at the time a genetic disorder is first considered, and which may have long-lasting psychosocial reverberations. Therefore, the advocate has a meaningful role beginning with evaluation and preparation, proceeding through presentation of findings, and continuing in follow-up contacts.

PSYCHOSOCIAL EVALUATION AND PREPARATION

Numerous characteristics influence a person's adaptive capacities. Although all significant areas need not be explored in depth, a skillful advocate can gain important information through observation as well as verbal interchange, even in a single interview, and identify relevant areas for additional exploration. Furthermore, he or she should remain attuned to these areas in subsequent contacts with the client. In this sense, evaluation is continuous as long as there is contact. If the interviews are carried out with sensitivity and convey understanding and acceptance of the client's individuality, the evaluation itself can be therapeutic.

Such interviews need not be rigidly structured, but attention should be given to the following considerations.

Motivation

Some people seek genetic counseling with a sense of purpose and clearly formulated questions. Others present themselves in passive and perplexed compliance with the advice of some authority figure. An initial task of the advocate would be to clarify what the client is seeking, because the issues that concern the client may be quite different from the issues relating to genetic risks.

Clients may be seeking information about their genetic endowment in order to develop a realistic sense of self:

> Dorothy A., 33 years of age and unmarried, applied for counseling on referral from her psychiatrist. Having 2 brothers with a crippling muscular disorder, she had been exposed in her early teens to an offhand statement that she should never reproduce because of her brothers' affliction. Her

struggle since then to reconcile herself to remaining single and childless caused grievous emotional trauma. She was now being encouraged to seek realistic information about the inheritance pattern of the disease, and to determine whether or not she carried the deleterious gene.

Clients may wish to resolve ambivalence within themselves:

Mr. and Mrs. B., a young professional couple, wished to have children, but struggled to weigh their personal rights against their obligations to society. Mr. B.'s father had Huntington chorea, so Mr. B. faced the possibility of being disabled by the disorder in 10–15 years, as well as the possibility that his children would be afflicted. They sought not only genetic information, but also help in reaching a need-fulfilling and socially responsible decision.

Clients may apply for help in resolving interpersonal conflict:

Mr. and Mrs. C. had a child with Down Syndrome. They were devout Roman Catholics and Mrs. C., again pregnant, declared that she would never consider an abortion. Mr. C. believed that his wife should have amniocentesis and that if the fetus were found to be defective, his wife would change her mind.

Clients may seek to resolve a grief reaction:

Mr. and Mrs. D's only child had cystic fibrosis. They had been referred by the child's physician, who believed they should avoid future pregnancies and hoped the geneticist would reinforce this. The couple, however, expressed an urgent wish for another child to replace the one they feared they would lose. A worsening of the child's condition had intensified their anxiety and grief. They longed to assuage their grief by planning another pregnancy: "We have to have one child who will complete his life cycle!"

Covert, as well as overt, motivation is often present. For example, some couples seek justification to avoid unwanted reproduction, perhaps in the face of family or peer-group pressures to bear children. There are also instances in which a couple, or one partner, wishes to legitimize abstention from intercourse.

In appraising motivation, the advocate should clarify not only the issues under consideration but also the client's expectations from genetic counseling. What contacts, questions, tests do the clients anticipate? Which of these do they fear, what answers do they expect?

Affect and Mood

The client's prevailing mood, the quality of affect, and the appropriateness of the affect to the ideas under consideration are highly relevant. Such information can be gathered informally during an interview, through observation of the client's motility, posture, facial expression, and tone of voice, as well as from the pace, flow, and content of verbal communications.

Significant qualities of affect. These include characteristics such as the range from variability to evenness, richness to paucity, intensity to flatness or blunting, as well as selective or pervasive ambivalence. Much affective quality reflects personality structure (eg, the hysterical personality may display intense and variable affect; the obsessive personality may display paucity of affect and pervasive ambivalence). These qualities may significantly influence the counseling experience. For example, the pervasively ambivalent client is likely to have difficulty using genetic information as a basis of decision making, and may need prolonged help to resolve his doubts and conflicts. The labile, histrionic client may become distraught and arouse discomfort in the physician or geneticist, who may be tempted to curtail further contact with the client.

Anxiety. Since genetic counseling contains an implied threat, the client can be expected to feel apprehensive or anxious.* The content of his fears should, however, be explored so that they can be both understood and resolved as fully as possible.

Furthermore, since anxiety interferes with the client's capacity to assimilate information, as well as his capacity to make decisions, its intensity and pervasiveness should be assessed in each contact. The severely anxious client may need frequent and extended contact to derive benefit from genetic counseling.

Grief and mood disorders. Many clients are actively mourning the actual or expected death of a family member from a possibly inherited illness. Therefore, clients may manifest sadness, pessimism, a sense of helplessness and futility, a lack of energy and interest, feelings of worthlessness and guilt. When such a constellation is observed, a differentiation between grief reaction, mood disorder, and a depressive personality style should be attempted.

There should be inquiry into the duration of the mood; any relationship between its onset and actual or expected bereavement. There should be inquiry concerning neurovegetative symptoms (disturbances of sleep, appetite, gastrointestinal function, and drive); cognitive disturbances (slowing of thought; impairment of concentration or memory); and suicidal ideation. Many health professionals are uncomfortable about mentioning suicide, fearing it may aggravate a client's emotional disturbance. On the contrary, open and tactful discussion of suicidal ideas generally affords relief and support to the depressed patient.

In the past, it was believed that grief and depression could be distinguished by duration: grief was self-limiting, depression was prolonged. This distinction had less value since it has been observed that acute depressions may be self-limiting; in contrast, grief may be prolonged when a loved one has a serious disease which runs an extended course, is severely crippling, is subject to remissions and exacerbations (blood dyscrasias), or has fluctuations of severity (cystic fibrosis). However, if the loss has already occurred and intense grief persists beyond 3 to 6 months, depression should be suspected.

As significant as duration of the mood is intensity of guilt and self-denigration. Most persons close to a seriously ill individual experience self-questioning or self-blame with respect to their responsibility for the illness and many suffer from guilt about hostile feelings toward the patient. However, self-accusation usually yields to self-forgiveness; guilt softens into regret.

---

*Apprehension is a response to perceived external dangers, whereas anxiety is a response to intrapsychic conflicts or threatening impulses and affects. Since the two states cannot readily be differentiated, the term anxiety will be used to denote both.

Unrealistic and persistent guilt may signify the characteristic self-loathing of depressive illness. If depression is identified, a sensitive judgment must be made about the wisdom of proceeding with genetic studies and risking further injury to the client's impaired self-esteem. The preferred course may be to recommend psychotherapy. When acute grief is being experienced, timeliness of the counseling should be evaluated just as carefully.

An occasional client may appear inappropriately expansive and euphoric, display unfounded optimism, deny realistic difficulties, and reveal a rapid flight of ideas. Although denial is a common defense, when it is observed in this constellation a manic disorder should be suspected.

Anger. Some persons react to threat with aggressive feelings and impulses. Genetic study of a family poses a threat to self-esteem and to significant relationships. Furthermore, anger is a component of mourning, and many clients are mourning ill or dead relatives. For both these reasons, clients may express hostility, either overtly or covertly concealed beneath a demeanor of appeasing compliance.

If anger is not manifest in facial expression or tone of voice, nonetheless it is worthwhile to give permission for its expression with a remark such as, "Many people in your situation would feel resentful." Anger seeks a target; it can destroy meaningful relationships and alienate medical staff. Only through ventilation can it be determined who serves as target: self, parent, spouse, offspring, a friend, God, doctor, or nurse. Extended help is often needed to safeguard these relationships.

It must be stressed that genetic counseling involves painful, intimate issues, and it is appropriate for the client to respond with painful feelings. It is the client's task to learn to deal with these feelings; it is the advocate's task to help him do so.

Severe blunting or inappropriateness of affect, pervasive anxiety, symptoms of affective disease, unremitting rage all warrant diagnostic evaluation by an experienced mental health professional to determine whether psychiatric intervention is needed, and whether this should precede or accompany genetic counseling.

Cognition

Even without formal mental status evaluation, an experienced interviewer can recognize certain cognitive characteristics that indicate whether a client has the capacity to use genetic information effectively or whether special help will be needed.

1. Pace of thought may vary along a continuum from the marked slowness signifying intellectual or depressive retardation to the flights of ideas that signifies severe agitation, mania, or schizophrenia.

2. Blocking, the sudden loss of ideational connections usually expressed by silence or the remark, "I forgot what I was talking about," may signify anxiety.

If severe and repeated, it may signify a psychogenic or organic thought disorder.

3. Conceptual qualities include profundity in contrast to shallowness, originality in contrast to stereotypy; abstractness in contrast to concreteness. Extreme sterotypy or concreteness, especially if inconsistent with the client's educational level, may signify psychopathology. In most cases, conceptual characteristics reflect an intellectual style that has been molded by inborn potential, personality development, and education. It is important to note these characteristics so that genetic information can be transmitted in terms that the client can comprehend.

4. Assimilation of information is also influenced by concentration and memory. These functions can be assessed informally by noting the client's capacity to recall significant past events, as well as by responses to the interviewer's comments and questions.

5. The client's realism and logic also influence the capacity to understand information and use it adaptively; that is, for problem-solving. Realism and logic reflect the client's capacity to grasp cause—effect relationships and abstract concepts and educational status and cultural background, which may foster either realism or primitive, magical thinking.

6. It is useful to evaluate the client's capacity for planning — the carrying out of trial actions in thought. Planning requires an orientation to the future, a capacity to delay gratification. Each of these components is influenced by existential states (eg, anticipatory mourning may constrict orientation to the future), by personality structure, and by cultural influences. An incapacity to plan effectively, or nonproductive, doubt-laden ruminations are indications for extended professional attention. In fact, any marked cognitive deficit or psychopathological characteristic (eg, severe blocking, retardation, racing thoughts, magical thinking) should be carefully evaluated.

Sense of Self

A client's capacity to cope with the knowledge that he or she carries a deleterious gene is strongly influenced by the sense of self, manifested through four interrelated aspects: body image, personal identity, self-valuation, and sense of mastery.

1. Body image has already been defined as the mental representations of the physical self. Body concepts may be distorted or realistic. The body may be the object of considerable attention and care,or subject to denigration and neglect.

2. Personal identity refers to the perception of oneself as a unique individual, separate from, but significantly related to others. In certain developmental phases such as adolescence or midlife, the sense of identity may become uncertain, accompanied by feelings of inner dishharmony and alienation. In psychotic states, the boundaries between self and nonself become blurred.

3. Self-valuation refers to the congruence or disparity between the self as per-

ceived and the self the person would wish to be, including physical self and self as a personality of significance within society.self-valuation may range from grandiosity through realistic self-acceptance to feelings of worthlessness.

4. Sense of mastery refers to an individual's confidence in the capacity to influence experiences and events. This may range from feelings of omnipotence through appropriate feelings of competence to a sense of being subjugated and overwhelmed.

Information about these four characteristics can be obtained by attention to the content and affect in the client's communications about the self, as well as observations of weight, grooming, carriage and clothing (keeping in mind the mores of the social group). Manifestations of distorted body image, precarious sense of personal identity, unrealistic self-valuation, or inappropriate sense of mastery indicate the need for great sensitivity in transmitting genetic information and careful follow-up.

Intrapsychic Defenses

Any among a wide range of psychic defenses may be employed to ward off unendurable information and the emotions associated with it. Some defenses are difficult to identify except in extended evaluation or psychotherapeutic relationship. Others, such as repression, denial, and isolation of affect can be recognized more easily by a perceptive interviewer; these are frequently observed when persons are confronted with unbearable medical realities.

1. The defense basic to most others is repression, which is the barring from consciousness of an idea, memory, affect, or fantasy. The operation is carried out unconsciously, and is thus outside of the person's knowledge and control. Repression is expressed as absence of awareness, or forgetting.

2. Denial is the rejection of a reality and its replacement in the mind with wish-fulfilling fantasy. It is expressed as disbelief or a distorted understanding that embodies substitute concepts.

3. Isolation of affect is repression of the emotion associated with an idea while the idea remains conscious. It is usually experienced as an absence of feeling related to a particular idea.

Even if such defenses are only temporarily employed, they may cause ill-feeling between client and medical staff unless they are recognized and understood. The client who has utilized repression may declare that the physician gave him scanty information, genuinely believing that the little he assimilated was all that he was told. The physician may respond defensively to what he perceives as unfounded criticism.

The "cool-as-a-cucumber" client, rational, devoid of emotional display (because of isolation of affect) may be one whose needs are neglected. He appears to assimilate information effectively, to cope competently. Unfortunately, the client or the family may subsequently be flooded with sealed-off feelings that were not released in manageable "doses," or feelings may "leak out" covertly and inappropriately.

Denial often serves as a red flag to medical staff who feel challenged to penetrate it: "He has to face facts!" Such professionals overlook the fact that denial serves to protect the client against incapacitating anxiety, depression, or despair and that it signals the client's need to confront painful issues at a tolerable pace.

The inevitability that clients will utilize defenses provides a central reason why genetic counseling must be a longitudinal process. The emotional impact of genetic findings may not be experienced until many months after they are presented. Staff and clients should be aware that professional help may be needed long after studies are completed.

Family Structure and History

The task of constructing and interpreting the genetic family tree is separate from the tasks of the psychosocial advocate. However, it is important for the advocate to know about family structure and history in order to understand the client's feelings and attitudes about family members who have been ill or died. There may be trust or hostility toward the medical caretakers of such relatives. There may be acceptance or self-blame associated with the illness or death. It is likely that such attitudes will be aroused again during discussion of genetic risks. Furthermore, unfinished mourning may be re-awakened:

> Mrs. E., the mother of an infant with cystic fibrosis, grieved with a duration and intensity disproportionate to her baby's mild manifestations of the disorder (mainly gastrointestinal, rather than pulmonary, with relatively longer life expectancy). Exploration of her despair revealed that throughout her childhood her own mother had been afflicted with incapacitating episodes of diarrhea. The mother's illness resulted in emotional deprivation of her daughter, who responded with sadness and rage. When the mother died of cancer, Mrs. E. was suffused with guilt related to her hostile feelings. Although Mrs. E's baby presented a different illness, the common denominator of bowel symptoms, as well as the sense of burden, produced overwhelming emotions in Mrs. E., which were related both to the present problem and the past experience.

The advocate should also assess present family relationships in terms of their potential for support as well as their vulnerability to strain. Clients may respond to the threat of a genetic disorder with angry protest ("Why *me?* It's not fair!") and with aggressive impulses that seek a target. Close family members frequently become targets. Members may engage in bitter recriminations, and the genetic information may be distorted to serve these needs:

> A young wife, Mrs. F., learning that her son's cystic fibrosis was inherited from her husband and herself, nonetheless lashed out bitterly: "It must be more on his side than mine because he's had 2 cases in his family and we've had none." Her parents, finding the idea of a "tainted" lineage unendurable, fully supported this position.

Family members may respond to the threat in individual ways which lead to alienation:

When Mr. and Mrs. G. bore a child with multiple defects caused by a chromosome abnormality, Mrs. G mourned openly. Fearful that she had "passed on" the defects, not wanting to know but fearing she must, she sought genetic counseling. Mr. G. refused to acknowledge the condition or to participate in counseling. He declared that the baby looked fine to him, and that if he couldn't see a defective condition it couldn't exist. He was impatient with his wife and gave her no emotional support.

Family members may have divergent beliefs about reproductive alternatives and come into conflict:

Sally H., the bright 16-year-old daughter of Roman Catholic parents, initiated contact and came to a genetics service with her parents in tow. Sally's brother suffered from Duchenne muscular dystrophy. Her mother believed that if Sally were proven a carrier, she must choose between two alternatives: avoidance of marriage and reproduction or marriage and submission to God's will thereafter. Sally renounced these alternatives, claiming that she could choose to practice birth control or to become pregnant, submit to amniocentesis and abort male fetuses. The mother–daughter conflict was profound and adversely affected every aspect of family life.

Religious Beliefs

An important component of the adaptation to stress is the search for meaning. Few find it tolerable to view tragedy as a chance event. Therefore, although the geneticist tries rationally to view genetic mutation or transmission as chance occurrences, few clients can at first accept this view ("Why?" is the urgent question). The client's interpretation of the meaning of a genetic defect may be strongly influenced by religious beliefs.

The defect may be seen as God's punishment for unacceptable thoughts, wishes, or deeds:

A young mother, Mrs. I., interpreted her baby's blood dyscrasia as punishment for the premarital intercourse which transgressed the teachings of her Church and family.

A father, Mr. J., considered his baby's Tay-Sachs Disease to be retribution for his earlier unwillingness to adopt a needy child at a time when he and his wife had believed themselves to have a fertility problem.

The condition may be interpreted as God's test or trial of the afflicted person or his parents. An individual may ward off resentment by believing himself to be specially chosen by God for his strength and capacity to care for himself or for his defective child.

It is relevant whether God is conceptualized as requiring unprotesting compliance, or whether personal feelings and individual choice are considered acceptable:

Mrs. K., the mother of a child with osteogenesis imperfecta, experienced severe distress because she believed that her resentment revealed an unwillingness to comply meekly with God's will and that this in itself was sinful.

Such beliefs and fantasies influence utilization as well as interpretation of genetic information. They influence the manner of coping with a child's affliction. For example, if parents see themselves as chosen by God to care for a defective child, consideration of institutionalization may be unacceptable, and such a suggestion may alienate them from medical staff. Religious beliefs also strongly influence attitudes concerning reproductive alternatives.

The strength of the client's Church affiliation is important. Not only may a clergyman be helpful in resolving conflicts related to theological doctrine, but also congregation members may provide a potentially supportive affinity group.

Ethnic Background

This influences attitudes toward a genetic defect as intensely as religious beliefs. For example, if a disorder is viewed by the ethnic group as an expression of evil in the afflicted person, acknowledgement of it may be taboo. There may be a culturally determined stance that defects must be denied.

Ethnic influences may mold attitudes toward reproductive choices as well as toward modes of responding to the birth of an afflicted child:

Mrs. L., a young Mediterranean mother, was a recent immigrant to the United States. She observed wistfully that had she remained on her native island, her baby with thalassemia major would have been given over to the care of the maternal grandmother, placed in a secluded corner of the cottage, and nourishment would have been withheld until the baby died.

In certain cultures, infanticide is practiced and accepted as humane and realistic. In recounting her story, this mother seemed to be expressing a wish.

It is important to determine if the client feels affinity with or alienation from his ethnic background. A sense of affinity with others sharing common values and attitudes about genetic defects will be a source of support. Alienation from ethnic and cultural roots exposes the client to inner conflict if he feels torn between divergent value systems.

Socioeconomic and Occupational Status

Peer groups of fellow workers, neighbors, and members of clubs or fraternal orders influence attitudes in ways similar to those derived from ethnic and Church affiliations. In addition, socioeconomic status affects the client's capacity to provide care for an afflicted child, expecially in terms of financial resources, health insurance coverage, and access to expert medical care.

Timeliness of Genetic Studies

Rarely is it justified to withhold genetic information from a client who requests it. However, it may be appropriate to postpone genetic studies, especially if other help is more urgently needed. For example:

Mr. and Mrs. M., married 5 years, had a healthy 3-year-old daughter. Mrs. M. had had multiple miscarriages and had experienced depressive reactions each time. She attempted to "fight off" depression with tranquilizers (possibly intensifying the depression). Her mother had experienced repeated "nervous breakdowns."

Mrs. M. declared that her daughter was a brat, had temper tantrums, and had a close relationship with her father that excluded herself. Mrs. M. could not enjoy her, and wanted another baby that would be hers. She believed she might currently be pregnant.

There was no known family history of inherited disorders, but because of the prior miscarriages the couple feared that the next baby might be defective. Were this so, they would want an abortion. They did not wish to adopt, nor had Mrs. M. been able to use contraceptives without disagreeable side effects.

Psychological intervention was clearly needed: evaluation of Mrs. M.'s depressive episodes and appropriate treatment, and consideration of therapy for the couple to help them clarify their wishes concerning reproduction and to strengthen Mrs. M.'s capacity to enjoy her daughter.

It was explained that amniocentesis could rule out only certain conditions, and could not be performed until later in the pregnancy. It was pointed out that in view of Mrs. M.'s longing for a baby and depressive reactions to the miscarriages, a decision to have a therapeutic abortion might be more difficult than presently supposed. It was suggested that a community mental health center would be the best initial source of help. After reassurance was given that Mrs. M. was not viewed as "crazy" but as troubled and in turmoil, the referral was accepted on the understanding that the M.'s could reapply for genetic counseling at a later time.

In such an instance, referral first to a separate facility for evaluation of emotional problems is indicated. A collaborative decision can be made with the therapist or counselor as to when genetic studies would be most helpful.

In other instances, referral may be indicated, but timeliness should be evaluated with the client. For example, if the client is mourning the actual or expected death of a loved one, genetic information might produce an emotional overload. Such a prospect should be gently but forthrightly discussed. If it appears that uncertainty and the fantasies that would substitute for knowledge would be more deleterious than information, the studies might best proceed. However, the client should be encouraged to postpone significant decisions based on genetic findings until his grief has abated.

One of the most critical aspects of timing concerns the counseling of children and adolescents. The case of Dorothy A., referred to earlier in this chapter, illustrates the damage that can result from adventitious information.

Dorothy A. was found to carry no deleterious gene. She had been needlessly burdened with a sense of impaired femininity, and had needlessly abstained from dating and mating. Even if correct genetic information and intensive psychotherapy were able to restore Dorothy's shattered self-esteem, she was by then at an age at which marriage was a more remote prospect and approaching the age at which the risk of other congenital defects might increase.

Withholding significant genetic information from youngsters is also risky. When a baby is born with a defective sexual apparatus (eg, Turner syndrome, testicular feminization) it is not uncommon for the physician to admonish parents, "You musn't let her know." Such advice tends to set in motion destructive sequelae. First, the caution itself conveys to parents the attitude, "This is so dreadful it shouldn't be talked about." Such a taboo will almost certainly reinforce the parents' guilt and anxiety. Just as grave, the interdiction against open discussion may interfere with communication between the parents or with other persons who might help the parents resolve their distress about the child. The taboo also fosters development of a system of secret-keeping in the family which may extend to other kinds of important information.

When a web of secrecy surrounds a child, the child inevitably senses from non-verbal cues that something is wrong. Without information, the child is likely to develop fantasies that may be more terrifying than the reality.

> Mary N., a 12-year-old with Turner syndrome, whose infertility was finally explained in a genetics clinic, sighed in huge relief and exclaimed, "Is that all? I thought it must be something much, much worse!"

Furthermore, secrecy may interfere with a child's sense of trust, a major foundation of a secure personality.

When should a child be told that the sexual or reproductive apparatus is defective? In our view, there is no ideal time to inform a youngster that he or she will be aberrant or unable to bear children. Nor is there an ideal time to inform the child that his or her body contains an unseen trait, a gene, that gives the child the potential of producing offspring who are ill, disabled, or who will die prematurely.

Informing a child is a longitudinal process. The first step is to help parents resolve their own feelings, since their attitudes will be transmitted with facts about the disorder. In the case of congenital defects, humane medical care should include such help during the post-partum period, and it should continue to be available. Even during the preverbal yerars, parents continually inform an infant about himself through the emotional qualities of their interactions with him.

During the period from approximately 3 to 6 years, children strive to develop a sense of sexual identity as girl-to-become-woman or boy-to-become-man. They inquire and should be informed in simple terms about sexual differences and reproduction. But there is much fluidity of boundaries between fact and fancy; the child only gradually develops a capacity for realism. There is also considerable concern about the intactness of the physical self. For these reasons, it is questionable whether information about an inborn disorder (unless it can be observed or felt) could be helpful to the child. More useful would be references to the fact that all persons are special in their own ways, and nowadays there are different ways to become a contented man or women. Some decide to have babies. Some have bodies not designed to bear children. Some adults may wish to adopt babies, or may choose other parenting roles, perhaps caring for children in their jobs. The door can thus be opened to further dialogue about the child's own potential.

By 8 or 9 years, most children have the intellectual capacity to understand more biological realities. Between then and puberty, sexual information begins to be assimilated with relative emotional neutrality. Facts about the child's special characteristics and potential for mating and reproduction may be accepted calmly. At 9 or 10 years, these issues are still quite distant and hypothetical, and may, therefore, be less threatening. Nonetheless, there is a risk that a genetic disorder will be interpreted as a badness inside, an evil influence, and this may arouse anxiety and guilt. The child will need help dealing with these feelings, as will the parents.

During puberty and early adolescence, the information (even if previously known) is likely to intensify the emotional turmoil typical of this developmental phase. This period is characterized by marked fluctuations in self esteem and fears of sexual inadequacy. That which was earlier accepted calmly may now arouse protest and misery. The information should not be withheld, but the youngster (and his parents) is likely to need much support in dealing with it.

In mid- or late adolescence, when mating and reproduction are imminent or existing realities, the information affects the young person's sense of adequacy. It may also influence interpersonal relationships.

In summary, a youngster suspected or known to carry a deleterious gene, or to be infertile, should have access to sensitive counseling that is adapted over the years to meet the child's developing cognitive potential and changing emotional needs. Parents should have access to professional help to enable them to deal constructively with the youngster's questions and emotional reactions.

Preparation for Genetic Studies

Psychological preparation for genetic counseling begins when the client considers seeking it. In the psychosocial evaluation, discussion of the client's personal concerns in itself furthers the preparation process.

In addition, however, the advocate should encourage the client to consider the feelings that may emerge as studies are carried out. The client should be helped to realize that extremely sensitive information will be needed; for example, data about consanguinous or out-of-wedlock mating and resulting offspring.* Defensive attitudes, resentment, feelings of shame may be aroused in kin as the family tree is constructed and relatives are faced with unwanted information about a "tainted" lineage.

The client should become aware of the likelihood that feelings of inadequacy and guilt may follow the discovery that he/she has a deleterious gene. This is not a matter of "programming" the client but, rather, or preparing him or her by giving reassurance that such responses are prevalent, and thus enhancing the person's capacity for self-awareness and self-mastery.

---

*In some instances, such information is more sensitive for staff with traditional attitudes about sexuality and reproduction than for clients espousing a more flexible morality.

PRESENTATION OF GENETIC FINDINGS

There is often value in including the psychosocial advocate in the conference(s) in which findings are presented to the client.

Supporting the Client's Understanding

From familiarity with the client, the advocate can note clues that the client is failing to understand information, needs repetition, or needs time for release of emotion. The advocate's presence may ease emotional tensions or facilitate continuation of the discussion after an emotional breakdown.

Safeguarding Self-Determination

Even when the geneticist wholeheartedly accepts the ethic of self-determination in his conscious thought, the client may sense unexpressed biases. The advocate should help counter-balance any such bias in the conference by tactfully encouraging open discussion of attitudes of all present toward sensitive matters. If the advocate has already assured clients of their prerogatives, this may enable them to be appropriately assertive in the session.

Such an occurrence took place with Mr. and Mrs. O. when the geneticist, believing he reflected both partner's wishes, supported Mr. O.'s opposition to having children. Mrs. O. stated with spirit, "You're not supposed to take sides." It then became apparent that the husband's "hidden agenda" had been to convince his wife that she should have no more children. In this case, self-determination led each partner toward opposing stances, and it was evident that continued marital counseling was needed.

The Issue of Burden

An individual's perception of the burden associated with a disorder significantly influences the use of genetic information for reproductive planning. Burden is perceived subjectively. One parent may view a brain-damaged offspring as a far greater threat to self-esteem, and to the potentiality for developing a satisfying parent—child relationship than a child with a life-threatening illness. Another parent may fear more the stigma and social ostracism related to a visible physical malformation.

Clients have varying levels of confidence in their capacity to cope with stress, whether the stress is that of restricting a child's diet (dealing with his protests without extreme guilt or anger), or that of enduring prolonged anxiety and grief when a child has a progressive, fatal condition.

Clients have varying degrees of assurance about their capacity to deal with the social and economic problems related to illness. They have variable access to sources of support in their families and communities.

The perception of burden is influenced by personality structure, value systems, socioeconomic realities, and by the extent to which the client is familiar with the disorder in question and is realistically aware of all that is involved in caring for an afflicted child.

The task of the advocate in this context is twofold: to listen attentively for clues to the client's perception of the disorder as burdensome, and to introduce discussion of stresses known to be associated with the disorder. The latter process must be carried out with great sensitivity, especially if the client has an affected child. It would be highly imprudent, for example, to overwhelm the parent of a child with cystic fibrosis with premature information about all the difficulties lying ahead, particularly if the parent is sustaining a need-fulfilling relationship with the child by denying the prognosis. It is essential to follow the pace of the client, testing out his readiness to explore various aspects of the illness with inquiries such as, "Had you thought about how a baby with this disorder might affect your family?"

Sensitive discussions should continue through follow-up: deepening a client's understanding of the burden a given disorder may impose, encouraging the client's own assessment of capacity to cope with this burden, fostering awareness of the potential influence of this burden on family relationships.

FOLLOW-UP

The alternatives available to a client who carries a deleterious gene can be complex. The physician or geneticist should explain medical procedures and genetic risks. The advocate should foster the client's understanding of feelings and attitudes about the available choices.

Accepting the Risk

A client may decide to do nothing to prevent pregnancy (leaving the outcome to nature or to God, in accord with beliefs) or actively seek pregnancy. Within ethnic or religious groups that proscribe contraception, either decision may be deemed appropriate. However, some criticism may be expressed by friends, relatives, or other associates. It may be helpful to alert the client to the uncomfortable feelings such criticisms could produce.

The client may need help in continuing to examine the issue of burden upon himself or herself and the family. If he or she already has an affected child, the advocate should encourage the client to consider whether he or she would be able to care for another baby, or whether the needs of the afflicted child would absorb so much time and energy that little would be available for a new baby or the marriage.

Understanding why it is important to have a child, what needs it would fulfill, what wounds it might heal, is essential for deciding whether to accept the genetic, social, and emotional risks described.

Contraception

Information about techniques of contraception is appropriately supplied by a physician or nurse. The advocate can help clients explore their attitudes in order to use contraceptives comfortably and effectively. If practicing contraception violates the dictates of the client's conscience, he or she is likely to feel guilt, and this may influence him or her to forget to use the contraceptive or to use it ineffectively.

The physician would consider medical indications in recommending a contraceptive, but may overlook personality characteristics which the advocate is better qualified to explore. For example, either a disorganized, forgetful woman or one with a history of depression is likely for quite different reasons to be a poor candidate for the pill. Some women feel aversion to touching their genitals and react against the diaphragm because of the self-manipulation it requires. Others object to the diaphragm because "planned sex" is less exciting or acceptable than spontaneous arousal. Some women shrink from the idea of the IUD, thinking of it as an alien object within themselves. Some men object because the condom requires an unwelcome interruption after they are aroused. Some believe it decreases penile sensitivity.

Sterilization

Sterilization is being sought with increasing frequency. Nonetheless, the idea arouses many fears. Unless a client is secure in his or her sense of sexual identity, there may be expectations that the procedure will result in diminished masculinity or feminity, or that the spouse will view the sterilized partner as less adequate. It has been pointed out that the wish to reproduce and the potentiality to reproduce are separate issues. Even if no more children as desired, a client may mourn the loss of fertility and grieve that the child-bearing phase of his or her life and marriage has ended.

A client may imagine that a child might die and he or she would then desire another child. The client may believe that a cure for the disorder in question will be found, making it safe to have more children. Some clients may consider that they might some day remarry and then wish for another child.

The family of an afflicted child is already stressed; sterilization may impose an emotional overload. The fears, needs, and wishes of each partner must be given careful consideration, and it must be ascertained that neither is denying the probable irreversibility of the procedure.

Interrupting Pregnancy

Abortion constitutes one of the most conflict-laden issues of our time, involving emotionally charged attitudes about the definition and meaning of life, about individual freedom and societal control, about relations between the sexes, and about the preservation of the species.

New methods of prenatal diagnosis make available new choices: whether or not to test for a defective fetus, whether or not to abort a defective fetus or one likely to carry a deleterious sex-linked genetic trait. An important concern that is sometimes minimized is the timing of abortion in relation to a procedure such as amniocentesis, which does not yield useful information early in pregnancy. At present, the client has little time between amniocentesis and abortion in which to make a complex decision. Furthermore, it must be made as the second trimester advances. Prenatal diagnosis may have been planned on the understanding that a defective fetus would be aborted. However, abortion may have an appreciably different meaning early in pregnancy, when the embryo is scarcely more than an abstract idea, than it has after fetal movement has been perceived. The time of "quickening" gives to many women their first awareness of the baby as a living being, and an interpersonal bond begins to be formed. Therefore, in the second trimester the decision about abortion may need thorough review.

Another special problem is presented when the fetus has the same disorder as a living child in the family. The idea of abortion may stir up repressed wishes that the ill child would die, and severe guilt and anxiety may result. The meaning of such an abortion for the ill child must also be considered. For example, it may strongly suggest to him that his parents wish that he had never been born, or hope that he will die.

Whatever choice is made, abortion is a complex issue. The possibility of ridding oneself of an unwanted, probably defective fetus may afford relief, but relief is likely to be mingled with grief at the loss of the healthy baby the parent wished to have had.

Artificial Insemination

In genetically appropriate instances, if a woman views pregnancy as a psychobiological experience of deep meaning and would feel deprived were it denied her, artificial insemination is a choice (this was the choice made by Mr. and Mrs. B.).

A couple should be encouraged to consider the significance of this in their marriage. The husband may view the procedure as an adulterous intrusion and may feel inadequate because his sperm are less desirable than those of other men. The wife may feel guilty for participating in this "unfaithful" act or may value her husband less. Such feelings may be ignored or denied at the time of decision-making, but they may emerge later. The couple should be apprised of this and encouraged to accept follow-up counseling.

Adoption

Adoption is often suggested to couples carrying deleterious genes. This is not always as facile as solution as is supposed. A couple whose resources are strained by a child with a serious disorder might not be considered good prospects as adoptive parents. Furthermore, the number of babies available fluctuates in proportion to demand. As safe, legal abortions become available, fewer unwanted babies are likely to be born. Furthermore, increasing numbers of unmarried parents are rearing their own children. On the other hand, there is widening acceptance of interracial adoptions. Since prospects for adoption are difficult to predict, it would be unwise for a couple to make a decision about reproduction on the assumption that adoption is an assured alternative.

Safeguarding Family Relations

In considering any of the choices discussed above, there may be marital or intergenerational conflicts. If need for professional counseling extends beyond the resources of the genetics service, referral to outside agencies should be effected.

Alternative Sources of Gratification

Boys have rarely envisioned parenthood as the totality of their adult experience, but this has been the expectation of many girls (although girls from small sectors of society have begun openly favoring goals other than motherhood because these seem to offer more potential gratification). It is constructive to acquaint all girls, but especially carriers of deleterious genes, with the variety of occupations that afford gratification of nurturant impulses (as well as other needs): medicine; nursing; and various therapies; education; child care; social work. Such professions are no less need-fulfilling for boys. Youngsters of either sex can also be encouraged to seek their sense of perpetuity through the building trades or creative arts.

It is also healing to foster such goals among older clients:

Mrs. O. whose husband opposed her wish for a fourth pregnancy after the death of a defective child, needed help not only in resolving her grief but also in filling existential emptiness. She had married young, had soon become pregnant, and had developed no interests outside of the home. Now her youngest (healthy) child had started school and Mrs. O.'s sense of significance was in jeopardy. It was learned that at the time of her marriage, she had set aside a wish to become a Licensed Practical Nurse. She was therefore encouraged to undertake volunteer work in the local hospital as a step toward deciding whether she still wished further training as a health professional.

CONCLUSION

The psychosocial needs and issues associated with genetic counseling are varied and complex. In addition to many reproductive decisions, clients may need to make major readjustments in their conception of themselves and their relationships to others and perhaps their total life styles.

Some clients may appear unable to assimilate and utilize genetic information constructively. In many such instances, a counseling "failure" can be averted if a necessary detour is made; that is, if the clients are first offered the psychotherapeutic services needed to enable them to confront painful facts and to use information realistically as a basis for decision making. If genetic counseling is to develop as a need-fulfilling human service, those engaged in the process must become sensitive to its psychosocial complexity. Whenever possible, a specially qualified professional person should collaborate with the geneticist or physician, serving as an advocate trained to evaluate the clients' social and emotional needs, and to help them accomplish the psychological tasks presented by genetic counseling.

SUGGESTED READING

Leonard CO, Chase GA, Childs B: Genetic counseling: A consumer's view. N Engl J Med 287:433–439, 1972.

Lieb J, Slaby AE: "Integrated Psychiatric Treatment." Hagerstown Md: Harper and Row, 1975.

McCollum AT, Gibson LE: Family adaptation to the child with cystic fibrosis. J Ped 77:571–578, 1970.

McCollum AT, Schwartz AH: Social work and the mourning parent. Social Work 17:25–36, 1972.

McCollum AT: "Coping With Prolonged Health Impairment in Your Child." Boston: Little, Brown and Co., 1975.

Olshonsky S: Chronic Sorrow. A response to having a mentally defective child. Soc Casework 43:190–193, 1962.

Prelinger E, Zimet CN: "An Ego-Psychological Approach to Character Assessment." New York: The Free Press of Glencoe. 1964.

Schild S: The challenging opportunity for social workers in genetics. Social Work 11:22–28, 1966.

Schild S: Social workers' contribution to genetic counseling. Soc Casework 54:387–392, 1973.

Schultz A: The impact of genetic disorders. Social Work 11:29–34, 1966.

Siggins LD: Mourning: A critical survey of the literature. J Psychoanal 47:14–25, 1966.

Taichert LC: Parental denial as a factor in the management of the severely retarded child. Clin Pediatr 14:666–669, 1975.

Tips RL, Smith GS, Lynch HT, McNutt CW: The "whole family" concept in clinical genetics. Am J Dis Child 107:67–76, 1964.

Turkow L, Lidz R: Psychiatric Considerations. Fertility Inhibition. In Hafez E, Evans T (eds): "Human Reproduction, Conception and Contraception." New York: Harper & Row, 1973.

12

Response to Genetic Counseling

Y. E. Hsia, BM, MRCP, DCH, and K. Hirschhorn, MD

INTRODUCTION

"Thank you, you have been very helpful, we feel better already."

It is gratifying for a genetic counseling session to end with an expression of gratitude and appreciation, but this can give a dangerously false sense of accomplishment to the genetic counselor. Outcome of genetic counseling should not be judged from immediate impressions or be based solely on whether subsequent children were affected or unaffected with a genetic problem [1, 2].

Some families are satisfied by reassurance and comfort, some seek enlightenment, some want practical support, while others demand nothing less than full cure and absolute guarantees of normality. Genetic counseling seeks to enlighten, and should be accompanied whenever possible by practical support, but may be more disquieting than comforting, and can never guarantee normality.

Many families with genetic disorders can be comforted and helped without being given any genetic information. For most genetic problems, the odds favor that a family's next child will be unaffected; conversely, if parents refrain from having any more children, obviously all genetic risks to progeny would be eliminated. Often, therefore, *absence* of genetic counseling would produce no harm and cause no grief. *Presence* of genetic counseling, on the other hand, can lead to confusion, anxiety, misunderstanding, or unfavorable outcome. In fact, incorrect genetic information may even turn out to be less harmful than right genetic information. How, then, can meticulously prepared genetic counseling be justified in place of giving simple comfort and casual advice? The answer is that families want to know and have a right to be informed.

This whole book is predicated on the presumption that genetic counseling demands thorough, skilled preparation and sensitive, lucid presentation. No proof exists yet that genetic counseling merits the time, effort, and training we claim it demands [3, 4]. Many individual families have been spared the recurrence of inherited tragedies by genetic instruction, and others have found relief following genetic reassurances, but some of these families might have had similar outcome without any genetic counseling [5]. Obviously, genetic knowledge would not have benefitted every recipient. To prove that genetic counseling is worthwhile, its effects in different situations have to be carefully assessed [3, 4].

Since genetic information will only be of value to those who are motivated enough to want it, sophisticated enough to understand it, and organized enough to utilize it, appraisal of genetic counseling has to consider who is likely to seek, to grasp, and to utilize genetic information. This necessitates studies of decision-making [6] (Chapter 10), psychological coping [7–9] (Chapter 11), reproductive planning [10] (Chapter 8), and resource utilization [11]. Prudent planners would be expected to make use of accurate genetic information, whereas heedless dreamers or impulsive gamblers would not become planners without drastic changes in attitudes and in behavior. Human nature is complex, inconsistent, and unpredictable; a wasteful spendthrift may plan carefully for his or her children, whereas a meticulously penny-pinching wage-earner might give no thought to procreative control. Furthermore, even the best laid plans may produce no results or unwanted results.

This chapter will examine the subjective reception of genetic information, objective measurements of its effects, and will suggest how appraisal of genetic counseling may improve services and support for families with genetic problems.

SUBJECTIVE RESPONSE

For any offered information to be used in personal decisions, it must be understood, remembered, believed to be true, and accepted as having personal relevance. Once accepted, the information may modify attitudes, alter plans, reinforce decisions, or stimulate action. For a family with a genetic problem, information may affect both non-reproductive coping and reproductive behavior.

Comprehension

Mr. & Mrs. A had an infant daughter with masculinization and severe electrolyte imbalance due to hormonal disturbances caused by the adreno-genital syndrome. They were told this was an autosomal recessive condition, with a one in four risk that any subsequent child would be affected (with masculinization in affected females). Their next child was a similarly affected daughter. They were very indignant, as they had expected three normal children before another would be affected. (After extensive re-explanations, they had a third affected daughter, but this time there were no recriminating claims of being misinformed.)

Every health professional has had similar experiences where patients had totally misunderstood apparently simple explanations [12, 13]. These are most apt to arise with statistical uncertainties and are to be expected in genetic counseling. Whatever the intended message, what was grasped by the listener need not correspond to what was told by the physician [2, 14–17]. However much a genetic counselor might blame the naivete of the counselee, the counselor's professional responsibility to explain is not fulfilled unless the explanation has been understood [18, 19].

Understanding demands attention, comprehension, and retention. These need freedom from distractions and release of undue tensions with careful preparation by the genetic counselor and sensitive presentation of the material. A written summary for the counselees may help ensure that information has been understood correctly [20]. For numerical risks, it often pays to rephrase predictions both in percentages and fractions, as well as in terms of being either unaffected or affected.

Retention

Mrs. B had been counseled that fetal diagnosis by ultrasonography could detect oligohydramnios and microcystic kidney disease, which had killed her previous infant. In her next pregnancy, she was convinced she had oligohydramnios, and was frantic since her doctor insisted that her condition could have many causes. Coincidental receipt of a follow-up enquiry from the geneticist reminded her (and the obstetrician) of what she had been told. Oligohydramnios was confirmed, she decided to have the pregnancy terminated, and the fetus was found to have severe microcystic kidney disease [21].

The genetic counseling given to Mrs. B was almost in vain, despite careful preparation and the issuing of an explanatory letter, since memory is fickle, but Mrs. B was reminded just in time by a routine follow-up enquiry.

Retention is especially unpredictable if a person is under strong emotional stress [9]. The minutest detail can sometimes be vividly recalled, or an entire episode can be totally forgotten. At times of medical crises, lengthy explanations are out of place and will rarely be remembered clearly. This is the time for simple words of comfort and reassurance (provided the reassurance is not false, because it can boomerang if it is remembered). This is also the time when explanations can be misunderstood, from partial retention of fragmentary facts, perhaps with totally distorted and garbled interpretations.

Mr. and Mrs. C were told at the birth of their child that the child's limb deformity could be fully corrected by orthopedic surgery. Eventually the child was found to have Larsen's syndrome with multiple joint dislocations and major visual handicap. It was difficult to make the parents understand that the visual problem was not correctable, and when they understood their child had incurable problems, they lost faith in all medical explanations or promises.

Belief

Belief requires faith both in the authority figure giving the information and in the substance of the information.

Belief in authority. When belief in the authority figure is misplaced, families with genetic problems are just as easily misled as those with concerns about cancer, mental illness, or any other handicap. Authority figures have led large followings into privations and even death, and faith healers have been flooded by adherents from among the worried, the ill, and the dying. These are powerful illustrations of how faith in an authority figure supercedes faith in objective facts.

The genetic counselor should try to discourage excessive reliance on himself or herself as an authority figure, but at the same time must establish some authority if the genetic facts are to be believed at all.

> Mr. D was from an ethnic and cultural minority with no traditional faith in Western medicine. In discussing medical facts with him, Dr. A, from a different ethnic group, was totally unaccepted. Dr. B, who was of the same ethnic minority, persuaded him of the validity of these facts by the argument "After all, you and I are both of the same culture."

This argument was unquestionably effective, but also undeniably dishonest, since persuasion was based on prejudice and not logic. More acceptable ways of establishing one's authority are by wearing badges of office, displaying diplomas and certificates, or by endorsements from referring physicians or colleagues.

Individual criteria for trusting an authority are irrational whenever they are founded upon personal or cultural biases. Mr. D rejected Dr. A solely upon racial grounds. Nonetheless, the objective of genetic counseling is to help a person or family with a genetic problem, and when one counselor will be more effective than another for whatever reason, it would be simpler to designate the first counselor as the authority figure for the sake of the counselee, and avoid confrontation on irrelevant issues in a counseling situation.

Undermining of authority. Authority can be undermined by conflict, confusion, or contrary experience. If there is conflict among the health professionals caring for a family, particularly within a genetic counseling team (see Chapter 13), this can undermine faith in the authority giving genetic information. This is one reason to refrain from overt criticism of other physicians or of previous medical care. Undermining of faith in any part of the care provided can raise doubts about all health care. Confusion can be caused if several authority figures give independent explanations, because minor discrepancies in their explanations can be greatly magnified in the minds of the recipients. There is a natural tendency to compare and contrast the different authorities, and this comparison is likely to be based on personality preferences at the cost of objectivity. Contrary experience occurs when a counselee's experience differs from what the authority has assumed or predicted. Irrelevant errors, such as forgetting a family's name or the sex of a child may seem unimportant, but can alienate the counselee; on the other hand, if a family has been led to expect one outcome and the actual outcome is different, this can cause the family to question anything else they have been told. The most notorious examples are related to life-expectancy and pregnancy outcome. Families may recount with triumphant glee how a patient has survived or achieved beyond a predicted limit, or may recall with disillusionment how an infant's sex was the opposite of what a doctor had promised.

In establishing an authority status, therefore, extravagant promises can backfire. In genetic counseling this should be forestalled by ensuring that counselees understand the limited certainty of genetic predictions. Similarly, physicians have to be warned about the limited accuracy of laboratory tests.

> Dr. E, an obstetrician, sent an amniotic fluid specimen to Laboratory A for chromosome analysis. The test report was that the chromosomes were normal female, 46XX. He had been given no cautioning about the possibilities of error. When a male fetus was born, the family lost faith in him and he vowed never to use Laboratory A again.

Belief in the content. Although acceptance of content is so predicated upon acceptance of an authority figure, genetic counselees should be encouraged to examine and judge information on its intrinsic merits. Information can be supported by published evidence, subjective experience, and logical criteria independent of reliance on authority.

Published evidence is valued especially by the highly educated, who can be given medical literature, which may be too frightening or technical for most lay readers. Brochure material produced by disease-related voluntary foundations can be useful, but is not always acceptable because of variable individual needs and inconsistent suitability of the material. Some of this material is confusing and misleading, while some is simple, clear, informative and reassuring. This material should be carefully assessed before it is recommended to families.

Subjective experiences from three sources, the counselee, the counselor, and other families with similar genetic problems, can also be very helpful. A counselee who has intimate familiarity with a chronic disability in a close relative knows far more about the impact of the disability than does the physician [22]. Experience with patterns of involvement and severity of a condition in relatives will bias a counselee very strongly toward the same patterns appearing in future generations. This bias may seriously hinder acceptance of information that is contrary to a family's prior experience. (On the other hand, appeal to prior experience, when a family has had normal as well as affected children, can be surprisingly effective reassurance of their obvious ability to have normal children.)

A counselor's prior experience can be a very persuasive credential for his acceptance as an authority figure. Many counselees enquire, often hesitantly but sometimes bluntly, about how many times a counselor had seen their particular problem before. Obviously they will have more confidence in the authority of someone who has had extensive experience than in someone who had never seen that problem before.

Outside testimony, from someone who has had personal experience with the same problem, can be a potent argument for acceptance of information. This approach has been used most effectively in chronic disease or rehabilitation counseling, and could be equally effective for a genetic problem from a patient or parent group. The dangers of using such a witness arise from biases of the volunteer or alienation of the counselee caused by personality conflicts with the volunteer, so no one volunteer will prove suitable for all counselees with a particular problem.

Use of logical criteria by counselees depends very much on the individual's capacity to weigh abstract concepts, but even the most unimaginative, unsophisticated person can be helped to see logical analogies with concrete life examples. For example, the variable sexes of children in different families can serve to illustrate predicted 50-50 odds.

Acceptance

Even when information is believed, it may not be accepted because of personal convictions of unique immunity or unique vulnerability. These are often based on past personal experiences (see Chapter 10).

> Mrs. F had had two children with X-linked recessive muscular dystrophy. She said she understood that the risk for her next son would be fifty-fifty, "but with my luck, my next one will be affected, too." She refused to contemplate having any more children.

When counselees' attitudes are immutably pre-set by non-genetic opinions and beliefs, then incompatible genetic information may be rejected even when fully understood.

> Mr. G, who was deaf from birth, stood up at a meeting for the deaf, after a talk on genetics, and affirmed (in sign language) "We all know that the reason children are born deaf is because their parents laughed at deaf people." There was general agreement with this viewpoint, and the argument that many people who had scorned deaf people still bore hearing children, failed to convince this audience.

> Mrs. H, from South-East Asia, had one son with a clawhand deformity. After she had seen many physicians and other health professionals, she finally confided to an Asian interviewer that she knew the cause of her son's malformation was her touching a toy crab when pregnant.

Partial acceptance. Genetic information includes considerations of cause, effects on the affected, possible treatment, expected complications, predicted risks to relatives, and reproductive options such as fetal diagnosis (see Chapter 1). Acceptance of a portion of this information by an individual or a couple need not imply acceptance of any other portion.

The most frequently rejected portions are the offers of options related to artificial insemination or adoption, and the most controversial option is that related to fetal diagnosis with its implied endorsement of intentional abortion (see Chapter 9).

The responsibility of genetic counseling is to include careful explanations of all relevant areas of a genetic problem for a family. Whether a family chooses to accept or reject any part of the explanation is a separate issue. The genetic counselor should be concerned with this issue only to the extent that rejection might be due to faulty presentation, and should be reconciled to selective acceptance of genetic options by a family.

Utilization

Acceptance of genetic information is determined by the interaction of a person's subjective attitudes toward the information, its manner of presentation, and its content. Skillful, sensitive presentation can enhance a person's acceptance of genetic facts, but may not influence how this information would be utilized [23].

Utilization, the extent to which genetic information is applied, should be the ultimate criterion for judging the value of genetic counseling. Application of knowledge requires that it be retained and accepted, used in the making of decisions, and then the carrying out of these decisions, with or without alteration of prior attitudes and behavior (see Chapters 7, 10).

Response to genetic counseling can result in utilization of genetic information both for non-reproductive purposes, in coping (see Chapter 11) and for reproductive purposes, in pregnancy planning (see Chapters 8, 9).

Non-reproductive coping. This entails a person's response to stress, which may be adaptive or maladaptive [24]. For a family with a genetic problem, non-reproductive stresses could arise from physical and mental disabilities with their consequences, fear of potential complications, or psychological damage to self-esteem [25]. How a person copes with these stresses is determined by personality, emotional status, and — to a certain degree — by knowledge [7–9]. Genetic information can facilitate the coping process by enhancing knowledge and promoting a person's perception of control over his or her own fate, because fear of the unknown too often exaggerates real threats to a family's health or future. Non-reproductive coping with a genetic illness differs little from coping with non-genetic illnesses [26], except for the threat a genetic illness poses to present and future relatives. This can undermine a person's self-esteem because the threat is seen to be inherent and internal, an intrinsic imperfection in a person's self.

Emotional. Emotional attitudes to genetic information are powerful forces determining acceptance or rejection of genetic information. By their nature these attitudes are irrational, and may resist appeals to reason. Since these attitudes fluctuate with time and are labile, success of genetic counseling can be critically dependent upon its timing and manner of presentation (see Chapter 1). Once genetic information has been grasped and retained it can facilitate realistic resolution of grief, anxiety, and psychological disturbances (see Chapter 11), whereas without accurate knowledge, a realistic attitude toward a genetic problem would not be attainable. When genetic reality is unpleasant, knowledge may impair a person's emotional ability to cope, so when a person's defense mechanisms are unrealistic, forceful intrusion of genetic information can be harmful [9, 27].

Emotional responses to genetic counseling will evolve with time as a person's emotional status changes. Therefore immediate effects of genetic knowledge on coping may fade without reinforcement, or without psychological support for dealing with emotional stresses. If a person's own resources are inadequate, long-term psychological counseling may be needed [9, 28].

When emotional attitudes become reconciled to genetic realities, then a person with a genetic problem can use genetic knowledge to help cope with practical problems [29].

Practical. Genetic problems can demand many practical responses from families, including adherence to recommended medical management [30], cooperation with detection of the problem in relatives [31, 32], constructive use of physical and mental resources to minimize handicaps, and adjustment of home environments for dealing with social aspects of a genetic problem. These practical demands would differ for each condition, and generally would depend more upon what can be done for the condition medically and nonmedically than upon whether the condition happens to have a genetic basis.

Coping with non-reproductive aspects of genetic problems are more significant than reproductive aspects for many families, because the non-reproductive aspects can be overwhelming, and often are of paramount importance to families. Genetic counseling can provide families with crucial information related to the cause, course, and management options for genetic problems which are relevant to non-reproductive coping.

Among constructive responses to genetic counseling are more realistic acceptance of the physical and mental limitations of a genetic handicap, more intelligent and responsible adherence to treatment plans, rejection of unorthodox health regimens, and channeling of energies into more constructive personal and community activities. These improved adaptations can all take place in the absence of genetic knowledge, but would be facilitated and expedited by the timely acquisition of appropriate genetic information.

Reproductive Planning

When there is a substantial risk of a handicapping genetic disorder, knowledge about this risk and its consequences should be a key factor in shaping the plans and hopes of a family about future children. This is the primary objective of genetic counseling [33].

Siblings and offspring of patients with disabling or disfiguring disorders are often fearful of having children, and are also often shunned by potential suitors.

The way families' attitudes toward reproduction are influenced by genetic information depends on the flexibility of these attitudes, which can have very complex components (see Chapter 8), and on how they view the genetic risk. When attitudes about having children are rigid for cultural or personal reasons, genetic knowledge can still affect how comfortable and secure families might feel about their attitudes; more flexible attitudes can be strongly influenced by genetic factors, but attitudes that are too evanescent will prevent genetic counseling from serving any useful purpose. Furthermore, hopes and fears related to child-bearing are modified by changing circumstances, so the persuasiveness of genetic information can vary considerably with time.

Desires about children must lead to decisions and actions for any substantive outcome to follow. Genetic information about reproductive options can contribute to these decisions prior to conception, or after conception.

Prior to conception. Marriage partnerships are generally based on romantic or mundane material considerations, and rarely on the specific genetic endowment of a person. Nonetheless, suitability for marriage as viewed by oneself or judged by others can be strongly influenced by genetic assumptions. Lay proscriptions against marrying into a family with mental disease or favoring a marriage partner of healthy stock are no sounder genetically than choosing mates by race ancestry.

> Miss J had always been fearful of getting married because her Caucasian mother had told her that her father was of a dark race. When she understood that there was very little probability of a child's complexion being much darker than that of either parent, this removed a major misapprehension about genetic threats to her unborn children.

Genetic information can be of great value in correcting misunderstandings and alleviating excessive fears held by relatives of these patients, but altering the attitudes of potential suitors depends on better genetic education of the general public, as few will seek or can be given genetic counseling about prospective mates until they have become serious suitors.

Accurate genetic information can damage a person's attractiveness as a marriage partner. Very unfortunate consequences of parental screening projects are the depressing ego-deflating effects that knowledge about being a carrier has on many individuals, and the stigmatization of identified carriers by others (see Chapter 14).

In the context of giving genetic counseling to a family, the implications for unmarried relatives must not be forgotten, as their responses to genetic information may seriously hamper their self-images, social activities, and future lives.

> Mr. K, a young Black student who refused to participate in a sickle cell screening project, said that he did not want to be tested, but if a girlfriend became pregnant and had a baby with sickle cell anemia, he would definitely have no more relationships with her.

When a couple has a casual consorting relationship, they may accept pregnancy, but would rarely seek genetic information. Few people would feel responsibilities about genetic risks without first developing a firm commitment for parenthood.

Before any pregnancy, or even at their premarital visit to their physician, couples may seek genetic information related to real or fancied genetic risks. Their response to genetic information would necessarily be in the absence of personal experience with child-rearing, and often without intimate knowledge about a genetic condition in question. Families who have already had a handicapped child or adult would base their decisions on their own exposure to the handicapping condition, and would tend to become more strongly deterred by a genetic threat, but with remarkable exceptions.

> Mrs. L, a cheerful young mother, had the Marfan syndrome. She was in a plaster cast for two years as an adolescent because of scoliosis, which finally needed a spinal fusion operation. She neither was deterred by the 50-50 risk for a child inheriting the Marfan syndrome, with similar risk of scoliosis, nor by the danger pregnancy might pose to her own health and life. She felt the ordeal she had as a teenager was quite bearable, and the risk to her in pregnancy was worth taking. (Her husband, however, disagreed vehemently.)

Choices open to a fertile couple regarding pregnancy are limited to allowing pregnancy, deferring pregnancy, sterilization, and alternative parenting options. Decision as to which of a couple is to be sterilized is rarely based merely on genetic status. Occasionally for dominant or sex-linked conditions, one partner can be designated as the one carrying the genetic risk, and this may persuade that person to be sterilized. Sterilization, once done, is essentially irreversible, but the other two choices are subject to change. Allowing pregnancy implies a willingness to accept any known genetic risk (or intention to have fetal diagnosis) and may result from a deliberate, careful weighing of the odds, a dismissal or denial of the risk, or a willingness to gamble (see Chapter 10). Deferring pregnancy can be for a multitude of reasons: personal, financial, or social, and does not necessarily imply any use of genetic information. Even when the deferral is for genetic reasons, it may equally indicate full intention to have a pregnancy in the near future, the putting off of a final decision, or relinquishing of all hopes for a pregnancy.

Alternative parenting options should be mentioned when giving genetic information to parents, although these are frequently rejected outright or found not acceptable by many couples. Artificial insemination is being conducted in a legal hiatus with ill-defined medical controls [35, 36], and has received little public support or acceptance. Nonetheless it does allow biological parenthood for the mother. Artificial enovulation and in vitro fertilization are controversial topics attracting much attention, but are not yet practical or safe enough to be recommended without major reservations. Adoption procedures are tedious and demanding, while adoptive children may be unfulfilling for some parents.

Mr. M, from a Mediterranean culture, had lost two children from severe congenital heart disease. He interrupted a genetic counseling session, conducted via an interpreter, to say in broken English "I want son . . . flesh of my flesh."

Other alternative parenting options include sublimation of parenting drives in teaching, volunteer activities with children, and fostering needy children. Some people derive immense gratification from these alternatives to biological parenthood, and these should be strongly encouraged from an early age for people who are infertile, though they will not satisfy everyone. Finally, it must be recognized that genetic risks may cause break-up of marriages, or engender extramarital affairs. It is doubtful whether a genetic factor alone is ever solely responsible for divorce, but if a marriage is unstable, the stresses related to a genetic disorder can aggrevate dissension and polarize the attribution of fault [37]. Some people find subtler solutions.

Mrs. N, whose first child had phenylketonuria, was not nearly as worried as her husband or the physicians about the risk of phenylketonuria for her next child. When the doctors announced to her that tests had shown the second child was unaffected, she said she knew there had been no risk because her husband was not the father. (If she had been terribly unlucky, the different father of her second child had about 1 chance in 70 of being a carrier too.)

After conception. Once pregnancy has occurred, parents still have several options related to genetic risks. They can choose to terminate the pregnancy, to continue the pregnancy, or continue the pregnancy with fetal testing.

Time constraints exist for these choices. Terminating the pregnancy in the first trimester is simpler, whereas mid-trimester abortions are more difficult technically and more of an ordeal psychologically as well as physiologically for the pregnant woman. Genetic reasons to terminate a pregnancy would apply to every pregnancy for a particular couple, and would be the same reasons as for avoiding a pregnancy. Hence, deciding to terminate a pregnancy would only occur after contraceptive failure, change of mind, or new information. When people have few qualms about the abortion issue and regard intentional abortions as a valid alternative to contraception, abortion to avoid a genetic problem may be an easy decision to make. If, however, new genetic information is obtained for the first time during pregnancy, and a couple has ambivalent feelings about abortion, choosing to abort can be a distressing ordeal (see Chapter 9). In early pregnancy a woman has to adjust to body and attitudinal changes. The sudden intrusion of genetic threats, plus urgent pressures to make life or death decisions about her fetus before the pregnancy has progressed too far, can create intolerable tensions for her. These tensions can impede wise, rational use of genetic knowledge. Whenever possible, families should be encouraged to seek answers to genetic questions before pregnancy [38].

Keeping a pregnancy in the face of known genetic risks can also be very distressing. Fears that a child will be afflicted can never be allayed until after birth, and doubts about pregnancy outcome can be magnified by genetic knowledge. For these reasons, although genetic counseling may be very important in early pregnancy to inform families about practical options, later in pregnancy the same information has no immediate practical value, and may only serve to disturb. Since ability to consider genetic information dispassionately may be compromised at this time, late pregnancy is not a good time to give genetic counseling.

Fetal diagnosis. The concept of fetal diagnosis for genetic disorders is relatively new, and is still unfamiliar to many. In learning about its applicability to their genetic problems, most families have little notion about its hazards, limits to its accuracy, and what it involves (see Chapter 4). Whatever practical knowledge a couple may have before pregnancy, reinforcement and reexamination of the option to undergo fetal testing in early pregnancy is advisable when the immediacy of the procedure will raise new questions. Because the procedure is not without hazard, and an abnormal test result is generally regarded as justification for therapeutic abortion, some couples for whom this test is applicable would reject it outright, some would decline having the test after careful consideration [39, 40], and some may refuse to believe an abnormal test result or to face abortion when confronted with this ultimate choice [41]. The experience of having amniocentesis can raise many doubts and anxieties in a person's mind [42], so these may well modify how a person views genetic risks. With time, as some mothers will be having repeat amniocentesis for several pregnancies, their experiences with previous amniocenteses will determine how they feel about undergoing the procedure again [43, 44] (see Chapter 9).

> Mrs. O had lost a brother and had a son with Duchenne muscular dystrophy. She had had two subsequent pregnancies monitored by amniocentesis; in both pregnancies the fetus was male and she elected to abort because of the 50-50 risk. In her next pregnancy, however, even when told (over-optimistically) [45] that fetal diagnosis for muscular dystrophy appeared possible, she decided against amniocentesis, because she could not countenance the deliberate destruction of yet another fetus.

OBJECTIVE RESPONSE

Measures of response to genetic information are of critical interest to all concerned with genetic counseling, because the usefulness or harmfulness of genetic knowledge can only be judged by objective observations of how it affects behavior. Justification for genetic counseling, its continuation, expansion or modification has to be based on studies of the efficacy of genetic counseling in conveying knowledge, in influencing decisions, and assessment of whether the ultimate outcome is beneficial [1, 3, 4, 46].

The importance of objective studies in response to genetic problems lies not just in the fascinating observations of human behavior, but in whether the studies can guide genetic counseling practices in the future. The many opinions, recommendations, and disputes about who should give genetic counseling [47], how it should be given [19, 33, 48], and what resources should be invested in its practice [49, 50] can never be resolved without careful evaluation of objective studies [1].

Because responses to genetic information are highly personal and liable to change with time, interpreting observed effects of genetic knowledge must be done cautiously, and with reference to relevant studies conducted in other disciplines [3] (see Chapters 7, 9, 11).

Early anecdotal accounts of response to genetic knowledge [51] were followed by reports emphasizing extended family studies [52], emotional and psychological factors [53], measures of reproductive outcome [54], of fertility patterns [5], estimations of effects on disease incidence in future generations [55] and comparisons of severity with risk [2]. Subsequently, there has been a flood of studies on genetic counseling [3, 4, 16, 17, 20, 29, 38, 46, 56], on the effect of specific disorders on families, including dominant [57, 58], recessive [2, 15, 16, 32, 34, 59, 60–62], sex-linked [38, 63, 64], multi-factorial [65–73] and chromosomal diseases [2, 13, 25, 74–77].

Knowledge

Acquisition of knowledge about a genetic problem is an interactional process (see Chapter 1) that requires the health professional to have the genetic knowledge [29, 47, 49, 50, 78, 79], to have adequate communication skills and effective interchange with the persons seeking genetic information [12–14, 18, 19, 80–82], and recipients to be motivated and receptive (see Chapters 10, 11).

Without understanding and retention of genetic facts, there would be no genetic knowledge and no possibility that decisions and outcome can be influenced or guided by this knowledge. Possession of knowledge is no guarantee that this knowledge will be used wisely (see Chapter 1) but genetic information must be known before it can be of any use.

All measures of genetic knowledge have shown that genetic counselees retain incomplete command of genetic facts [2, 3, 15, 16, 20, 25, 29, 32, 34, 38, 43, 44, 46, 54, 63, 71–73], but with care and attention to the psychological as well as educational aspects of genetic counseling, genetic counseless can be given a better grasp of genetic facts [70, 73].

Attitudes

Attitudes toward illness in oneself or in a loved one would be basically the same, regardless of whether the cause might be genetic or not [7, 8, 83–88]. There are stages of shock, denial, and grief — often complicated by withdrawal, anger, or depression – followed in due course by adaptive adjustments (Chapter 11). A person's passage through these stages can be helped by sympathetic, supportive intervention [89, 90]. For genetic disorders, there are direct implications for procreation as well as health, so reaction to a genetic problem affects attitudes toward both reproduction (Chapter 8), and health behavior (Chapter 7).

Attempts to probe the attitudes of persons with genetic concerns may fail because of their reluctance to reveal their private feelings or because of their limited self-awareness about their own true feelings. Behavior outcome is easier to observe, but the underlying forces motivating persons with genetic problems are much more complex and subject to fluctuations.

In view of the notorious difficulties in studying family attitudes toward health [8, 9, 23, 24, 26, 30, 31, 83, 90] or reproduction in general [91] (Chapter 8). appraisal of these attitudes in relation to genetic threats has to be carefully planned [1–4, 15–17, 20, 25, 27, 29, 34, 38–40, 42–44. 46, 56–58, 70–73, 75–77, 83]. Although such studies are fraught with pitfalls, nonetheless there is a great need for valid objective measurements of these attitudes and of how genetic counseling may modify them.

The crux of genetic counseling is to improve these attitudes, to make them more realistic, more rational, and, hopefully, more constructive. Eventually, justification for genetic counseling and judgment of how genetic counseling might best be delivered has to be based upon how families' attitudes might be benefited by genetic information.

Decisions

How a person makes decisions, and whether a particular item of information has influenced that decision, are very complex questions. Decision-making by trained physicians is not necessarily always rational [92, 93]. It is therefore not surprising that many decisions made by families with genetic problems appear irrational to observers [46].

Decision-making is a private subjective process [94] strongly biased by personal attitudes (see Chapters 7, 10) that can only be objectively observed when the decisions are manifested in outward behavior. This means that while measures of genetic knowledge are quantifiable and can be quite reliable, measures of attitudes and decision-making process can only be based on subjective opinions about how genetic information has influenced attitudes and decisions.

Attitudes and decisions are dependent in large part on personality strengths and resources, so even when someone attributes an attitude or decision to the influence of genetic facts, there can be no certainty that this opinion is based on valid insight. Controlled observations on statistically adequate populations [73] are almost impossible for genetic problems, because of the relative rarity of each genetic disorders, the great variability in their risks and consequences, and the complex behavioral factors that cause each individual to respond differently to the same genetic problem.

A formal decision-analysis schema has been proposed to help families decide whether to accept fetal diagnosis [95]. This is an interesting application of decision theory which has yet to be evaluated in field trials.

Outcome

Outcome of genetic counseling, or objective response to genetic information, are manifested in non-reproductive adjustments and in reproductive behavior.

Non-reproductive. Non-reproductive adjustments of attitudes, and coping behavior in response to the consequences of a genetic problem, can be studied in the same way that non-genetic health behavior and sickness behavior can be studied (see Chapter 7). Adaptive behavior may become more realistic when a genetic problem is better understood, but better understanding may be a result of rather than a cause of improved adaptation. Knowledge can dispel guilt and fears, leading to better capacities to cope, but objective evidence of how knowledge produces behavioral changes are difficult to assess.

Reproductive. Reproductive actions and outcome have two distinctly different portions, the first is intention to have a child or refrain from having a child, and the second is whether the intended outcome had successful fruition. In response to a known genetic risk, a couple may decide upon a given course of action that leads to unintended results. A wanted pregnancy may never come, or an unwanted pregnancy can arise accidentally [3] (see Chapter 8). Also, because genetic predictions can never guarantee normality, a low-risk for abnormal pregnancy outcome still involves *some* risk that the outcome could be unfavorable.

Studies of reproductive outcome after genetic counseling [5, 17, 54] have served to confirm that genetic predictions are reasonably accurate, but do not measure the influence genetic information made to reproductive decisions, or whether these decisions were rationally made or not.

SUMMARY AND CONCLUSIONS

Response to genetic counseling is highly subjective and individual. When a family seeks genetic information, a health professional is obliged to try to give accurate, balanced information in as effective and sensitive a way as possible, to help that family to a better understanding. The aim of genetic counseling is to confer understanding, so that a family can better anticipate and better adjust to practical consequences of a genetic problem, and also plan more wisely and realistically about whether to undertake any future pregnancies, with or without the option of fetal diagnosis.

Objective measures of response to genetic counseling are essential for justification of the time, talent, and resources spent in genetic counseling. Measures of genetic knowledge can be accurate and objective, but give no assessment of the usefulness of genetic information. Observations of attitudes and behavior can document familes' practical needs and can record their adjustment to a genetic problem, but do not necessarily indicate what influence genetic knowledge may have had.

Limited scope and validity of measuring objective responses to genetic counseling should not lead to abandonment of attempts to appraise its value. On the contrary, carefully designed interdisciplinary prospective studies may indicate how genetic information should be given and when familes benefit from genetic knowledge.

ANNOTATED REFERENCES

1. Murphy EA: Clinical genetics: Some neglected facets. N Engl J Med 292:458–462, 1975.
   A brief lucid tabulation of what we have neglected to find out about use and usefulness of genetics.
2. Leonard CO, Chase GA, Childs B: Genetic counseling: A consumers' view. N Engl J Med 287:433–439, 1972.
   A comparative study emphasizing the importance of disease severity from the consumers viewpoint.
3. Hsia YE: Approaches to the appraisal of genetic counseling. In Lubs H, de la Cruz F (eds): "Genetic Counseling." New York: Raven Press, 1977, pp 53–81.
   A discussion of multi-disciplinary approaches.
4. Godmilow L, Hirschhorn K: Evaluation of genetic counseling. In Lubs HA, de la Cruz F (eds): "Genetic Counseling." New York: Raven Press, pp 121–130, 1979.
5. Sultz HA, Schlesinger ER, Feldman J: An epidemiologic justification for genetic counseling in family planning. Am J Public Health 62:1489–1492, 1972.
   The procreative practices of families were found to be influenced more by past experiences than by the size of genetic risk.
6. Cohen J: The psychology of gambling. New Sci 68:266–268, 1975.
7. McCollum AT: "Coping With Prolonged Health Impairment in Your Chld." Boston: Little, Brown & Co, 1975.
   A sensitive supportive book for parents by an experienced social worker.
8. Burton L: "The Family Life of Sick Children." London: Rutledge and Kegan Paul, pp 65–78, 1975.
9. Rainer JD: Psychiatric considerations in genetic counseling. In Porter IH, Hook EG (eds): "Service and Education in Medical Genetics." New York: Academic Press, 1979.
   An excellent review of the psychiatric stresses met by families with genetic problems.
10. Hass PH: Wanted and unwanted pregnancies: A fertility decision-making model. J Soc Issues 30:125–165, 1974.
11. Chan JL, Hsia YE, Oglesby AC, Wright PM: "Genetic Needs Assessment for Hawaii." June, 1978. Special Report for Health Services Administration, US Department of Health, Education and Welfare, 1978.
12. Freemon B, Negrete VF, Davis M, Korsh BM: Gaps in doctor-patient communication: Doctor-patient interaction analysis. Pediatr Res 5:298–311, 1971.
13. Raimbault G, Cachin O, Limal JM, Eliacheff C: Aspects of communication between patients and doctors: An analysis of the discourse. Pediatrics 55:401–405, 1975.
    Disturbing examples of families' misunderstandings of medical explanations about the Turner syndrome.

14. Waitzkin H, Stoeckle JD: The communication of information of illness: Clinical, sociological and methodological considerations. Adv Psychosom Med 8:180–215, 1972.
    A lucid analysis of the process of learning medical information.
15. Sibinga MS, Friedman CJ: Complexities of parental understanding of phenylketonuria. Pediatrics 48:216–224, 1971.
16. Carter CO, Evans K, Norman A: Cystic fibrosis genetic counseling follow-up. In Mangos JA, Talamo RC (eds): "Fundamental Problems of Cystic Fibrosis and Related Diseases." New York: Intercontinental, 1973.
17. Reynolds B DeV, Puck MH, Robinson A: Genetic counseling: An appraisal. Clin Genet 5:177–187, 1974.
18. Bennett AE (ed): "Communication Between Doctors and Patients." (Nuffield Provincial Hospital Trust) London: Oxford University Press, 1976.
19. Kelly PT: "Dealing With Dilemma: A Manual for Genetic Counseling." New York: Springer-Verlag. p 143, 1977.
    A brief sensitive discussion of practical considerations in delivery of genetic counseling.
20. Hsia YE: Choosing my children's genes: Genetic counseling. In Lipkin M, Rowley PT (eds): "Genetic Responsibility." New York: Plenum Press, 1973.
21. Hsia YE, Berman R, Uemura HS: Fetal diagnosis of infantile microcystic kidneys. Pediatr Res 13:420, 1979.
22. Anon: Having a congenitally deformed baby. Lancet 1:1499–1501, 1973.
    A brief elequent personal experience.
23. McKinley JB, Dutton DB: Social-psychological factors affecting health service utilization. In Mushin SJ (ed): "Consumer Incentives for Health Care." New York: Prodist, 1974.
24. Livsey CG: Physical illness and family dynamics. Adv Psychosom Med 8:237–251, 1972.
25. Gayton WF, Walker L: Down syndrome: Informing the parents. A study of parental preferences. Am J Dis Child 127:510–512, 1974.
    See also reference 62.
26. Simons RC, Pardes H (eds): "Understanding Human Behavior in Health and Illness." Baltimore: William and Wilkins, p 718, 1977.
27. Antley RM: Variables in outcome of genetic counseling. Soc Biol 32:108–115, 1976.
28. Tsuang WT: Genetic counseling for psychiatric patients and their families. Am J Psychiatry 135:1455–1475, 1978.
    A good review of genetics for psychiatrists.
29. Clow CL, Fraser FC, Laberge C, Scriver CR: On the application of knowledge to the patient with genetic disease. Progr Med Genet 9:159–213, 1973.
30. Lasagna L (ed): "Patient Compliance." Vol 10 of "Principles and Techniques of Human Research and Therapeutics." Mt Kisco: Futura Publishing, p 162, 1976.
31. Zola IK: Studying the decision to see a doctor: Review, critique, corrective. Adv Psychosom Med 8:216–236, 1972.
    An excellent analysis of attitudes and motivations.
32. Beck E, Blaichman S, Scriver CR, Clow CL: Advocacy and compliance in genetic screening. N Engl J Med 291:1166–1170, 1974.
33. Fraser FC: Genetic counseling. Am J Hum Genet 26:636–659, 1974. The formal report and recommendations of a Committee of the American Society of Human Genetics.
34. Stamatoyannopoulos G: Problems of screening and counseling in the hemoglobinopathies. In Motulsky AG, Ebling FJG (eds): "Birth Defects: Proceedings of Fourth International Conference." Amsterdam: Exerpta Medica, pp 268–276, 1974.
    Disturbing social stigmatizations and misunderstandings following heterozygote detection in an Old World culture.

35. Curie-Cohen M, Lutrell L, Shapiro S: Artificial insemination by donor in the United States. N Engl J Med 300:585–590, 1979.
    A review of practices and outcome with recommendations.
36. Behrman SJ: Artificial insemination and public policy. N Engl J Med 300:619–620, 1979.
    An editorial comment.
37. Martin P: Marital breakdown in families of children with spina bifida cystica. Dev Med Child Neurol 17:757–764, 1975.
38. Emery AEH, Watt MS, Clack ER: The effects of genetic counseling in Duchenne muscular dystrophy. Clin Genet 3:147–150, 1972.
39. Hsia YE, Leung F, Carter LL: Attitudes toward amniocentesis: Surveys of families with spina bifida children, 1974, 1977. In Hook EB, Porter IH (eds): "Service and Education in Medical Genetics." New York: Academic Press, 1979.
40. Finley SC, Varner PD, Vinson PC, Finley WH: Participants' reaction to amniocentesis and prenatal studies. JAMA 238:2377–2379, 1977.
42. Elias S, Mahoney MJ: Prenatal diagnosis of trisomy 13 with decision not to terminate pregnancy. Obstet Gynecol 47:75s–76s, 1976.
42. Fletcher J: The brink: The parent-child bond in the genetic revolution. Theolog Studies 33:457–485, 1972.
    Thoughtful presentation of interviews with several couples undergoing amniocentesis by a sensitive, scholarly ethicist.
43. Robinson J, Tennes K, Robinson A: "Amniocentesis: Its impact on mothers and infants. A 1-year follow-up study. Clin Genet 8:97–106, 1975.
44. Blumberg BD, Golbus MS, Hanson KH: The psychological sequelae of abortion performed for a genetic indication. Am J Obstet Gynecol 122:799–808, 1975.
    Reports of interviews of several couples after termination of pregnancy post-amniocentesis, uncovering considerable unresolved psychological stress.
45. Ionasescu V, Zelleger H, Cancilla P: Fetal serum-creatine-phosphokinase not a valid predictor of Duchenne muscular dystrophy. Lancet 2:1251, 1978.
46. Shaw MW: Review of published studies of genetic counseling: A critique. In Lubs HA, de la Cruz F (eds): "Genetic Counseling." New York: Raven Press, pp 35–52, 1977.
47. Peterson ML: Should generalists provide genetic counseling? In Bergsma D, Hecht F, Prescott GH, Marks JH (eds): "Trends and Teaching in Clinical Genetics." New York: Alan R. Liss for The National Foundation–March of Dimes, BD:OAS XIII (6): 171–185, 1977.
48. Headings VE: Alternative models for genetic counseling. Soc Biol 22:297–303, 1975.
49. Childs B: Perspectives in medical genetics. In Bergsma D, Hecht F, Prescott GH, Marks JH (eds): "Trends and Teaching in Medical Genetics." New York: Alan R. Liss for The National Foundation–March of Dimes, BD:OAS XIII(6): 131–138, 1977.
50. Rimoin DL: The delivery of genetic services. Ibid pp 171–185.
51. Reed SC: "Counseling in Medical Genetics." Philadelphia: Saunders, 1955.
    A most readable early anecdotal review of families given genetic counseling.
52. Tips RL, Smith GS, Lynch HT, McNutt CW: The "whole family" concept in clinical gentics. Am J Dis Child 107:67–76, 1964.
53. Lynch HT, Krush TP, Krush AJ, Tips RL: Psychodynamics of early hereditary deaths. A Am J Dis Child 108:605–610, 1964.
54. Carter CO, Roberts JAF, Evans KA, Buck AR: Genetic clinic: A follow-up. Lancet 1:281–285, 1971.
    Report of whether genetic risks had deterred hundreds of counseled families from procreation.
55. Mayo O: On the effects of genetic counseling on gene frequencies. Hum Hered 20:361–370, 1970.

56. Emery AEH, Watt MS, Clack E: Social effects of genetic counseling. Br Med J 3:724–726, 1973.
57. Langsley G, Wolton RV, Goodman TA: A family with a hereditary fatal disease. Arch Gen Psychiatry 10:647–652, 1964.
    Attitudes and adaptations in a family with autosomal dominant pre-cancerous von Hippel-Lindau disease.
58. Lynch HT, Harlan WL, Dyhrberg JS: Subjective perspective of a family with Huntington's chorea. Arch Gen Psychiatry 27:67–72, 1972.
59. Childs B, Simopoulos AP (eds): "Genetic Screening." Washington, DC: National Academy of Science – National Research Council, 1975.
    A most important report of all aspects of this topic.
60. Crocker AC, Cullinane MM: Families under stress: The diagnosis of Hurler's syndrome. Post Grad Med 51:3:223–229, 1972.
61. Edwards JH: Genetic counseling in cystic fibrosis. Lancet 2:919, 1973.
62. Gayton WF, Friedman SB, Tavormina JF, Tucker F: Children with cystic fibrosis. I. Psychological test findings of patients, siblings and parents. Pediatics 59:888–894, 1977.
63. Hutton EM, Thompson MW: Carrier detection and genetic counseling in Duchenne muscular dystrophy: A follow-up study. Can Med Assoc J 115:749–752, 1976.
    An excellent survey of the experience in a long-established clinic.
64. Swinburne L: A measure of acceptance: Patients' attitudes to hemophilia. Lancet 1:1048–1049, 1977.
65. Freeston BM: An enquiry into the effect of a spina bifida child upon family life. Dev Med Child Neurol 13:456–461, 1971.
66. Walker JH, Thomas M, Russell IT: Spina bifida – and the parents. Dev Med Child Neurol 13:462–472, 1971.
67. Tew BJ, Payne B, Laurence KM: Must a family with a handicapped child be a handicapped family? Dev Med Child Neurol 16:Suppl 32:95–98, 1974.
68. Tew B, Laurence KM: Some sources of stress found in mothers of spina bifida children. Br J Prev Soc Med 29:27–30, 1975.
69. Dar H, Winter ST, Tal Y: families of children with cleft lips and palates: Concerns and counseling. Dev Med Child Neurol 16:513–517, 1974.
70. Rozansky GI, Linde LM: Psychiatric study of parents of children with cyanotic congenital heart disease. Pediatrics 48:450–451, 1971.
71. Kupst MJ, Dresser K, Schulman JL, Paul MH: Improving physician-parent communication. Some lessons learned from parents concerned about their child's congenital heart defect. Clin Pediatr 15:31–41, 1976.
72. Reiss JA, Manashe VD: Genetic counseling and congenital heart disease. J Pediatr 80:655–656, 1972.
73. Halloran KH, Hsia YE, Rosenberg LE: Effect of genetic counseling for congenital heart disease in a pediatric cardiac clinic. J Pediatr 88:1054–1056, 1976.
    A small controlled prospective study.
74. Smith DW, Wilson AA: "The Child With Down's Syndrome (Mongolism): Causes, Characteristics and Acceptance." pp 106, Philadelphia: Saunders, 1973.
    A valuable small monograph for health professionals and parents.
75. Antley MA, Antley RM, Hartlage LC: Effects of genetic counseling on parental self-concepts. J Psychol 83:335–338, 1973.
76. Humphrey Mrs. HH: Down's syndrome in the family: A personal perspective. In Lipkin M, Rowley PT (eds): "Genetic Responsibility." New York: Plenum Press, pp 69–70, 1974.
    A grandmother asks doctors to be thoughtful and caring.
77. Pueschel SM, Murphy A: Assessment of counseling practices at the birth of a child with Down's syndrome. Am J Ment Defic 81:325–330, 1976.

78. Childs B: A place for genetics in health education, and vice versa. Am J Hum Genet 26: 120–135, 1974.
79. Hsia YE, Bucholz KK, Austein CF: Genetic knowledge of Connecticut pediatricians and obstetricians: Implications for continuing education. In Hook EB, Porter IH, (eds): "Service and Education in Medical Genetics." New York: Academic Press, 1979.
   A questionnaire survey of knowledge and attitudes of practitioners.
80. Leventhal H, Fischer K: What reinforces in a social reinforcement situation – words or expressions? J Pers Soc Psychol 14:83–94, 1970.
81. Werner A, Schneider JM: Teaching medical students interactional skills. N Engl J Med 290:1232–1237, 1974.
82. Sasz TS, Hollender MH: A contribution to the philosophy of medicine: The basic models of the doctor-patient relationship. In Millon T (ed): "Medical Behavioral Science." Philadelphia: Saunders, p 432, 1975.
83. Drotar D, Baskiewicz A, Irvin N, Kennell J, Klaus M: The adaptation of parents to the birth of an infant with a congenital malformation: A hypothetical model. Pediatrics 56:710–717, 1975.
84. Natterson JM, Knudson AG: Observations concerning fear of death in fatally ill children and their mothers. Psychosom Med 22:456, 1960.
85. Friedman SB, Chodoff P, Mason JW, Hamburg DA: Behavioral observations in parents anticipating the death of a child. Pediatrics 32:610, 1963.
86. Kubler-Ross E: "On Death and Dying."New York: MacMillan, 1969.
87. Fischoff J, O'Brien N: After the child dies. J Pediatr 88:140–146, 1976.
88. Lewis E: The management of stillbirth: Coping with an unreality. Lancet 2:619–620, 1976.
   A deeply thought-provoking plea to help mothers grieve.
89. Heffron WA, Bommefaere K, Masters R: Group discussions with the parents of leukemic children. Pediatrics 52:831–840, 1973.
90. Kaplan DM, Smith A, Grobstein R: Family mediation of stress. Social Work 18:60–69, 1973.
91. Beach LR, Townes BD, Cambell FL, Keating GW: Developing and testing a decision aid for birth planning decisions. Organ Behav Hum Perf 15:99–116, 1976.
92. Todres ID, Krane D, Howell MC, Shannon DC: Pediatricians' attitudes affecting decision-making in defective newborns. Pediatrics 60:197–201, 1977.
93. Schwartz WB: Decision analysis: A look at the chief complaints. N Engl J Med 300:556–558, 1979.
94. Slovic P, Fishhoff B, Lichtenstein S: Behavioral decision theory. Ann Rev Psychol 28:1–39, 1977.
95. Paulker SP, Paulker SG: Prenatal diagnosis: A directive approach to genetic counseling using decision analysis. Yale J Biol Med 50:275–289, 1977.
   A detailed decision-model for couples to use in weighing pros and cons of whether to opt for amniocentesis.

13

The Process of Genetic Counseling

Ruth L. Silverberg, MSSA, ACSW, and Lynn Godmilow, MSW, ACSW

INTRODUCTION

The process of genetic counseling itself has not been studied or examined in depth. Years of study and research have gone into exploration of the scientific aspects of human genetics and more information is being gathered that could be of benefit to many persons as individuals. Learned theologians, ethicists, and lawyers are exploring the questions on how this knowledge can be used in a democratic society in a legal, moral and ethical way and are identifying some of the potential pitfalls [1—4]. Genetic counselors themselves are beginning to evaluate the effects of genetic counseling [5—14].

Our concerns in this chapter are very pragmatic: to explore the most appropriate process by which individuals or families can be given genetic information, in regard to their personal genetic makeup and their own personal reproductive decisions. Shakespeare said it beautifully in Henry VI: "For many men that stumble at the threshold are well foretold that danger lurks within."

THE SYSTEM AND GENETIC COUNSELING

Needs of the Client

In discussing an interacting process such as genetic counseling, we must start with the needs of the client [15]. In the absence of such needs, why spend millions of dollars on research and education of health professionals? To aid people who need medical help is the "raison d'etre" of all of the other areas of a health care system. Are services structured with this clearly in mind or are we so far from reality that clinical work is seen as secondary to research and teaching? We need to examine whether all of the laboratories, offices, and highly skilled, well-educated professionals are actually in tune with the purpose of their being, which is to bring better health care to those who need it [16].

A family or individual seeks genetic counseling for a variety of reasons. One family may believe in anticipatory planning and wish to know what the risks are for having a child with a genetic handicap. Another family may come to the doctor to find out what their symptoms mean and receives genetic counseling as a byproduct of diagnosis. Many patients come to specialized genetic counseling services with the statement "I don't know why I'm here; my doctor sent me." Expressions of need are not always verbalized or even consciously realized. Some patients who say they do not know why they have come may indeed not have been told, or may be denying or misinterpreting the information their doctors have given them. The woman seeking a reason not to procreate may be able to verbalize this feeling, or may prefer to cover it over by protesting how much she really wants a baby. She may then show unexpected relief when told she has a high risk for a child with a problem.

The importance of assessing the motivation and needs that bring a client in for counseling cannot be stressed enough. Information about motives should be elicited from the patient but should also be solicited from the referral source. A genetics counselor should not be surprised if a couple, when told they can bear healthy children, are disappointed rather than joyful. We obviously must not project our values onto the people whom we are trying to help. Patients seeking genetic counseling often have very definite but unrealistic expectations about what can be offered them in terms of information or intervention (eg, by prenatal diagnosis). Often patients have no concept of what will be involved in establishing the diagnosis of a particular genetic disease or how long the diagnostic process will take. All too frequently the patient has seen a number of medical specialists and consultants and has been referred to the geneticist as a last resort.

It is imperative from the start to ascertain the family or patient's expectations from genetic counseling, and to clarify how these needs and expectations may or may not be met.

Needs of the Service

A medical genetic service can include professionals from many different health-related fields and specialities. A genetic service usually is composed of a variety of professionals or paraprofessionals who have different interests, goals, and philosophies. Certainly while all are dedicated to the provision of good medical and clinical care for patients, there are other needs, spoken and unspoken.

If the team members can openly discuss and identify their needs and goals and integrate these into the provision of clinical service, the needs of both patients and the service can usually be met. Team members share the common goal of helping patients with the diagnosis and treatment of genetic problems. For members of the team who never meet a patient, this may seem a very remote goal. This goal can be personalized by making opportunities for these workers to meet with concerned families. This is a very effective way of promoting mutual respect. Physicians, geneticists, social workers, nurses, psychologists, dieticians, medical students, and religious counselors all approach families in different ways, with varied values and professional orientations as well as personal biases. The importance of mutual respect and understanding of the goals and efforts of each group and the conflicts this generates must be moderated by someone in authority. Research and teaching are two major components of university-based genetics centers. If the patients can be helped to understand these components and to see that they may enhance the service and help to provide valuable information to further medical understanding of the very problems with which they themselves are concerned, mutual respect and cooperation can result. If the attitude of the service is one of respect for the client and if efforts are made to assess and meet his needs, the contract for services and cooperation can be made without any hidden agendas. The needs of of the service can actually enhance the ego of the client in a time of stress, if well-handled. In addition, workers such as dieticians, social workers, nurses, and receptionists can be much more effective and helpful if their roles are interpreted positively to the patients. This can save the physicians time and be of benefit to the families who can make use of diverse sources of help to meet their particular needs. The reverse is also true: These specialists can reinforce the work the physician does or undermine it by a negative attitude.

Three Models of Genetic Counseling

Whether counseling is done in a private physician's office or a large medical center, it is an evolving process influenced by three different operational models: traditional, educational, and psychotherapeutic [17, 18].

1. Traditional: Patient-physician model. In this model, when the patient has what he understands to be an illness (see Rosenstock, this volume), he comes to his doctor for help, and the physician prescribes a course of treatment which may or may not include advice on procreation. This is clearly a directive approach. A spouse is not necessarily included until the point that information is given. When the doctor recognizes the particularly delicate needs of a concerned patient and the long-range significance of these needs, he will respond traditionally as the health advisor for his patient. After determining the extent of the problem and its possible solutions, he will talk with his patient and with other affected family members about the genetic risks and the options that he recommends for them. In this model the counselor uses his knowledge of the patient and family to help choose the best option for them.

2. Nondirective Educational Model. The first, and by far the most widely promoted model, is the non-directive approach.

In this model a counseling team is usually the rule and the process is seen as educational from the first contact. Relevant background information about genetics is given early in the relationship. The patient or family is provided with all the facts about the problem: diagnosis, prognosis, identification of family members at risk, magnitude of risk, alternatives with regard to future reproductive behavior, etc. Explanations are given for why various tests are recommended. The goal of self-determination is seen from the start. When all of this information is understood, the client is encouraged to make his own choices. The assumption is that such decisions will reflect the values and needs of the family and not necessarily those of the counselor or those of society. An integral part of this educational process is respect for individual differences and the psycho-social components of the situation. The counselor endeavors not to let his or her own personal value system impinge on the right of a family to self-determination. The need to give emotional support to families who are receiving stressful information is recognized and efforts are deliberately made to provide it.

3. Psychotherapeutic model. In this model, the patient is seen as an individual under stress with inner conflicts requiring resolution. Genetic counseling is seen as an opportunity to provide an emotional growth experience for the participants. Feelings are probed and worked through as part of the counseling process. This model requires a long-term involvement and a counselor trained and skilled in psychotherapy. It also requires that families who come seeking genetic information wish to involve themselves in a psychotherapeutic process.

Regardless of which model is followed, attention should be focused on consensus and continuity. All involved personnel must be aware of and comfortable with the model espoused, or they may work at cross-purposes. In the directive traditional model, the patient is advised to follow one course; in the nondirective model, he is provided with options; in the psychoterapeutic model, he is helped to explore and resolve his subliminal stresses. There are ethical and practical ways of giving people the help they need in making procreative decisions via all three models.

From our viewpoint as social workers, however, whose professional responsibility is to help clients find their own solutions among the available alternatives, the non-directive approach seems to be the most valid for genetic counseling. We believe the value system of the patient should be the determining force, not that of the counselor. We see genetic counseling as an educational process based on communication and support through which the patient will be able to make appropriate use of the information provided. Recognition of the client's right to self-determination is a presupposition, but when the client becomes a patient in a medical model, this right may be neglected in confusion between directive and nondirective counseling. In the psychotherapeutic model, which can only be practiced by trained therapists, emphasis is placed on recognition and resolution of inner conflicts. It is mandatory not only for all members of a medical genetic team to adopt a unified approach and also for them to make this approach clear to the referring physicians and other involved health professionals, so that the patient will receive reinforcement and support when they return to the primary physician.

STAGES OF GENETIC COUNSELING

Preparatory

In any of the above models, the first consideration of the counselor must be the readiness and receptiveness of the counselee. Following this assessment, genetic counseling is a process which occurs in several stages. Basically these include 1) the setting of a contract about what is sought and what will be provided; 2) the establishment of the diagnosis; 3) provision of information, ie, the formal counseling, encompassing discussion of the diagnosis, prognosis, persons at risk, magnitude of risk, possible reproductive options, and the possible outcomes of each option; 4) decision making, ie, the arrival by the patient or family at a decision about which option to choose; 5) reinforcement of this decision; and 6) monitoring of the results, ie, assessing the usefulness of the service to the persons served with identification of successes and failures so that unproductive aspects of the service might be modified.

1. The contract. An informal contract should be offered to the family relating to the nature of the process in which they are engaging. There must be understanding by all parties about what examinations, laboratory tests, and historical data are necessary. Discussion of what diagnoses are being considered should be entered into judiciously and with a sense of timing. Financial cost of the process is important and should be discussed fully at the outset, together with possible means of meeting these expenses (ie, health insurance or third payees).

Resistance may appear in this early stage of seeking help. The ambivalence people have when they approach something that may be traumatic must be taken into account. Broken appointments, refusal of important procedures, questions about the credentials of the involved professionals reflect this resistance and should be understood by the individuals initially in contract with prospective clients. Perhaps the family is not ready to deal with information of this kind. Perhaps one member is and another is not. Coercion by family or physician may be ill advised. The counseling effort may be wasted if this resistance is not confronted and worked through before continuing to another stage. If denial of the problem is too great and resistance cannot be overcome, it may be wise to defer counseling. The counselor and or the counseling team need to have awareness of the dynamics of human behavior and the defenses that come into play when a person feels threatened by potentially stressful news or emotionally charged information. To approach the giving of genetic information without senstivity to the psychosocial milieu which patients bring to such situations is unrealistically wasteful and futile. Each family is unique, and some information about the attidues of family members is a necessary element in preparing to counsel them.

2. The diagnosis. Accurate scientific knowledge of the medical problem and it's genetic aspect is a most important preparatory stage. Because so many genetic disorders are rare and complex, it is often necessary to review the medical literature. This is particularly true in genetics, a field that is acquiring new knowledge at such a very rapid pace. The time it takes for material to appear in the literature is frequently so great that a telephone inquiry of researchers and their most recent findings may sometimes modify counseling information. A physician who tells a family that they have a high risk of having a malformed child can do irreparable harm if that statement is not based on sound data. A social worker or nurse or other team member who gives well-meaning reassurance that is not compatible with reality puts vulnerable recipients at risk of considerable emotional damage. The giving of information, even at its least complex level, may be presented with overtones, biases, and value judgments that can create unnecessary difficulties for the patient

3. Provision of information. When the preliminary work has been completed, the information can be communicated to the family. The time and place of this communication can affect what is heard, what is understood, and how the information is subsequently used by the recipients. It is totally unacceptable to follow a meticulous diagnostic workup with a casual approach to the actual transmission of the genetic information. A 15-minute discussion in a hospital corridor or a brief telephone call may be expedient, but we cannot dignify such methods by calling them genetic counseling. Adequate transfer of information needs planned, uninterrupted time, at least one full hour, in a setting that is comfortable for clients and counselor. Intrusion by observers, unless welcomed by the counselees, can militate against adequate communications.

In addition to providing information, good communication must include the opportunity for patients to ask questions. Counselees should be encouraged to show feelings, express opinions, and reveal ignorance with no embarrassment. Judgmental remarks or attitudes shown by the counselor toward anyone present or not present is very unprofessional and can hinder the objectives of counseling.

Where people choose to sit and their posture, affect, and other nonverbal communication should be noted. The words used in genetic counseling can have strong influence on the layman who feels like a stranger in a foreign land. The psychosocial advocate can be most helpful at a counseling session by helping to reinterpret what is said and by enabling family members to raise questions or express differences in feelings (see Chapter 11, this volume). Emotionally charged words and judgmental attitudes can intrude upon communication because they disturb concentration, making it impossible for the listener to hear what comes next.

The words which most commonly cause problems are those that are judgmental in essence, such as "good," "bad," "right," "wrong." If we believe that a family has the right to self-determination we should make an effort, however, difficult, to avoid judgmental attitudes when we discuss this highly personal and frequently threatening material. The most glaring, albeit unintended error of this kind in our experience was the lapse of a highly qualified, kindly physician who told a group of parents of retarded children that their children's problems were probably due to "poor protoplasm." Even if this were a scientific fact and a well-meaning supportive explanation, it was a cruel and unnecessary statement, impugning the basic humanity of the children's biological makeup. Counselors should develop insight into their choice of words, manner of speaking, and responsiveness to inquirers. In addition, it is important for them to appreciate the distance which separates their scientific discipline and rationality from the average counselee who has a very different frame of reference. Use of technical jargon or discussion of unfamiliar concepts without explanation can destroy the counseling process.

4. **Decision-making process.** It becomes very quickly apparent in genetic counseling that a simple prescription does not suffice (as if it ever could in any good medical practice). The diagnosis is frequently complex, treatment (if necessary) is long, and decisions to be made about procreation are subject to many variables. People do not always behave in expected or rational ways. Some people come for counseling seeking a way to have healthy offspring; others surprisingly come looking for a reason not to have children at all. Because it is not socially acceptable at present, those seeking reasons against having children frequently mask their true motives. Still others are sincerely seeking facts on which to base a rational decision. To some a 25% risk factor is very low, and to others 1% may be too high (see Pearn, this volume). Attitudes toward a visible deformity and physical or mental retardation are different for each family. Cultural and emotional factors contribute to the vast attitudinal differences in people seeking genetic counseling. To one couple, a visible deformity would seem to be intolerable; to another, a serious physical handicap might be something they can cope with, whereas a mentally defective child would be an unacceptable source of great grief.

Members of the counseling team have some influence on the decision-making process from the first telephone inquiry. A family can be made to feel comfortable with their right to make their own decisions, or to feel uncomfortable or guilty because their feelings and needs meet with disapproval from the experts. This does not mean that the couples or individuals being counseled will not ask for or even demand opinion and advice from anyone they consider to be an expert. Their internal conflicts over a difficult decision would make this a natural reaction. (At a later date, if things do not go well, someone else can be blamed.)

The nonjudgmental attitude is particularly important for certain topics about which there is public controversy, such as abortion. The wrong words or attitudes can be most destructive to people going through crisis. Professionals need to examine their own biases in order to relate in a nonjudgmental way towards clients. In any genetic service, there may be professionals who have six children and others who believe strongly in zero population growth. There are staff members active in the women's movement, campaigning actively for the right of abortion on demand, and others who are active proponents in antiabortion groups. In order not to let our own personal prejudices influence the counseling process, we need to recognize these biases and strive to separate them form our professional responsibilities. If we do not strive to convey a nonjudgmental attitude, patients may be overly influenced by the attitudes of a counselor or confused by the lack of agreement among the team members.

We have seen a geneticist who was personally against abortion provide magnificiently balanced nonjudgmental information to a patient due to have an abortion. Once he had brought his own feelings to a conscious level and recognized the importance of self-determination for his patient, he was able to give unbiased information and appropriate professional support without antagonizing or upsetting his patient.

In a nondirective counseling situation, the counselee needs to be helped to weigh the alternatives in light of his or her own life-style and to make a decision consistent with it. Such a process can be enhanced by a social worker or other psychosocial advocate because their training is specifically for this purpose. If a physician does not wish to provide this type of support, a family service agency or clinical social worker can be of great help.

5. Reinforcement and follow-up. Follow-up and reinforcement must be integral parts of any genetic counseling process. Families may need to hear genetic information many times before they can actually understand the concepts or can accept the reality. From the outset, it must be made clear that the counselor will not slam the door once the formal counseling session is over, but that the patient or family are free, and even expected, to return with further questions or for further discussion at any time. The content of much genetic information is quite complex even for a well-educated and sophisticated patient. If emotional blocks to understanding exist, patients may need to hear the facts many times and in many ways before the blocks are removed.

Methods of follow-up can include telephone calls, further interviews when indicated or written material. An invitation to return without additional charges is an extended helping technique. Even if very few counselees use it, the self-selection process makes those few the most needful, and it seems important to provide this kind of opportunity.

It has been repeatedly demonstrated that a detailed letter summarizing the counseling for the patient is greatly appreciated, as it can be shared and used to refresh or correct recall of what was said. Families tell us that such letters become tattered with handling. They share it with extended family, clergymen, family counselors, schoolteachers, and other doctors. Sending a copy of such a letter to referring physicians will make them aware not only of the facts, but of how the facts were interpreted and communicated to the family.

Should improved tests or other new information become available, follow-up is needed to update families' knowledge of their problem or perhaps to offer new treatment. Often genetic services follow follow patients medically because they also provide ongoing management for various types of genetic disorders. In this situation, the whole process of adjustment to the illness, and awareness of its future course and meaning to the patient and his family, can be dealt with over a longer span of time. A primary physician offering counseling for the patient can continue to reinforce or help resolve feelings about the counseling as needed. For those who are sent to a genetic service for a short-term contact, special provisions have to be made for meaningful follow-up. For some, close cooperation with their community doctors is of great value; for those who have no such doctor or frequently change their source of medical care, this would not suffice.

Raising a handicapped child [21] or living with the threat of a possible handicap can be a tremendous burden for a family to carry, and frequently a parent group can share the strain, boost the morale, and funnel energies into cooperative, mutually beneficial activities. Dangers arising from groups can be seen in the spreading of misinformation or overidentification with negative elements in other families. An example of a group that seemed to be of harm to the members was a cystic fibrosis group that had at one point been supportive for its members, but had reached a stage wherein each death of another child threw the entire group into deep mourning. Experienced social workers and psychologists, familiar with group work, can help to steer or even terminate groups of this kind.

Fund-raising activities can also serve a purpose apart from the money they raise. For some people, they provide a healthy outlet for dealing with feelings of helplessness; for other families this does not work, and coercing them into activity of this kind by making them feel guilty can be destructive.

6. Evaluation of genetic counseling. To monitor the activities of a genetic counseling service, its goals and objectives have to be clearly stated [22].

A genetics service might well incorporate ways of monitoring itself. While national guidelines are being developed, it would be helpful to gather data on ways to help people by assessing what actually happens to families who receive genetics counseling. The methods of this kind of measurement would have to draw heavily from the social scientists. Follow-up questionnaires, in-depth interviews with families, attitude scales and sociologic data are useful tools for this kind of study. Methods of measuring subjective satisfaction with the counseling, although difficult, would be far more comprehensive than the measurement only of how many high-risk families did or did not have children. This kind of data might result in more realistic goal setting by the counselors.

In nondirective counseling, the goal is to provide the patient or family with all possible information about the genetic aspects of a problem: family members at risk, magnitude of risk, options for future procreative behavior, etc. In addition, support must be made available to families during their difficult decision-making periods. To evaluate the effectiveness of such a goal, the critical questions are whether genetic information was conveyed in a way which enabled the patient or family to make a decision appropriate for them. We cannot and must not measure effectiveness by placing a value judgment on the nature of the decision reached by a family.

Despite a clear intention to provide nondirective counseling, centers which have attempted to evaluate their own effectiveness have often fallen into the trap of measuring their success by whether or not a family decision seemed rational to the counselor. In other words, despite the intention to encourage self-determination in the decision-making process, most counselors have a hidden agenda. When looking at the results of their counseling, their criteria were whether or not a family behaved according to their own precepts. All of us have our biases and prejudices and cannot avoid nonverbal transmission of them to some extent. We can, however, attempt to recognize these biases in advance and suppress them as much as possible. Certainly when examining the outcome of counseling, we must recognize that these decisions are extremely personal ones which cannot be measured by the standard of what we would do in a similar situation. Evaluation of the nondirective counseling process must be based on whether a patient or family comprehended the counseling facts and used them in their decision making. Some effort must also be directed towards determining if the family felt that the counseling service was supportive [23].

In the directive situation, it is far easier to measure or evaluate effectiveness. One needs only to determine if the patients followed advice or not. In this situation, use of the options offered would indicate that the counseling was successful.

Mr. and Mrs. A were referred for genetic counseling when their first child, a 4-month-old son, was admitted to hospital for diagnostic evaluation of muscle weakness. Tests established a diagnosis of Werdnig-Hoffman disease, a recessively inherited problem with progressive deterioration, weakness, and eventual demise. (Brain function is not affected and prenatal diagnosis is not possible because the basic biochemical defect is unknown.)

Mr. and Mrs. A had an excellent marriage based on honest openness, love and a mutual desire for a large family. They were devastated by the diagnosis and especially distraught about the genetic implications for future progeny.

The A's were told that there were four options for them in terms of future parenthood: 1) not to become parents, 2) adoption, 3) artificial insemination with donor sperm; 4) acceptance of a 25% recurrence risk in future pregnancies.

It was clear that the first option was totally unacceptable to this couple, and they dismissed it from consideration. Initially they were enthusiatic about artificial insemination with donor sperm. Over a period of several months, however, as they discussed this between themselves and with the genetic counseling social worker, they decided that psychologically they would not be able to accept such a child as their own. This eliminated option No. 3. For the next several months they examined the issue of adoption. They contacted adoption agencies, private adoption resources, and other adoptive parents. They continued to discuss their feelings with each other and with the social worker. Finally, they came to the conclusion that they were not able to accept an adopted child as their own and thus elminiated option No. 2.

At this juncture, at age 11 months, their son died. Almost immediately Mr. & Mrs. A decided to go with option No. 4. Mr. A put the final decision quite succinctly: "The worst that will happen is that we will have another beautiful baby whom we will love and who will love us and whom we will lose before he or she is a year old." Thus this couple decided that they could live with the burden of another affected child if necessary, and were willing to risk a 25% probability of having that happen.

A pregnancy was conceived almost immediately, which unfortunately resulted in the birth of a daughter who was also affected with Werdnig-Hoffman disease, and who also died at age 11 months. After their daughter's death, Mr. and Mrs. A reexamined their options and chose adoption. They have since adopted two healthy children and Mrs. A has had a tubal ligation.

Can we judge that we failed in counseling because they had a second affected child? We think not. Mr. and Mrs. A did not think we failed them. They fully comprehended and understood the counseling. They carefully thought through and worked through each option and made the decision that was right for them in the context of their needs and goals and the limits of their endurance at that time.

The importance of evaluating the effectiveness of genetic counseling should not be minimized. It is imperative for us to determine if we are reaching the goals we set for ourselves and if not to determine why not, so that we can modify the process accordingly. Evaluation is important for either nondirective or directive counseling, and some comparisions need to be made between methods.

SUMMARY AND CONCLUSIONS

Genetic counseling can be offered in many different settings, by various professionals, in a variety of different approaches. Regardless of who provides the counseling and under what auspices and in what manner it is offered, the process requires several basic components in order to be successful.

The needs and goals of the patient or family must be clearly spelled out and coordinated with the needs and goals of the counselor. A counselor should decide whether the approach will be directive or nondirective, and the chosen philosophy must be adhered to consistently for each patient by all involved.

Competent determination of medical history and pedigree, careful physical examination, reliable laboratory tests, and the establishment of an accurate diagnosis are essential before counseling can be given. Insight into the psychosocial and cultural orientation of the family to be counseled can optimize the communication process.

The formal counseling must be done carefully and with close attention to use of terms, with explanations of difficult biologic and medical concepts in language understandable to the client.

Reinforcement by written review of the counseling, telephone contacts, and in-person follow-up are valuable. Provision of support services and professional help in working through the decision-making processes are important additions to the formal counseling. Judicious collaboration with other professionals and paraprofessionals can enhance the counseling process.

Evaluation of the counseling process and its effectiveness, as well as comparison between the directive and nondirective approaches, needs to be carefully conducted, and changes made wherever appropriate. Only by constant examination of what we are doing and what effect it is having can we continue to upgrade the quality of a new and important aspect of medical care.

REFERENCES

1. Milunsky A, Annas GJ (eds): "Genetics and the Law." New York: Plenum, 1976.
2. Harris M (ed): "Early Diagnosis of Human Genetic Defects: Scientific and Ethical Considerations." Fogarty International Center Proceedings, No. 6, 1972.
3. Fletcher J: The brink: The parent-child bond in the genetic revolution. Theor Stud 33:457–485, 1972.
4. Reilly PR: "Genetics, Law, and Social Policy. "Cambridge: Harvard University Press, 1978.
5. Emery AEH, Watt MS, Clack E: Social effects of genetic counseling Br Med J 1:724–726, 1973.
6. Tips RL, Lynch HT: The impact of genetic counseling upon the family milieu. JAMA 184: 183–186, 1963.
7. Antley MA, Antley RM, Hartlage LC: Effects of genetic counseling on parental self-concepts. J Psychol 83:335–338, 1973.
8. Leonard CO, Chase GA, Childs B: Genetic counseling: A consumers' view. N Engl J Med 187:433–439, 1972.
9. Reynolds BDV, Puck MH, Robinson A: Genetic counseling: An appraisal. Clin Genet 5:177–187, 1974.
10. Carter CO, Evans KA, Roberts JAF, Buck AR: Genetic clinic: A followup. Lancet 1:281–285, 1971.
11. Hsia YE, Silverberg RL: Genetic counseling: How does it affect procreative decisions? Hosp Pract 8:52–61, 1973.
12. Emery AEH, Watt MS, Clack ER: The effects of genetic counseling in Duchenne muscular dystrophy. Clin Genet 3:147–150, 1972.
13. McCrae WM, Burton L, Cull AM, Dodge J: Cystic fibrosis: Patients' response to the genetic basis of the disease. Lancet 2: 141–143, 1973.
14. Rosenstock IM, Shaw MW: The evaluation of genetic counseling: A committee report. Public Health Rep 92:332–335, 1977.

15. Hall J: The concerns of doctors and patients. In Hilton B, Callahan D, Harris M, Condliffe P, Berkely B (eds): "Ethical Issues in Human Genetics. New York: Plenum, 1973, pp 23–32.
16. Murphy A: Clinical genetics: Some neglected facets. N Engl J Med 292:458–462, 1975.
17. Capron AM, Lappe M, Murray RF, Powledge TM, Twiss SB (eds): "Genetic Counseling: Facts, Values and Norms." Birth Defects Original Article Series (In press).
18. Headings VE: Alternative models for genetic counseling. Social Biology 22:297–303, 1975.
19. Fraser FC: Survey of counseling practices. In Hilton B, Callahan D, Harris M, Condliffe P, Berkely B (eds): "Ethical Issues in Human Genetics." New York: Plenum, 1973, pp 7–13.
20. Taichert L: Parental denial as a factor in management of a severely retarded child. Clin Pediatr, Vol 14, pp 666–668, 1975.
21. McCollum A: Coping with prolonged health impariment in your child. Boston: Little, Brown, 1975.
22. Hsia YE: Appraisal of genetic counseling. In Lubs HA, de la Cruz F (eds): "Genetic Counseling." New York: Raven, 1977, pp 58–81.
23. Hsia YE: Parental reactions to genetic counseling. Contemp Obstet Gynecol 4:99–106, 1974.

14

Genetic Screening

Marc Lappé, PhD

INTRODUCTION

The enlightenment of a target population about an unfamiliar genetic problem is the challenge to genetic counseling in any genetic screening program [1, 2].

There are three basic groups of genetic screening programs [1, 3–5]. In *presymptomatic* screening, an individual potentially affected with a genetic disorder is sought before the disorder becomes evident symptomatically. The objective here is to identify such individuals in time to initiate preventive treatment before irreversible damage has been done. Phenylketonuria (PKU) testing of newborn infants is the archetype of presymptomatic genetic screening, but childhood screening for visual and hearing defects [4] and adult screening for diabetes, glaucoma, or hypertension [5] can all uncover previously unsuspected preclinical disorders of genetic origin. With few exceptions, there is no conceptual or operational difference between screening for a genetic disorder or screening for any non-genetic medical disorder [5].

In *parental* screening the objective is to help prospective parents determine whether a future child is at risk of a genetic disease. Tay Sachs testing [6], sickle cell carrier testing, and also testing of pregnant mothers for α-fetoprotein (for neural-tube malformations [7–10], or for fetal chromosome abnormalities, [11–13], are all examples of parental screening. Parental screening is not unique to genetic disorders, since premarital detection of blood group incompatibilities, venereal diseases, or prenatal detection of microbial infections are analogous situations.

In *research* screening, the objective is to collect data for eventual determination of applicability for presymptomatic or parental screening, but the participants can only be given unproven information of doubtful interpretation. Testing for hyperlipidemia in childhood [14], of XYY males at birth [15], for Huntington

295   © 1979 Alan R. Liss, Inc.

chorea in adolescence [16], or prenatal detection of hemoglobinopathies [17] are all examples of research screening. Many of the issues raised by these studies are not peculiar to genetics, but the basic issue of informed consent is complicated by the psychological impact of learning that one may have a genetic disorder [18].

Additionally the issues are totally different among these three types of screening.In the first two (presymptomatic and parental), individuals to be tested will likely have had no prior personal experience condition in question, and they need to be made aware of the condition and the risks to themselves. Only then can they decide whether to participate in the testing program. Those unaffected, possibly affected, and definitely affected each have to be given a clear understanding of the results of the tests, the implications to themselves, and what actions are open to them. In the third type, research screening, there is an even greater responsibility to forewarn the target population that data collected would be inconclusive although possibly frightening [18, 19].

Hence genetic counseling must be an essential component of any type of genetic screening program [1–3]. Counseling can provide the critical link between medical knowledge and rational personal action. There are ever-present chances that test results gleaned through screening programs will be ignored, denied, suppressed, rejected, misunderstood, or overinflated, so the counselor has a key responsibility both as a proposer of test participation and as an interpreter of test results.

The task of the genetic counselor within the context of screening programs differs radically from traditional forms of genetic counseling, both in terms of counselee experience and counselee motivation [19]. Most individual families seeking genetic counseling are strongly compelled by the distress or anxiety accompanying the discovery of a genetic problem affecting a family member, often a severely handicapped newborn infant. They are seeking, retrospectively, means to anticipate or prevent recurrence of the problem. With screening, on the other hand, a central coordinated community progect is seeking, prospectively, means to identify affected individuals or parents with high genetic risks to progeny, by convincing or compelling members of a large normal population to submit to testing [1, 6]. Hence the counselor's previously reasonable expectation, that his client *wants* genetic information, is clouded by conflicting motivations and desires.

In the screening situation, a person may have been tested unwittingly, unwillingly, or with total misunderstanding of what the test can or cannot reveal. This chapter will discuss issues related to the quality of the tests, the responsibilities of the testing program, the rights and requirements of individuals being tested, and societal concerns and obligations. It should be kept in mind that a screening program, if poorly designed or operated or not backed up by adequate counseling services, can do more harm than good [2].

Technical Considerations

Any individual or agency operating a screening program must be deemed responsible both for the quality of the testing and for the quality of the information being given to individuals being tested [16]. This means that at least moral accountability for the quality of the tests is assumed by a physician or health professional recommending or promoting a screening program, and that whoever provides genetic testing must also provide adequate informational services. The person giving genetic counseling as part of a screening program, therefore, should be familiar with the nature of the tests being employed, their accuracy, limitations, interpretations [20].

As a general rule, the population being tested should be told of the limits to the proposed tests as part of an "informed consent" procedure [21]. Such procedures, where they exist, will provide clients with an appreciation of the nature and limits of information they may receive from the screening tests *before* results are obtained.

Acceptability

The test has to be one that causes minimal inconvenience, discomfort, or hazard to individuals being tested and should be also reasonable in cost. This entails using tests that require simple collection, proccessing, and storage procedures, backed up by an efficient record-keeping system as well as a satisfactory testing technique [22, 23]. Safety cannot be taken for granted. When testing for PKU, the heel-prick necessary to draw an adequate sample of blood from the infant has, on rare occasions, caused bone injury, tissue infection, and other complications. Similarly, pregnancy screening for abnormal fetuses in alpha fetoprotein-positive mothers by amniocentesis appears to carry a finite risk of precipitating an abortion [24].

Accuracy

Technically, a test can be tuned to different levels of sensitivity and reliability. Conceptually, virtually all tests measure a quantity that has a normal range, with abnormal results that exceed the normal range.

A test is *sensitive* if it can detect a wide difference between levels in different individuals. The test is *consistent* if it yields closely reproducible results when used repeatedly. The test is *reliable* when there is minimal technical variability and narrow biological variation among normal individuals. Even when a test is technically and biologically accurate, it still may lack adequate *specificity* if the range of normal values is wide. Consider a test to measure blood phenylalanine for detecting PKU: While one in 15,000 infants can be expected to have abnormal blood concentrations of phenylalanine due to PKU, if there is also one chance in 15,000 that a normal infant may yield a similar test result because of inaccuracy, insensitivity, or statistical variability of the normal range (over six standard deviations from the mean for a Gaussian distribution), then half of all abnormal test results will be from normal unaffected infants. In actuality, test results for PKU are often ambiguous because of other causes of abnormal blood phenylalanine levels and retesting and follow-up are necessary to ensure a precise diagnosis [3, 25].

Ambiguity

Depending on the test, it is quite possible for the assay to measure substances other than that intended [3, 22, 25]. Microbiological assays can be confounded by infected specimens or by antibiotic therapy; tests for certain body constituents are interfered with by various medications; some tests measure a group of substances, such as tests for sickle hemoglobin. By the summer of 1976, 40 states had sickle cell screening programs, with over 250 screening centers offering one or another of the proliferation of commercially available diagnostic tests for hemoglobin S; some of these cannot distinguish hemoglobin S from other abnormal hemoglobins (see Table I), an untenable situation from a medical standpoint [26].

False Negatives

If a test is insufficiently sensitive, technically inaccurate, clerically mislabeled, or biologically inconsistent, an affected individual may be missed by the test. In testing for PKU, false negatives have occurred from administrative errors (see Chapter 15) or by testing too early, before blood levels of phenylalanine have become elevated [3, 27]. Whatever the risk that false negatives might arise, it is the responsibility of a genetic screening program to minimize these risks, and the genetic counselor has a moral if not a legal obligation to warn prospective participants of limits to detectability. A program that uses suboptimal procedures so that a proportion of positive subjects is missed is inadequate. In general, false positive tests of the condition in question are preferred to false negative ones, because follow-up can be arranged [1–3, 20, 22, 23, 25].

False Positives

Any individual detected by testing as being possibly affected or abnormal may be falsely identified, and it is desirable both to reduce the fasle positive rate to a minimum and to rely heavily on confirmatory tests before labeling any individual with a definite diagnosis. A counselor who negligently passes on misleading data from such tests to clients is legally and morally derelict. For example, if a couple should act on faulty information in a way which results in injury (eg, a misdiagnosis of predicted sickle cell disease in future children leading to attempted fetal blood sampling and a miscarriage), the counselor may be subject to lawsuit [28] (see Chapter 15).

Whenever an individual is told that a test result is ambiguous or abnormal, anxiety is bound to be provoked. Therefore a prudent measure would be to forewarn all prospective participants that false positive results may be obtained which will necessitate confirmatory tests.

Confirmatory Testing

Except for tests with absolute reliability and unequivocal interpretation, screening programs should have built-in arrangements for confirmatory testing [2, 3, 6,

TABLE I. Factors Affecting the Accuracy of Solubility Tests for Hemoglobinopathies*

A. Patient-factors leading to false-positive results
   1. Dysglobulinemia
   2. Recent transfusion
   3. Hyperlipidemia
B. Patient-factors leading to false-negative results
   1. Anemia (hemoglobin less than 7 gm/100 ml)
   2. Recent transfusion
   3. Age at testing (newborns and infants less than 6 mo. of age)
C. Practitioner-factors leading to inaccurate test results
   1. Failure to perform hematocrit or hemoglobin assay
   2. Failure of conduct electrophoresis
   3. Use of improper reagents (eg hydrous instead of anhydrous potassium salts, potassium salts, poor grades of saponin)
   4. Improprer use of reagents (eg prior to reaching room temperature)
   5. Improper preparation of blood samples
   6. Failure to run controls
   7. Measurement errors
   8. Interpretation errors

*Adapted with permission from Schmidt and Wilson [26]. "Accuracy" as used here means both precision and reproducibility.

22]. Even when a screening test has a high false positive rate, if it can identify a small segment of a population as being at high risk for a given condition, it can focus confirmatory tests in an effective and efficient way, provided the people so identified are not unduly alarmed or harmed by being singled out.

Client Expectations and Screening

Different screening programs will likely differ in how they arouse expectations for genetic advice, information, or other help. A client's conceptual orientation toward genetic information will be shaped largely by the nature of the education program that accompanies screening. Prescreening pamphlets, brochures, or briefings are powerful determinants of the mindset of the target population, conceivably an-antagonizing some, confusing some, leaving others passive or undecided, and only motivating a fraction of the population to participate. If the program is presented as offering positive, real-life options to parents who want to have a child free of genetic disease, as in the case of some Tay-Sachs screening programs, then carrier parents entering postscreening counseling will be better prepared to discuss realistically the problems associated with prenatal diagnosis and selective abortion.

In contrast, if participants have not been adequately prepared or have persistent misconceptions about test results, identified carriers of parental screening programs may be frightened, depressed, or otherwise upset at learning their test results. At least for Tay-Sachs programs, prospective parents can be offered the option of prenatal diagnosis. For sickle cell screening, the only options presently available are artificial insemination or nonreproduction, neither of which may be acceptable.* Presenting these options in the absence of adequate education (for participants and planners) may understandably raise the specter of genocide in the minds of some participants.

Even when screening is predominantly for research, as in prospective studies or data-gathering programs, counseling should not be neglected, for it may be precisely in such programs that the counselor's special skills and services are most needed to help participants understand the meaning of test results [29].

For example, screening programs for a complex class of disorders in lipid or triglyceride metabolism may generate considerable anxiety in the screened population. Initially, such programs are almost certainly "research" in nature in that they are designed to determine the as-yet-unknown sequelae of different genetically based lipid or triglyceride disorders. Many of these disorders are associated with an increased risk of heart disease and early death [30]. At-risk parents whose children are invited to participate in such programs will therefore require counseling so that they can handle their fears and anxieties. Although this type of screening begins as presymptomatic screening, it becomes parental screening of a special kind, in which usually one of the parents not only is a carrier but also is genetically affected. The increased risk of coronary vessel disease and ancillary consequences of the atherosclerosis that accompanies type II disease are problems that require scrupulous and careful counseling, since they threaten not only the health of future children, but also the life plans of an affected parent [20].

Purposes Served by Screening Programs

To understand the relationship between counseling and screening, it is desirable to appreciate the objectives of the various forms of screening. Genetic screening programs may be instituted to serve a range of related but not mutually exclusive purposes (Table II).

Signers of a 1972 document that enumerated these purposes agreed that priority should be given to those programs that provide health benefits to families or individuals [29]. In view of these cosigners, the value of screening programs that are limited to data-gathering and research procedures would be enhanced by adjunctive health services. "Eugenic" screening programs were considered unfeasible and unjustified to the extent that they arbitrarily constrained the reproduction of genetically specified individuals but not other members of the populace who may also carry deleterious genes. Future restrictions of individual lives and invasions of privacy in reproductive choice were considered largely medically unsubstantiated and unjustified on the grounds that they did not constitute a legitimate excercise of the police powers of the state. It is well to keep in mind that genetic counseling is currently unlicensed and unregulated and could readily be turned to

*Research on prenatal tests for hemoglobinopathies using fetal or placental venipuncture will make such diagnoses possible, but likely more risk-laden than simple amniotic fluid sampling. Use of restriction enzymes on amniotic fluid cells to elucidate base sequence changes indicative of aberrant globin chain synthesis is a more promising avenue of research.

TABLE II. Purposes Served by Screening

A. Education –	To provide reliable information to a couple or person regarding their genetic status by which they can make informed reproductive decisions.	
B. Research –	To contribute knowledge about the population frequency or birth incidence of medically significant genotypes and/or to establish the extent of human genetic polymorphisms.	
C. Public Health –	To reduce the incidence or burden of genetic disease through prenatal diagnosis and selective abortion or through early detection and treatment of affected individuals.	
D. Eugenic –	To reduce the frequency of deleterious genes in the population through constraints on reproduction of carriers.	

the services of interests that would identify eugenic or population limitation ends as legitimate primary goals for counseling. Nevertheless, whereas some genetic counselors concur that attention to potential deterioration of the gene pool is desirable, few if any would advocate eugenic measures to improve the pool.

TYPES OF SCREENING PROGRAMS

Prescriptive Screening

The traditional form of medical screening, which is intended to find cases at risk for disease before damage is done, is well known and requires little emphasis here [4, 5]. In prescriptive screening, tests are used pre-emptively for case-finding with the intention that medical intervention will head off the sequelae of incipient disease. Usually, the test picks out a critical level of a well-understood biochemical indicator of later disability (eg, the Guthrie test for raised plasma phenylalanine levels), after which treatment may be instituted. Prescriptive screening is therefore primarily for case-finding and therapy. Its health benefits are usually calculable, and, except where these conflict with the costs of the program, they are recognized as the key rationale for conducting the screen. Where reasonable therapeutic benefits *can not* be expected in genetic screening, the program should neither be termed "prescriptive" nor presented in a manner that implies that medical benefits are forthcoming.

Prospective Screening

In prospective screening, tests are used experimentally to determine if a given marker or other identifying characteristic is associated with disease or disability. In the design of prospective studies, otherwise indistinguishable but marker-identified at-risk persons are followed longitudinally in parallel with normal cohorts to determine if the indicator in question is in fact associated with an increased risk of morbidity. Most prospective screening is therefore initially a nontherapeutic form of experimentation.

In a prospective study, the first group of subjects may thus be subjected to unnecessary testing, stigmatization, or anxiety. Frequently, as in the case of prospective screening of newborns, or children for muscular dystrophy [31], hyperlipidemia [14], hypertension [32], schizophrenia [18], or chromosome imbalances [15, 33], preemptive therapies may be nonexistent or purely experimental. Hence, the screener is engaged in an excercise to obtain information likely to be critical to *future* at-risk populations, but he cannot offer the promise of a therapeutic intervention to his present subjects. When genetic screening programs contain research objectives — as distinct from therapy — they should be labeled as such, so that the participants' expectations are tempered and participation can be based on meaningful informed consent.

Retrospective Screening

In retrospective screening, older individuals with a genetic or chromosome marker that is suspected of being associated with disease or disability (eg, an extra Y chromosome) are sought with the expectation that the causal relationship can be traced. As a form of research screening, retrospective screening faces difficulties in case selection and research design (eg, adequate control populations) that may compromise the validity of its results. Often an indeterminate portion of the marker individuals may have died or become otherwise inacessible at the time of the screen, so that random selection, the standard requirement for surveys of this kind, will be difficult to achieve. These and other objections are among those cited in the controversy over XYY screening where prospective screening was considered the only valid way to establish the relationship, if any, between institutional prevalence and behavioral deviancy [15, 33].

Because of difficulties in design, research screens that are set up to determine the incidence and nature of a given condition retrospectively are inferior to those that monitor newborn populations for incidence statistics. In the instance of population prevalence studies in adults, however, acceptable informed consent procedures are more easily devised than in newborn prospective studies. In the latter type, a satisfactory role for the counselor has been ill-defined, and the public health justification for screening is less persuasive than where newborn populations are being screened with the promise of realizable therapies.

Multiphasic Screening

In multiphasic screening, the objective is generally to use one or more samples of body fluids to ascertain a profile of critical metabolites or other substances that might indicate a genetically based predilection for disability. The Massachusetts metabolic screening program is a representative example [22].

In Massachusetts circa 1973–1975, some 15 different genetic abnormalities were sought from blood or urine specimens taken from the newborn. The Massachusetts program used three separate tests:

1. An umbilical cord blood sample taken at birth to screen for potentially lethal disease like galactosemia, where the earliest possible detection is vital.

2. A peripheral blood sample taken soon after dietary protein has been introduced (usually 2–4 days after birth).

3. Urine samples taken when the infant is 3–4 weeks old.

The utility of the last approach is because separation and identification of compounds in urine by paper chromatography can identify abnormalities of membrane transport that would be missed if only the blood were examined. Approximately 260,000 urine tests were done each year, an average of about three tests per patient. The "extra" testing was required to establish the significance of any "abnormal" result by eliminating false positive results due, for example, to bacterial contamination. A number of consecutive positive tests were required for confirmation of a metabolic disorder requiring further investigation.

In its current form, the Massachusetts program screens 85,000–90,000 infants per year and detects 30–35 infants with some metabolic disorder, of whom about 60% subsequently manifested clinically significant disease [22]. The Massachusetts program cost about $200,000 per year, or about $1.75–$2.00 per infant screened. About 80% of the program's annual budget came from a federal grant (Children's Bureau, U.S. Health Services and Mental Health Administration); the remaining 20%, from the Massachusetts Department of Public Health, and individual payments.

Recent technical developments in biomedical engineering are beginning to make mass multiphasic testing appear more feasible. Automated tests are available to detect at least eight significant metabolic disorders: PKU, maple syrup urine disease, homocystinuria, histidinemia, valinemia, galactosemia, and arginiosuccinic aciduria (and nongenetic neonatal hypothyroidism). While some current tests rely on bacterial growth inhibition assays of the Guthrie type, other developments that would facilitate automation are on the horizon.

Gas chromatography [34], centrichromatography [35], thin-layer chromatography [36], and chemical ionization mass spectrometry [37], coupled with computer diagnosis, have made feasible quantitative analyses of biologically important compounds at the nanogram (10^{-9} gram) level. The use of stable, nonradioactive isotopes promises to permit safe and quantitative means of follow-up screening for rare disorders. For example, nonradioactive amino acids can be used in conjunction with gas chromatography and mass spectrometry to define a number of disorders of leucine and tryosine metabolism, (eg, propionicacidemia, isovalericacidemia, and maple syrup urine disease [38]. In view of the recent demonstration of apparently effective dietary treatment of these disorders [20], this may prove an extremely valuable technique. Obviously, the genetic counselor should be aware of these developments in order to anticipate increasing demands for his or her services.

Antenatal Screening

Antenatal screening will allow the detection of a serious defect or chromosome structural abnormality at a time (14–20 wk) when abortion is feasible. This type of screening presents the greatest challenge to a genetic counselor. The medical literature has increasingly dealt with the utility and versatility of prenatal diagnosis for the detection of chromosomal anomalies, a variety of single gene defects [39–41], and neural tube defects [7–10]. Most of these diagnostic procedures entail amniocentesis and may ultimately obviate the need for all but confirmatory intrauterine diagnosis. The U.S. collaborative study on amniocentesis, involving over 1,000 cases, has shown this technique to be reasonably safe [22]. Following any successful amniocentesis procedure, unfavorable information about the fetus would afford the parents and attending physicians specific data that could be used as a basis for an abortion decision.

Down syndrome screening. It is common now at major medical centers for pregnant women past the age of 35 to be offered amniocentesis because of the increased risk of bearing a child with a chromosome abnormality (specifically Down syndrome) in this age group [40, 41]. A formal proposal for such chromosome screening, beginning with women over 40 and gradually becoming a routine part of prenatal care for all pregnant women, has already appeared [13], and according to the NIH Record of August 27, 1974, has been strongly endorsed by the then acting director of the National Institute of Child Health and Development.

Maternal blood. Maternal blood testing has been used to detect women at risk for Rh antigen sensitization and thereby to anticipate fetal hemolytic disorders. This has been supplemented by the development of a blood test that measures a serum fraction indicative of neural tube defect in the fetus. Pioneered by Brock and his colleagues in the early 1970s [42, 43], this test for α-fetoprotein has been developed to the point where it allows a rapid initial screen of high-risk populations (eg, populations with an inordinately high incidence of affected births [44]. A confirmatory test for abnormally elevated α-fetoprotein in the amniotic fluid allows for the high suspicion of spinal cord defect. Problems of interpretation of what constitutes a diagnostic concentration of this protein remain, however, and should alert the counselor to mistaken diagnoses, since there seems to be a finite, albeit small, false positive rate, as well as a false negative rate, for amniotic fluid α-fetoprotein, as well as post-amniotic tap fetal loss [24].

Abortion. The outcome of prenatal diagnosis is statistically weighted toward the positive for most of the women who undergo it. The news is usually reassuring, and the pregnancy can then proceed. It is important to remember, however, that until recently the chief purpose of prenatal diagnosis was to afford couples the option of abortion of an affected fetus. There may be a rare case in which prenatal daignosis will be done for information purposes only, to help a family prepare for a coming ordeal, but, by and large, affected fetuses will be aborted. In fact, in the early period of development of amniocentesis it was forcefully argued that such a test — expensive and risky — should not be done unless the woman had agreed in advance to abortion if the test were positive (John Littlefield, personal communication, September 1972).

Conditions for which prenatal diagnosis is available encompass a wide range of severity, and it is probable that all these conditions may not be regarded equally as candidates for abortion. It may be possible to get wide social argreement on abortion for a disease that is irrevocably fatal and whose course is exceptionally pathetic, such as Tay-Sachs. But that agreement can begin to break down, depending on the nature of the condition under consideration. Should one routinely abort for Down syndrome? A formal proposal for universal prenatal diagnosis in hopes of eliminating this condition has been proposed [13], but it is by no means certain that everyone would agree, given its range of severity, and the differences with which mental retardation is regarded in various cultures.

The dilemmas grow more difficult as we move into the area of treatable conditions. Since some palliative therapy is available for XXY boys will manifest Klinefelter syndrome at puberty, should they be aborted? What about hemophilia? For this, antenatal selection entails abortion of all male fetuses, affected or not, yet it could be reasonably well controlled, providing resources — blood and money — were available [45].

Choices are murkier still when considering conditions where the risk of a behavioral disorder (such as XYY) is largely unknown, or where the disability is not life-threatening (as in Turner syndrome), or where questions solely of parental preference are involved (like gender).

Indeed, widespread acceptance of prenatal diagnosis, which seems almost inevitable, makes it critical that these issues be throughly explored by prospective and practicing genetic counselors. The question of setting any limits for prenatal diagnosis should be posed now. What diseases generally warrant abortion? Should the availability of treatment matter? Should the expense of treatment matter? How much freedom should parents — or the profession — have, to decide what is and is not an abortable condition? What about possible legal issues such as suit for "wrongful life" or physician or counselor failure to inform at-risk couples about the availability of testing?

For the moment, access to prenatal diagnosis is limited by the fact that it is being done largely at major medical centers, but that situation shifts daily. Will it be available only to the knowledgeable and well-off? Are physicians obligated to provide it to anyone who asks, or can pay, no mattter what the reason? How can the field be expanded in an orderly fashion that will maintain the current reasonable safety record without depriving millions of women of its possible benefits? How will severity and treatability of conditions affect access?

ETHICAL AND SOCIAL PROBLEMS IN SCREENING

Several critical issues in screening design and purpose are relevant to genetic counseling. Chief among these are 1) the relationship that the screening program bears to realizable benefits to the individual; 2) community involvement in program design and operation; 3) the nature of access to screening information; 4) the existence of mechanisms for informed consent; 5) the protection of subjects; and as a separate but related issue; 6) the legal safeguards afforded the practioner and his subjects.

People who are enlisted into screening programs have a right to expect a clear explanation of potential hazards and benefits of therapies prior to their enrollment. Where the program is experimental, as in the hyperlipidemia screening programs initiated in New York State and Massachusetts, the participant should be informed of the initially limited nature of the benefits he may expect. Prospective screening and research screening therefore, both require close communication among the planners, practioners, and subjects engaged in the screening enterprise. It is here that genetic counseling assumes an ancillary role above and beyond the traditional one of relaying medical information after the fact.

The counselor should be knowledgeable about existing therapeutic options which can be offered after screening. An intending participant needs information concerning risks and benefits from the screening as part of the informed consent procedure. The counselor is also responsible for assuring that the programs provide adequate safeguards for voluntary compliance, confidentiality, and privacy.

Even here, ethical problems arise, as when a participant refuses to share information about a serious genetic risk with relatives. A case in point is hemophilia A, in which screening can detect some 95% of women who carry the gene on their X chromosome. Nondisclosure to female relatives at high risk of carrier status constitutes a major ethical problem for the counselor, whose first allegiance is traditionally to the screened individual. Beyond active persuasion of the subject, the counselor would probably exceed legal precedents if he or she breached the confidentiality of the doctor—patient relationship.

CONCLUSIONS

The role of genetic counseling in screening programs is critical whenever the objective of the screening includes the uncovering of medically significant data. The skilled communication of that data to the screened person is what gives genetic screening its utility and justification. Because of differences in expectations and confidences in medical practitioners among different screened populations, the willingness of participants to receive, understand, and act upon genetic information may be expected to differ radically. A strong understanding of the power differentials that exist between the professional and lay communities juxtaposed in screening programs is a prerequisite to adequate counseling [46].

The counselor must expect and be able to handle distortions of understanding of screening program objectives or the perceived relationship of screening information and medical care. In the critical role of a person who controls the information flow between the two communities, the counselor has a special obligation to ensure that the testing systems and followup procedures that exist in screening centers give his or her clients accurate information, and that they identify at-risk persons correctly.

The coordination of medical services in screening requires an adequate counseling staff. The importance of the counseling function in screening makes it critical that counselors form the backbone of that staff. Ideally, genetic counselors should be involved in the planning, coordination, and running of all genetic screening programs. Without them, the knowledge gained from screening may be worse than no knowledge at all.

REFERENCES

1. Childs B, Simopoulos AP, (ed): "Genetic Screening". Programs, Principles and Research. Washington, DC: National Academy of Sciences, 1975.
2. Reilly PR: Mass neonatal screening in 1977. Am J Hum Genet 29:302–303, 1977.
3. Committee on Genetics: Screening for congenital metabolic disorders in the newborn infant: Congenital deficiency of thyroid hormone and hyperphenylalaninemia. Pediatrics 60:389–404 (Suppl) 1977.
4. North AF (ed): Screening in child health. Pediatrics 54:608–640, 1974.
5. Whitby LG: Screening for disease. Lancet 2:819–822, 1974. See also ibid: pp 880–883, 939–942, 996–998, 1057, 1061, 1125–1127, 1189–1191, 1245–1248, 1305–1309, 1364–1369, 1434–1436.
6. Kaback MM, Zeiger RS, Reynolds LW, Sonnenborn M: Approaches to the prevention and control of Tay-Sachs disease. Progr Med Genet 10:103–134, 1974.
7. Emery AEH, Eccleston D, Scrimgeour JB, Johnstone M: Amniotic fluid composition in malformations of the central nervous system. J Obstet Gynecol Br Com 79:154–158, 1972.
8. Allan LD, Ferguson-Smith MA, Donald I: Amniotic-fluid alphafoetoprotein in the antenatal diagnosis of spina bifida. Lancet 2:522–525, 1973.
9. Milunsky A, Macri JN, Weiss RR, Alpert E, McIsaac DG, Joshi MS: Prenatal detection of neural tube defects. Am J Obstet Gynecol 122:313–315, 1975.
10. Nadler HL: Present status of the prevention of neural tube defects. Pediatrics 55:751–753, 1975.
11. Steele MW, Breg WR: Chromosome analysis of human amniotic-fluid cells. Lancet 1:383–385, 1966.
12. Milunsky A, Atkins L, Littlefield JR: Amniocentesis for prenatal genetic studies. Obstet Gynecol 40:104–108, 1972.
13. Stein Z, Susser M, Gutterman AV: Screening programme for prevention of Down's syndrome. Lancet 1:305–310, 1973.
14. Chase H, O'Quin J: Screening for hyperlipidemia in childhood. JAMA 230:1535–1537, 1974.
15. Borgaonkhar DS, Shah SA: The XYY chromosome male – or syndrome. Progr Med Genet 10:135–222, 1974.
16. Klawans HL, Paulson GW, Rimmel SP, Barbeau A: Use of L-DOPA in the detection of presymptomatic Huntington's chorea. N Eng J Med 286:1332–1334, 1972.

17. Kazazian H: Prenatal detection of hemoglobinopathies. N Eng J Med 292:1125–1126, 1975.
18. Romano J: Reflection in informed consent. Arch Gen Psych 3:129–135, 1974.
19. Sorenson JR: Some social and psychological issues in genetic screening. In Bergsma D, Lappé M, Roblin RO, Gustafson JM, (eds): "Dimensions of Screening". BDOAS 10:165–184, 1974, New York: Stratton Intercontinental Book Co.
20. Milunsky A: "The Prevention of Genetic Disease and Mental Retardation". Philadelphia: Saunders, 1975.
21. Fletcher J, Roblin RO, Powledge TM: Informed consent in genetic screening programs. In "Dimensions of Screening". BDOAS 10:137–144, 1974.
22. Levy HL: Genetic screening. Adv Hum Genet 4:1–104, 389–394, 1973.
23. Nitowsky HM: Prescriptive screening for inborn errors of metabolism. A critique. Am J Ment Defic 77:538–550, 1973.
24. Chamberlain J: Human benefits and costs of a national screening programme for neural tube defects. Lancet 2:1293–1296, 1978. [See also pp 1287 and 1297–1298.]
25. Scriver CR: Screening, counseling, and treatment for phenylktonuria: Lessons learned – a precis. In (Lubs HA, de la Cruz F eds): "Genetic Counseling". New York: Raven Press, 1977.
26. Schmidt R, Wilson SM: Standardization in detection of abnormal hemoglobins. JAMA 225:1225, 1973.
27. Holtzman NA, Mellits ED, Kallman C: Neonatal screening for phenylketonuria. II. Age, dependence of initial phenylalanine in infants with PKU. Pediatrics 53:353–357, 1974.
28. Green HP, Capron AM: Issues of law and public policy in genetic screening programs. In D. Bergsma (ed): "Dimensions of Screening".BDOAS 10:137–144, 1974. New York: Stratton International Book Co.
29. Lappé M, Gustalson JM, Roblin RD: Ethical and social issues in screening for genetic disease. N Engl J Med 286:1129–1132, 1972.
30. Slack J: Risks of ischaemic heart disease in familial hyperlipoproteinaemic states. Lancet 2:1380–1383, 1969.
31. Annotation: Screening the newborn for Duchenne muscular dystrophy. Br Med J 1:403–404, 1975.
32. Garbus SB, Garbus SB: Guidelines for blood pressure mass screening projects. South Med J 68:279–286, 1975.
33. Witkin HA, Mednick SA, Schulsinger F, Bakkestrøm E, Christiansen KO, Goodenough DR, Hirschhorn K, Lundsteen C, Owen DR, Philip J, Rubin DB, Stocking M: Mental Retardation in XYY and XXY men. Science 193:547–555, 1976.
34. Hardy JP, Ksrin SL: Rapid determination of twenty amino acids by gas chromatography. Anal Chem 44:1497–1498, 1972.
35. Karasek FW, Rasmussen PW: Separation and identification of multi-component mixtures using centrichromatography mass spectrometry. Anal Chem 44:1488–1490, 1972.
36. Ersser RS: Some simple and rapid thin-layer chromatographic methods for clinical purposes. Biochem J 122:35–37, 1971.
37. Mee JML, Korth J, Halpern B, James LB: Rapid and quantitative blood amino acid analysis by chemical ionization mass spectrometry. Biomed Mass Spectr 4:178–181, 1977.
38. Rosenberg LE, Tanaka K: Amino acidemias and organic acidemias. The Year in Metabolism, 1976.
39. Dorfman A (ed): "Antenatal Diagnosis". Univ of Chicago, 1972.
40. Milunsky A: "The prenatal Diagnosis of Hereditary Disorders". Springfield, IL: Charles C. Thomas, 1973.

41. Emery AEH (ed): "Antenatal Diagnosis of Genetic Disease". Edinburgh: Churchill, Livingstone, 1973.
42. Brock DJH, Bolton AE, Scrimgeour JB: Prenatal diagnosis of spina bifida and anencephaly through maternal plasma alphafoetoprotein measurement, Lancet 1:767–768, 1974.
43. Brock DJH: Antenatal diagnosis of spina bifida and anencephaly. In (Lubs HA, de la Cruz F, eds): Genetic Counseling. New York: Raven Press, 1977, pp 225–239.
44. Hagard S, Carter F, Milne RG: Screening for spina bifida cystica: a cost-benefit analysis. Br J Preven Soc Med 30:40–53, 1976.
45. Annotation: Costing cryoprecipitate for haemophilia. Br Med J 2:123, 1975.
46. Lappé M, Brody JA: Genetic counseling: A psychotherapeutic approach to autonomy in decision-making. In Sperber MA and Jarvik LF (eds): "Psychiatry and Genetics", New York: Basic Books, 1976, pp 129–146.

15

Genetic Counseling: A Legal Perspective

Philip Reilly, JD

INTRODUCTION

Recent developments in genetic diagnostic technology, particularly the antenatal detection of chromosomal disorders, growing professional and public awareness of hereditary disease, and the availability of safe, legal abortions (at least to those who can afford them) have created a hospitable climate for genetic counseling. This new procedure is being stimulated by a steady growth in patient demand.

As it expands rapidly, practioners are reevaluating their role in helping clients make decisions that often have profound implications for their lives. Working in a new field, without the security of tradition, without a formal code of ethics, sometimes without definitive facts and often without special counseling skills, a physician or a nonmedical genetic counselor has little guidance to determine what action is appropriate in a particular case.

Naturally, values closely held by the counselor, especially the allegiance he feels to his clients, and the web of experience that supports those values, shape his conduct. As he deals with the delicate ethical issues that may arise, the counselor often practices situation ethics [1]. During the past few years a number of genetic counselors, troubled by their responsibilities, have interpreted their concerns as legal questions. To the extent that law is a set of rules, codified by legislators or fashioned by judges, to which people can adhere, it offers some measure of guidance.

I offer here a legal perspective on genetic counseling. Although the practice is new, most of the applicable legal principles are old. For two centuries, courts have been determining the nature of the relationship between a professional person and his client. The resulting cases constitute the body of malpractice law, from which several general rules of conduct may be abstracted. First, I shall briefly discuss the legal nature of the standard of care owed by a professional to his client. Among the traditional duties of a physician are three of relevance to the genetic counselor: the duty to take a medical history, the duty, in certain circumstances, to refer a patient; and the duty to keep up with developments in a field. I shall then explore questions concerning the use and misuse of confidential data. Quite rightly, these are the questions about which counselors are most concerned. Another issue in which counselors may be interested is the scope of their liability for a counseling misadventure. Courts are just beginning to adjudicate malpractice actions in this field, but I shall discuss these few cases.

There are several legal issues which impinge on genetic counseling, but which I will not discuss here. The rapid elevation of a right-to-privacy to constitutional status had a profound impact on genetic counseling, because that right protects a woman's decision to undergo an abortion. Ample literature is available for persons wishing to study this subject [2–4]. The requirement that conduct of physicians be premised on the informed consent of patients has ramifications for the manner in which counselors handle sensitive data. I treat this subject in a cursory fashion here, but exhaustive treatments have been undertaken by others [5, 6]. Neither shall I explore the legal problems associated with amniocentesis [7]. Finally, I will not discuss the complex question of whether genetic counselors should be licensed.

THE ROLE OF THE PROFESSIONAL

The Notion of a Fiduciary

The decision by an individual to consult a member of a profession is premised on the assumption that the professional possesses knowledge, skill, and power beyond the ken of the layman. It is not merely differential access to special knowledge, or the possession of special skills, however, that has stimulated the evolution of a distinct legal attitude toward the conduct of professionals. Many people in our society (plumbers, carpenters) provide services that they perform with much greater expertise than the average person. Most failures of persons to perform properly a promised service is not considered to be malpractice. Although it is difficult to demarcate the boundary precisely, professions differ from occupations by the magnitude of the task which the professional is called upon by his client to perform. Professionals are frequently asked to act in ways that may profoundly affect the lives of their clients.

The essence of the relationship between a doctor and his patient is its fiduciary nature. Technically speaking, a fiduciary is a person who has agreed to manage a trust, but the term has been expanded to cover any situation in which it is understood that one person has undertaken to protect the primacy of the interests of another. Thus, the fiduciary cannot "serve himself first and his beneficiary second" [8]. Applying the term more specifically, it has been said that a "physician must act in good faith for the utmost benefit of his patient" [9]. Although the assumptions of requisite skill and due care in its exercise are essential, it is the expectation that the professional will be loyal to the overall interests of the client that lies at the heart of the relationship [10].

The Standard of Care

For the purposes of this chapter, I will assume that the legal nature of genetic counseling is analogous to the traditional legal view of medical responsibility. The duty owed by a physician to a patient who has engaged his services is articulated as a standard of care. The precise nature of that standard is determined on a case by case basis. The plaintiff in a malpractice action must prove four major elements: that a standard of care can be established covering a specific constellation of facts; that the standard was breached; that the breach proximately caused foreseeable injuries; and that compensation is required. The manner by which a standard of care is established in a malpractice action is significantly different from traditional tort cases such as automobile accidents. There the defendant is held to the standard of the "reasonable man" (a concept that embodies the law's search for universal rules). The professional performance of a defendant physician is usually measured against the performance expected of other doctors in the same community who offer similar services. Similarly, the liability of a specialist usually can only be established through expert testimony form specialists in the same or a similar community. This standard of measurement, known as the "locality rule," is being replaced by a national standard (that is experts can be imported from other, different communities). There are three main reasons for this change: it is often difficult for the plaintiff to obtain expert witnesses to establish local standards of practice; virtually all doctors now have access to the latest medical advances through contact with colleagues and through journals; and board certification is on a national basis. The national rule will probably lead courts to require an even higher standard of performance of specialities, including genetic counseling.

It is not the purpose of this chapter to provide a general primer on medical malpractice law (several are available) [11, 12]. Nonetheless, it may be help to identify several duties discussed in law that are of special relevance to genetic counselors.

The duty to take a medical history. Detailed medical and family histories are crucial to the accurate diagnosis of genetic disease and subsequent genetic counseling. The failure of a physician to elicit suffecient medical history to permit a complete assessment of a person's health can be negligence [13]. Several cases have involved the failure to uncover a history of drug allergy. Liability is limited to those situations where an appropiate history was not taken. If the patient provided erroneous information, liability may be correspondingly mitigated [14]. As we learn more about pharmacogenetics, it will become important to take a family history of drug reactions rather than merely a patient history. The patient is not, however, under a duty to offer information that has not been solicited. Given the pivotal role of family history in genetic counseling, it hardly need be stressed that failure to probe the past to distinguish between a de novo mutation and inherited disease would constitute negligence.

The duty to consult or refer. Due care frequently requires that a physician refer the patient elsewhere. Ther may be several reasons for this. The physician may be unable to make a diagnosis, unable to perform a procedure, unwilling to provide a service which violates his moral values (for example an obstetrician may refuse to perform abortions, but he ought not refuse to suggest a doctor who will provide that service). Although the duty to refer is well established [15], there may may be situations where physicians acting with due care would not recognize the need to refer [16]. Naturally. although no physician can be expert in the diagnosis and treatment of more than a small fraction of the many known genetic disorders, a patient with an undiagnosed condition, especially an infant, should trigger a series series of consultations (or referrals) that eventually might include a medical geneticist. Failure to do so may lead to a medical tragedy not only for the proband, but possibly for a subsequent child being similarly affected [17].

The duty to keep current. It is the duty to keep up with developments that offer the greatest problem for those persons involved in diagnosis of genetic disease. A leading case considers this very issue. Two pediatricians were sued for failing to diagnose phenylketonuria (PKU) in a young child with retarded development. The initial doctor-patient contact occurred in 1960, and further examinations took place over several years. The plaintiffs successfully used the testimony of persons expert in the diagnosis of PKU to argue that in 1960 a pediatrician should have been alert to that diagnosis, despite its relative rarity [18].

As this case suggests, the duty to keep up includes the duty to be aware of and to recommend or provide appropriate tests. For example, we may infer that obstetricians who are board-certified specialists are probably now under a legal duty to inform women about fetal diagnosis whenever they have an obviously increased risk for diseases that are detectable by the option [19, 20]. It is difficult to predict how strict the courts will be in applying this duty, but one recent case is provocative. The highest court in the state of Washington held opthalmologists liable for failure to diagnose glaucoma in a young woman. The case is remarkable because the jury, impressed by incontrovertible evidence of the rarity of glaucoma in a person under forty, and the obvious medical consensus not to test for the disorder in young people. found the physicians not liable. However, on appeal the higher court reversed, in effect finding all opthalmologists negligent for failure to screen any patient with visual field defects routinely for glaucoma, regardless of age. Behind the court's reasoning was the fact that the usual glaucoma test is simple, rapid, inexpensive, and safe. Thus, the court usurped the role of the physicians to delineate the precise nature of the duty to screen for glaucoma [21].

As screening tests evolve, there may develop a corresponding duty for certain specialists to order them, even though the chance of finding an affected person is very unlikely. Given the vast array of genetic disorders, their rarity, and the highly technical nature of many tests, it would not be wise or practical to impose a blanket duty on the medical profession. It is already possible that a physician treating patients who have a higher ethnic risk for a genetic disease (eg, sickle cell anemia, Cooley's anemia, Tay-Sachs disease, and the neural tube defects) already has a duty to counsel them about the disease and available screening tests. Similarly, the substantial risk that a pregnant woman with hyperphenylalaninemia will bear a brain-damaged child suggests that obstetricians should routinely perform the low cost, simple phenylalanine test during a prenatal visit (just as they test for Rh incompatability).

New diagnostic technology raises two problems: 1) which patients should be tested? and 2) how much reliance should be placed on the results? Genocopies pose special problems for genetic counselors. Should a newborn baby with skeletal deformities consistent with achondroplasia be subjected to radiological examination? If the infant in fact has diastrophic dwarfism (transmitted as an autosomal recessive), an erroneous diagnosis of achondroplasia could be misleading for future childbearing plans. The risk of recurrence for the parents may be 1 in 4, not the 1 in 10,000 to 1 in 100,000 for an infant with achondroplasia. In situations where diagnostic tests can definitely distinguish phenocopies or genocopies, failure to employ them provides a possible basis for a lawsuit if a misdiagnosis is made. However, if the diagnostic error has been caused by a rare variant, the physician or nonphysician counselor may be comforted by a tradition of legal deference to the uncertainties of such diagnoses.

Reliance on biochemical parameters as indicators of genetic disease can never be absolute. The phenylketonuria testing experience [22], the inherent risk of

false positives and false negatives in all screening (see Chapter 14) and the
potential for test perturbations by unusual environmental factors all urge
cautious interpretation. The genetic counselor must be alert to follow up borderline results. If a false positive diagnosis results in improper treatment to the patient,
then liability might ensue. Perhaps the greatest danger of a false negative is in antenatal diagnosis. The birth of an affected infant after a reassuring diagnostic test
could certainly give rise to a malpractice claim. Similarly, the abortion of an unaffected fetus could, if discovered, also stimulate a lawsuit. When test results are
difficult to interpret, it is prudent to discuss the uncertainties with the client.
Of course, the patient with inconclusive findings should be urged to undergo retesting whenever appropriate.

There are no published decisions that discuss liability for errors in genetic screening tests of prospective parents to assess the risk of bearing a child with a recessive
disease. In one unreported case, a child with thalassemia major sued a hospital for
negligence. The father had been diagnosed to have thalassemia minor. Before she
became pregnant, the wife was screened to determine if she also was a carrier; the
results were negative. Fifteen months later an affected child was born. Subsequent
use of a more refined test revealed that the mother was a carrier [23].

Several principles may be abstracted from case law that are probably applicable
to genetic diagnoses. First, failure to utilize the appropriate diagnostic test may
constitute negligence [24]. Second, misdiagnosis alone does not lead to liability
unless the erroneous diagnosis in fact causes damage to the patient [25]. Thus, a
false negative diagnosis of carrier status for a genetic trait probably would not lead
to liability, unless it was relied upon and an affected child was born. Third, a diagnosis of a nonexistent disease (false positive) could lead to liability if the patient
received unnecessary treatment (eg, sterilization or abortion) [26].

The great diversity of contexts in which genetic counseling may be offered complicates the problem of developing uniform standards of care for this new activity.
Consider these possibilities. A physician may engage in casual genetic counseling
with those few patients that he recognizes to be at special risk for some disorder.
An opthalmologist may uncover the first signs of a genetic disease, such as incipient retinitis pigmentosa in an asymptomatic patient, and become the initial source
of genetic data, A pediatrician might hold himself out as an expert genetic counsel-
or, despite his lack of subspecialty training. Of special importance is the widespread
use of a team approach to genetic counseling now favored at large medical centers
[27]. It would be virtually impossible to expect individual practioners to match
some aspects of the care provided by the "teams." The team as a whole will em-
body a high degree of expertise, yet a nonmedical team member, such as a social
worker, while discussing the impact of a genetic problem with a family, may be
hardpressed for genetic and medical information (see Chapter 11).

In determining the standard of care, courts will be strongly influenced by the
profound dilemmas faced by the client. As they do with all specialists, the courts

will expect genetic counselors to adhere to a high standard of care. Certainly, physicians who offer genetic advice without adequate knowledge do so at their peril. Similarly, all members of a genetic team, despite the fact that some are not scientific or medical experts, will be judged by a high standard of performance. Needless to say, everybody who is a member of a counseling team is a potential defendant in a malpractice case (including a physician-geneticist directing a genetic team, who may not have had substantial contact with the client, but is responsible for the services rendered by those under his supervision).

THE COMMUNICATION OF INFORMATION

Counseling the Client

The task of the genetic counselor is the acquisition and analysis of genetic data followed by communication to and interpretation with the client. It is sometimes quite difficult to explain to the counselee the statistical risks for future pregnancies and the potential burden (economic, emotional, and physical) of the specific disorder so that it is comprehended and retained (see Chapters 10, 11, this volume). This is especially true if the individual has yet to absorb the shock of an unexpected malady affecting his or her child. The future reproductive decisions of the couple will depend on adequate comprehension, so the counselor should not lose sight of the fact that in his attempts to "explain" the data, he may also convey his own philosophical and ethical values, which are not necessarily in tune with those of the counselee. It is even more dangerous, however, if excessive caution over abuse of professional discretion hampers the counseling process. A cold, objective explanation, scrupulously nondirective, may simply force a counselee to turn elsewhere for more supportive help. There is no easy answer to this problem. I believe that the courts will recognize that counseling is a dynamic process in which decision-making is the product of participation by two (or more) human beings – one striving to help the other(s) to deal with very difficult problems.

Informed consent. The problem of truth-telling has to be considered in the context of informed consent. Space does not allow detailed review of how this concept evolved. Although case law on informed consent dates back to the turn of the century, only during the past decade has it emerged as a new and major element in consumer rights. The patient is a health care consumer, often seeking elective (nonermergency) care. Physicians are debating the depth and breadth of information to be imparted to a patient, prior to securing consent for any diagnostic study or treatment. Although the courts continue to increase the doctor's duty of disclosure, they have remained sensitive to a physician's dilemma in balancing the patient's right to know against the disconcerting effects some information may cause. The broad outlines of physician conduct delineated in a leading case,

Canterbury v Spence, could influence judicial analysis of the genetic counselor's duty to disclose:

To the physician, whose training enables a self-satisfying evaluation, the answer may seem clear, but it is the prerogative of the patient, not the physician, to determine for himself the direction in which his interests seems to lie. To enable the patient to chart his course understandably, some familiarity with the therapeutic alternatives and their hazards becomes essential.

A reasonable revelation in these respects is not only a necessity, but, as we see it, it is as much a matter of the physician's duty. It is a duty to warn of the dangers lurking in the proposed treatment, and that is surely a facet of due care. It is, too, a duty to impart information which the patient has every right to expect . . . [29].

Traditionally, the duty to disclose medical facts has been measured against the standard of the "reasonable" physician. As I have stated, expert testimony is used to determine what is commonly disclosed by other doctors in the area. Some courts have used a different criterion: the duty of disclosure considered from the perspective of the patient. What information is material to a reasonable person who must make a choice? This formulation tends to reduce dependence on the testimony of medical experts. As this standard becomes adopted—it is now being advocated by courts in about one-third of the States—physicians will be further restricted in their right to act as custodians over information on behalf of their patients [30].

If the analogy of genetic counseling to medical counseling is valid, then it is reasonable that a genetic counselor should, in some instances, be able to withhold information in the best interests of his counselee. There are at least two serious objections to permitting genetic counselors the same latitude in censoring information that has been allowed to clinicians. First, the right of a physician to withhold relevant information has usually been considered in the context of a presurgery scenario [31]. In this acute situation, patient anxiety might only complicate therapeutic efforts, hence a valid consent may sometimes be secured upon something less than complete disclosure. As medical intervention becomes less immediate, the physician has less latitude in disclosure. Where there is no imminent "treatment," as in much genetic counseling, disclosure rules are more stringent. A second more obvious reason for holding genetic counselors to full disclosure is founded on both philosophical and practical grounds. The ethic of self-determination and the privacy of family life place clear primacy on decision-making with those individuals who who must live with its consequences. Although many counselors in attempting to honor the autonomy of their patients, may prefer to adopt a passive posture — that is, not to influence decision-making — they will often be asked, "What should I do?" While it is not improper to answer that question, the patient should first be made familiar with all the relevant facts. To side-step direct requests for aid in decision-making may be just as unethical as imposing personal bias. Skilled team members with ample time can help a couple reach a decision instead of leaving them with just cold facts.

Both counselors and laymen react differently among themselves to the risks and burdens of genetic disease. Most people, but certainly not all, would condone abortion of a fetus with Down syndrome (see Chapter 10, this volume). When a fetus has Turner syndrome or sex chromosome mosaicism, however, the decision to abort might be considerably more difficult. Some couples at risk for bearing a child with an autosomal recessive disease will consider the one in four risk to be very high; others will regard the odds as three to one in their favor. Of course much depends on their perception of the burden associated with the particular disorder [28]. When a counselor is asked to help people reach a decision in the face of known risk, it is appropriate for him to stress that he has no special expertise or personal experience in predicting the impact of an affected child on a particular family.

The problem of non-paternity. Fortunately, truth telling in genetic counseling rarely needs to be curtailed. The most troublesome problem about truth telling arises when genetic information suggests nonpaternity. Perhaps as many as five percent of children born in wedlock are from an adulterous union. What legal problems are evoked by this situation? When a couple engages the services of a genetic counselor, he owes the same duty to each partner. Thus the traditional practice of discussing this problem with the woman may involve the counselor in a breach of duty to the husband. It is tempting to draw upon recent abortion law decisions [32, 33] to argue that the right of a woman to control her childbearing activities implies that she has a greater interest in genetic counseling than the man, but this is a tenuous legal position. The information may be of material consequence to the husband if it determines whether his children have a genetic risk, particularly if he should change marriage partners. Alternatively, resolution of this problem may be found in a public policy argument. Preservation of a marriage by resolving feelings of accusation or guilt is a fit subject for participatory counseling, but when the counselor has access to information that he believes could destroy a marriage, he may be justified in withholding it. The usual practice of informing the woman of the facts first makes the most practical sense, yet such a practice may eventually provoke a lawsuit by an outraged husband. I believe that societal interest in the integrity of the family would insulate the counselor from liability. Further, it might be extremely difficult for the husband to prove that he was injured in a manner that required compensation. Of course, to convey the facts and develop their implications, by telling the whole truth to both parties, may be looked upon as undesirable by counselors, but it leaves no grounds for liability.

Nevertheless, there may be situations in which the decision to convey facts revealing nonpaternity could lead to a successful lawsuit against the counselor. At least one case has occurred where counselors advised the mother of an infant with sickle cell disease that her husband was not the father of the child. After she repeatedly denied nonpaternity, the counselors conducted a repeat test on the husband. They found that, in fact, he did have the gene for sickle cell anemia, but that only

about five percent of his blood contained hemoglobin S — substantially below the
expected value [34].

The unexpected chromosome. Another aspect of truth telling about which
counselors are concerned involves information derived from an antenatal diagnosis. Occasionally, (up to 1 in 600 male fetuses) chromosomal studies performed
on amniotic fluid taken from a woman over 35 will reveal the presence of an extra
Y chromosome. Much uncertainty surrounds the implications of this finding for
the health or life of the infant [35]. It does appear that persons with an XYY
karotype are slightly more likely to be incarcerated at some time in their lives
than are XY males. I should stress that the reasons for this are unknown [36].
Despite the fact that a counselor may believe that the extra Y chromosome is not
sufficient reason to terminate a pregnancy, he should share this fact and the
current medical controversy with his client. Although to do so may alter the childbearing plans of the woman, there is now a clear legal trend favoring such disclosure. The same difficulty arises from other abnormal test results of uncertain
significance found in fetal diagnostic procedures or in genetic screening programs.

The Disclosure of Confidential Information to Third Parties

As all members of the health professions know, the principle of confidentiality has been revered for centuries. For our purpose it is interesting to note the
change in the statement of that principle since ancient times. The Hippocratic
Oath reads:

> Whatever in connection with my professional practice, or not in connec-
> tion with it, I see or hear, in the life of men, which ought not to be spoke of
> abroad, I will not divulge, as reckoning that all such should be kept secret.

Recently the American Medical Association restated the duty in this way:

> A physician may not reveal the confidence entrusted to him in the course
> of medical attendance, or the deficiencies he may observe in the character
> of patients, unless he is required to do so by law or unless it becomes neces-
> sary in order to protect the welfare of the individual or of the community [37].

Clearly the modern version is more cognizant of the reality of overriding social interests that may compromise the principle.

Confidentiality is an elusive legal concept. It is distinctly different from the
legal notion of a privileged communication. In many states there are laws that prohibit doctors from testifying in court about the medical history of a patient unless
the patient has authorized that testimony [38]. Of course, the privilege statute does
not apply when the doctor is directly involved in the case. Although few state laws
specifically protect patients' medical records, in many states a medical license can
be revoked for an inappropriate breach of confidence. For example, Alabama for-
bids the "willfull betrayal of a professional secret" [39]. In New York, regulations
drafted by the Commission of Education define unprofessional conduct to include:

"The revealing of facts, data or information obtained in a professional capacity relating to a patient or his records without first obtaining consent of the patient or his duly authorized representative, except if duly required by a court of competent jurisdiction." The courts have tended to interpret these laws to find a government intent to protect the privavy of medical information [40].

The genetic counselor deals with information that most clients regard as private. Naturally, the counselor should be expected to honor the safekeeping of that data. However, on occasion the counselor may feel very strongly that a limited disclosure to third parties is appropriate, even against the wishes of his client. For example, the diagnosis of hemophilia in a young boy alerts the counselor to the possibility that the mother's female relatives could also be carriers. Of course, in the vast majority of cases, the mother will be eager to contact appropriate relatives. There may be situations where, because the family is divided sharply over issues like abortion, the client might be unwilling to permit other persons to be informed. What course should the counselor steer? A small body of case law supports the right of a physician to make a limited disclosure of confidential data when a superior interest is clearly served. So far, these cases are too few and too scattered to provide a strong legal argument.

Several fairly recent cases consider the notion of waiver. It may be that actions taken by the patient prohibit him from subsequently objecting to a limited disclosure by the physician. In Clark v Geraci the plaintiff had consulted a doctor for treatment of conditions caused by his abuse of alcohol. Further, he sought letters from the doctor for his employer (the Federal government) to explain multiple absences. When the physician, against the instructions of his patient, finally informed the employer that the underlying cause was alcoholism, the man was fired. The patient then sued the doctor for breach of confidentiality [41]. In rendering a judgement for the doctor, the court raised the question of supervening interest. "Was the duty to divulge the employee's weakness which conceivably, could be used to rid the government of a worthless servant and thereby save public funds, greater than the duty to maintain a confidential professional· communication?" This question went unanswered as the court chose to decide the waiver issue. As the court put it, because the patient had asked the doctor to tell part of the truth, he could not be stopped from telling the rest. Similarly, it has been held that patients have no cause of action against a doctor who divulged confidential data to a life insurance company [42]. The parents lost control of that information when they filed a claim for their child's death and agreed to an investigation, which prompted the insurance company to interview the doctor.

Other courts have been quite protective of the principle of confidentiality. For example, in a case again involving disclosure to an insurance company, the court stated bluntly: The unauthorized revelation of medical secrets, or any confidential communication in the course of treatment, is tortious conduct which may be the basis for an action in damages" [43]. In 1974, the Supreme Court of Alabama, reversed a lower court ruling that had held that a disclosure by a doctor to a patient's employer was valid [40].

Although the case law on improper disclosure of confidential medical data is not very helpful, it does offer some guidance. First, the notion that supervening social interests may validate disclosure is sometimes acknowledged [41]. Second, it appears that courts will be much more wary of a disclosure that merely poses a threat to a patient than of one that is primarily intended to help innocent third parties, who may themselves be injured if the disclosure were not made [44–46].

Indeed, there may actually be a duty to disclose when the life or health of a third party is endangered. In Tarasoff v Regents of the University of California, the Supreme Court of California ruled that psychotherapists had a duty to warn a person about threats made against her life by a patient during a counseling session [47]. The assertion that a physician may have a special obligation to nonpatients has been given its most extreme statement by the Supreme Court of Iowa [48]. A person who had been injured in an automobile accident sued the driver and his physician, claiming that the doctor erred in not advising his patient, who had a history of seizures, to stay off the roads. The court held that the plaintiff should be given the opportunity to attempt to prove that the doctor was negligent in not advising his patient to give up his license, and that negligence was the proximate cause of the accident. These two cases do not constitute a trend, but they do indicate, unfortunately, that there is no precise legal explanation of the obligations owed by a physician to his patient and to the general public.

No court has yet been asked to decide whether the decision of a genetic counselor to alert relatives of a client about the risk of bearing a child with severe genetic disease constitutes a supervening interest. Recently, a Committee convened by the National Academy of Sciences considered this question in the context of parental genetic screening. The Committee concluded:

Under current law, genetic screeners would be ill-advised to contact relatives without the screenee's consent in view of the sparse case law support for a 'public health' exception to the confidentiality rule [49].

Given the uncertainty of case law, the best solution is for clients to be told that information acquired from or about them could be important to other family members and should be shared with them. If the counseling is offered by clinics that use consent forms, it would be helpful to add a sentence that requests approval of limited disclosures to appropriate blood relatives. If the counselor unilaterally contacts a relative of the counselee, he may be liable to a tort action for invasion of privacy. About forty states now recognize invasion of privacy as a basis for tort liability. Substantial money damages can be awarded upon proof that the invasion caused mental anguish. Some of these states require malice, but in others, mere willfulness can be sufficient ground for recovery. Among several meanings of the common-law notion of privacy, is that a person has a right to be free from "public disclosure of private facts." A possible defense in such cases is the argument that the disclosed facts were matters of legitimate public concern.

In those rare cases where a counselor has compelling genetic information which the client refuses to communicate (for example, when one or more relatives may be affected with a condition that would benefit from treatment, or that poses a serious genetic risk to progeny), I would believe counselors should breach the principles of confidentiality and make the disclosure. In so doing they run only a small risk of legal action. Further, the risk of bearing a child with a serious genetic disease probably constitutes a sufficient public interest to justify his act. Of course, this may be a moot point, since conselors often cannot reach other relatives without the cooperation of the client.

LIABILITY OF GENETIC COUNSELING

Four events that could trigger a malpractice action against a genetic counselor are 1) a failure in the counseling process itself; 2) the wrongful communication of confidential information to third parties; 3) an irrevocable medical intervention (abortion or sterilization) based on erroneous data; and 4) the birth of a child with a genetic disease after a diagnostic error.

The possibility of a lawsuit brought by clients because they are dissatisfied with the way in which they were counseled is remote. The task of defining what constitutes an adequate standard of performance in counseling and of proving that the standard was breached in a way that caused actual harm to the client is exceedingly difficult. The only situation, short of malicious actions by a deranged person, that might provoke such a suit would be an incorrect assertion of nonpaternity made to the husband. I have already discussed the problem of lawsuits generated by disclosure to third parties.

When lawsuits are provoked by unnecessary medical interventions, the plaintiff's task is to show that 1) the diagnostic data upon which he had reason to rely was incorrect; 2) the physician or counselor is not shielded from liability by known variabilities in test results or treatment outcome; and 3) real injury was suffered In such cases, many factors will determine the extent of damages. For example. a 36-year-old woman without children who has undergone an unnecessary abortion (due to an erroneous antenatal diagnosis) would have a stronger case than a woman who already had three children; similarly, the procreative history of a man undergoing an unnecessary vasectomy would be an influential consideration. To my knowledge no court has yet been asked to assess damages for loss of procreative power consequent to a genetic diagnostic error.

The Tort of Wrongful Life

The most important question of liability involves the birth of a child with a serious genetic disease. This has become known as the tort of wrongful life. At least four legal developments set the stage for such lawsuits: 1) the expansion of the right of an infant to sue for prenatal injuries; 2) the recognition that in certain circumstances the birth of a child could be a burden; 3) the abolition of laws prohibiting abortion; and 4) the rise of the doctrine of informed consent.

1) **Prenatal injuries.** At common-law, there has been no established cause of action for prenatal injuries [50]. The right of a child to recover for injuries in utero was first recognized about 1946 [51]. Today a substantial number of states recognize the right of a child to sue for injuries sustained during any part of gestation [52].

2) **Unwanted births.** The question of whether the birth of a healthy child could be a legally compensable event was first considered in 1934. The Supreme Court of Minnesota, denying recovery for a unsuccessful sterilization, held that whatever discomforts were associated with the birth of a child were more than balanced by the "blessing" that it brought to the family [53]. This remained the dominant view until 1967, when a California court held that a woman for whom a faulty tubal ligation had resulted in the birth of a ninth child had a valid cause of action for all physical effects and medical expenses [54]. The courts today are still divided on whether the birth of a healthy child should be compensable, but the trend is favoring the cause of action [55].

3) **Wrongful life.** The notion of a tort of wrongful life was first considered in 1963. An illegitimate child sued his father because of the stigmata associated with bastardy. The court, recognizing that a tort had been committed, nevertheless refused to award damages because of public policy considerations. The great fear was that a flood of litigation might ensue [56]. Three years later a legal commentator suggested that, because the plaintiff was forced to argue that he should never have been born, he had destroyed his legal standing for suing. The writer asserted that every claim in tort based on act or omission to which the plaintiff owes his life must fail, because it is impossible to compare existence to nonexistence [57].

Shortly thereafter, in a case of major importance to persons concerned with prenatal diagnosis, Gleitman v Cosgrove, the Supreme Court of New Jersey held that there was no valid damage claim against a physician who had told the mother of a malformed baby that a rubella infection during the first trimester would not harm her fetus. By a divided vote, the court held that neither she nor her affected infant could sue the doctor for withholding important information, because the mother had testified that, had she been informed of the risks of birth defects, she would have aborted the pregnancy, which at that time was illegal [58].

Of course this illegality of abortion greatly complicated the Gleitman decision. This certainly diminished the gravity of the breach of trust made by the physician. Nevertheless, this case has been sharply criticized on two grounds. First, the decision disregarded the most central principle of tort law—that a person who has been injured has the right to be compensated. Mrs. Gleitman had acknowledged that she would have obtained an abortion if she had known the risks of rubella to her fetus. (Despite their illegality, they were available in reputable hospitals.) By failing to inform her, he foreclosed that option. Second, the court asserted that it could not ascertain damages where the problem involved the difference between nonexistence and a life burdened with defects. Nonetheless, courts make similar subjective measurements daily in personal injury cases, for example, evaluating loss of vision. With the exception of a couple of cases that followed Gleitman, the problem of damages for prenatal injuries lay dormant until 1975.

In February 1975 the Texas Supreme Court considered Jacobs v Theimer, a case virtually identical to Gleitman v Cosgrove. The parents of a child born with severe congenital anomalies sued their physician for failing to inform them of the risks posed by a rubella infection during pregnancy. Breaking sharply from Gleitman, the court ruled that the doctor was under a legal duty to make a reasonable disclosure about the danger of rubella; that such a disclosure would not have made him an accomplice to a crime had the woman obtained an illegal abortion (the pregnancy occurred in 1969); and that damages covering "expenses reasonably necessary for care and treatment of the child's physical impairment" were not barred by public policy [59].

Although it is impossible to know exactly what influenced the judges most, there were at least three critical differences between the two cases. First, since Gleitman, the notion of therapeutic abortion had become much more acceptable; second, the principle of informed consent had become more widely embraced. Finally, in Jacobs the defective child was not named as a plaintiff. This circumvented some of the metaphysical objections. It allowed the court merely to focus on the familiar problem of compensating families for extraordinary medical costs.

Since the Jacobs decision, two New York courts have considered issues that probe the damage question more deeply. In Howard v Lecher, the parents of a young child who died of Tay-Sachs disease claimed that their doctor should have realized that their ethnic heritage put them at risk for bearing a child with this disorder and that he should have informed them about the existence of a blood test to determine their carrier status. Further, the plaintiffs asserted that they would have aborted the affected fetus [60].

The defendant did not appeal the first cause of action, which claimed damages for medical and funeral expenses. He did challenge a claim for suffering endured by the parents as they watched their daughter deteriorate. Finding that New York law restricts damage awards for suffering to persons directly injured, the trial court, agreeing with the physician that nothing he did harmed the parents, dismissed the cause of action. Although it was unnecessary, the court went further and approved the position taken in Gleitman that public policy precluded recovery for wrongful life. This foreclosed the possibility of adding a claim for pain and suffering on behalf of the estate of the deceased child.

The case was appealed all the way to the highest court in New York. The Court of Appeals, reversing an intermediate appellate court that had reversed the trial court ruling, held that the parents could not recover for mental suffering that they had endured during the illness. But, the high court did not exclude the possibility of bringing a cause of action for the mental suffering endured by the child [60].

A few months after the decision in Howard v Lecher, an intermediate level appellate court in New York handed down its ruling on another case involving assertions of malpractice in genetic counseling. In Park v Chessin parents of two children who had died of infantile polycystic kidney disease (an autosomal recessive disorder), acting as administrators of the second child's estate, filed a lawsuit that included a cause of action for the wrongful life of the child. They argued that the second infant would never have been conceived had they been warned of the risks inherent in pregnancy — risks that the doctor should have recognized after the birth of the first child. The judge, noting that the case was different from Howard v Lecher in that parents were not suing on their own behalf, found that the cause of action was valid. He suggested that a conditional, prospective liability attached when the child was born. Refusing to get immersed in metaphysical speculations about wrongful life, he asserted that the child's right to sue had grown out of its suffering, not its birth. This is the only judicial decision in the United States that has explicitly approved a cause of action for wrongful life [61].

Given the courts' new interest in protecting personal autonomy, the legalization of abortion and the first plaintiff victory in a "wrongful life" case, genetic counselors would be well advised to make a full and complete disclosure to the counselee of 1) the limits of the specific diagnostic technology 2) the therapeutic alternatives; and 3) the risks and burdens of the particular disease. They should be wary of diluting or softening harsh realities to assuage the anguish felt by their counselees.

SUMMARY

I have offered a general discussion of legal issues that may confront genetic counselors [62, 63]. Although the case law is sparse [64] and the future is uncertain, there has been international forensic concern about injuries to the unborn [65]. I believe that certain physicians (especially obstetricians and pediatricians) will be expected to recognize at least the more prominent problems encountered in medical genetics. Thus, an obstetrician is obliged to advise his older patients about antenatal diagnosis for chromosomal disease. In general, as time goes by, all physicians will be expected to be cognizant of at least some genetic problems.

I have identified some of the legal problems that surround use of confidential medical data. Although such information should be accorded the utmost respect, I reaffirm my belief that the physician or counselor who discloses a genetic fact to selected blood relatives, because it may be important to their health, runs a very small legal risk. This problem should be effectively handled by discussion during the first stage of the counseling process.

Most important, of course, is that patients be given an accurate genetic diagnosis and good supportive care. Then the malpractice risks of genetic counseling, which are quite small, can be further diminished.

REFERENCES

1. Fletcher J: "Situation Ethics: The New Morality." Philadelphia: Westminister Press, 1966.
2. Note: Abortion after Roe and Doe: A proposed statute. Vanderbilt Law Rev 26:823, 1974.
3. Byrn RM: Abortion amendments: policy in the light of precedent. St. Louis Univ Law J 18:280, 1974.
4. Vieira N: Roe and Doe: substantive due process and the right of abortion. Hastings Law J 25:867, 1974.
5. Capron A: Informed consent in catastrophic disease research and treatment. U Penn Law R 123:340, 1975.
6. Riskin L: Informed consent: looking for the action. Illinois Law Forum 1975:980, 1975.
7. Friedman JM: Legal implications of amniocentesis. Univ Penn Law Rev 123:92, (1974).
8. Meinhard v Salmon 249 NY 458, 164 NE 545 (1928).
9. Sevier R: The hazards of medical treatment: the duty to inform and the right to know. Proceedings of the ABA Section of Insurance, Negligence and Compensation Law 396, 1968.
10. Davidoff DJ: "The Malpractice of Psychiatrists." Springfield, Illinois: Charles C Thomas, 1973, p 46.
11. Holder A: "Medical Malpractice." New York: Wiley, 1974.
12. King J: "Medical Malpractice in a Nutshell," CV Mosby Co, St Louis: 1976.
13. Johnson v St Paul Mercury Insurance Company 219 So 2d 524, (1969).
14. Johnstone v Brother 12 Cal Rptr 23 (1961).
15. Benson v Dean 133 NE 125 (NY, 1921).
16. Holder A: Duty to refer patient to a medical specialist, J Am Med Assoc 204:281, 1968.
17. Manion v Tweedy 100 NW 2d 124 (Minn 1959).
18. Naccarato v Grob 384 Mich 248, 180 NW 2d 788 (1970).
19. Holder AR: "Legal Issues in Pediatrics and Adolescent Medicine," New York; Wiley, 1976, p 35.
20. Reilly PR, Milunsky A: Medicolegal aspects of prenatal diagnosis. In Milunsky A (ed): "Hereditary Disorders and the Fetus." New York: Plenum Press, 1979.
21. Helling v Carey and Laughlin 519 P 2d 981 (1974).
22. Holtzman NA, Meek AG, Mellits ED: Neonatal screening for phenylketonuria I. Effectiveness. J Am Med Assoc 229:667, 1974.
23. Mellis v Chicago Wesley Memorial Hospital (Illinois Cir Ct, Cook Co Docket No 701-15177 June 18, 1974).
24. Clark v US 402 F 2d 950 (CCA4 1968).
25. McBride v Roy 58 P 2d 886 (Okla 1936).
26. Bryson v Stone 190 NW 2d 336 (Mich 1971).
27. Fraser FC: Genetic counseling. Am J Human Genet 26:636, 1974.
28. Leonard B, Chase A, Childs B: Genetic counseling: a consumer's view. N Eng J Med 287:433, 1972.
29. Canterbury v Spence 464 F 2d 772 (DC Circ 1972).
30. Schneyer TJ: Informed consent and the danger of bias in the formation of medical disclosure practices. Wisconsin Law Rev 1976: 124, 1976.
31. Scott v Wilson 396 SW 2d 532 (1965).

32. Roe v Wade 410 US 113 (1973).
33. Planned parent of Central Missouri v Danforth 428 US 52 (1976).
34. Bowman J: Genetic screening programs and public policy. Paper presented at the WEB Dubois Conference, Atlanta, Georgia, December 15, 1976.
35. Borgaokar DS, and Shah SA: The XYY chromosome male – or syndrome? In AG Steinberg AG and Bear AG (eds): "Progress in Medical Genetics X." New York: Grune and Stratton, 1974, pp 135–222.
36. Witkin HA et al: Criminality in XYY and XXY men. Science 193:547–555, 1976.
37. Principles of Medical Ethics, Section 9, American Medical Association, 1957.
38. Waltz J, and Inbau F: "Medical Jurisprudence," New York: MacMillan, 1971, pp 287–291. 291.
39. Alabama Code, Title 46, § 257(21), 1973.
40. Horne v Patton 287 So 2d 824 (1974).
41. Clark v Geraci 208 NYS 2d 564 (1962).
42. Hague v Williams 37 NJ 328, (1962).
43. Hammonds v Aetna Casualty and Surety Co 243 F Supp 793 (ND Ohio 1965).
44. Simonsen v Swenson 164 Neb 224, 177 NW 831 (1920).
45. Curry v Corn 52 Misc 2d 1035, 277 NYS 2d 470 (1966).
46. Jacobson v Jacobson 207 App Div 238, 202 NYS 96 (1928).
47. Tarasoff v Regents of the University of California 118 Cal Reptr 129:529 P 2d 553, (1974 (1974).
48. Freese v Lemmon 210 NW 2d 576 (1973).
49. Committee for the Study of Inborn Errors of Metabolism: "Genetic Screening." Washington, DC: National Academy of Sciences, 1975.
50. Dietrich v Inhabitants of Northhampton 138 Mass 14 (1884).
51. Bonbrest v Katz 65 F Supp 138 (DDC, 1946).
52. Milunsky A, Reilly P: The new genetics: Emerging medicolegal issues in the prenatal diagnosis of hereditary disorders. Am J Law Med 1:71–87, 1975.
53. Christianson v Thornby 192 Minn 123, 255 NW 620 (1934).
54. Custodio v Bauer 59 Cal Rptr 463 (1967).
55. Troppi v Scarf 31 Mich App 240, 187 NW 2d 511, 1971.
56. Zepeda v Zepeda 41 Ill App 240, 190 NE 2d 849 (1963)
57. Tedeschi R: On tort liability for "wrongful life". Israel Law Rev 1:513, 1966.
58. Gleitman v Cosgrove 49 NJ 22, 227 A 2d 689 (1967).
59. Jacobs v Theimer 519 SW 2d 846 (1975).
60. Howard v Lecher 386 NYS 2d 460 (1976), 397 NYS 2d 363 (1977).
61. Park V Chessin, 387 NYS 2d 204 (1976), 400 NYS 2d 110 (1977).
62. Wright, E: Father and Mother know best: deferring the liability of physicians for inadequate genetic counseling. Yale Law J 87:1488–1515, 1978.
63. Reilly P: "Genetics, Law and Social Policy." Cambridge, Mass: Harvard University Press, 1977.
64. Lynch PM, Lynch HT: Genetic counseling of high-cancer-risk patients: jurisprudential considerations. Sem Oncol 5:107–118, 1978.
65. Carter G: Legal responses and the right to compensation. Brit Med Bull 32:89–94, 1976.

16

A Personal View of Genetic Counseling

Marjorie Guthrie

INTRODUCTION

Many of you know that my husband, Woody, father of my children, had Huntington Disease. I want to share with you some of our experiences in learning about Huntington and the experience other families have shared with me about Huntington. I hope these experiences will help genetic counselors understand some of the joys and sorrows in the lives of families with genetic problems.

I have been amazed at the uniqueness of each person's experience, and then on reflection I see many similarities. There are common threads of fears, anticipation of fears, concerns with how individuals at-risk might react to the diagnosis, how (or if) to tell a spouse or children, how to find a way to live with the diagnosis, and whether there will be treatments or a "cure." As I have often sat and listened to these people pouring out their concerns, I try to help by listening, encouraging them to explore their feelings, observing how they speak and what they leave out. Each one has his or her own story that "leaps out," once an opening is given, to share.

Sometimes, two persons come together, a husband and wife, a mother and daughter, and reveal thoughts to each other that have been hidden a long time.

I find that someone capable of understanding and sharing things that are difficult to say can help a family face the reality of what might or might not happen with the threat of Huntington Disease. I do not consider myself a professional counselor. When someone comes to me we just talk together. Hopefully, I help by sharing my own feelings and how I have found strength. Out of all this, I, too, am helped and am finding my way. It is not a constant routine, but one that changes from person to person. As I look back, there have also been changes from year to year in my thinking as well as those with whom I speak.

HUNTINGTON IN OUR FAMILY

Early Recollections

Let us go back and begin with my earliest recollections about Huntington and see how I came to where I am today.

In the early 1940's, I was a professional dancer. When I first met Woody, I found him to be a shy yet strong, creative, child-like fun person. He had a kind of innocence and yet when he looked at you, his gaze was direct and complete. His body, in comparison with most of my dancer friends seemed awkward but strong and sinewy. He had the coloring of the earth itself, and one had the feeling that he had slept upon the ground many nights. He carried his guitar everywhere he went, hanging on his back. Sticking out of his breast pocket, one could see a few sharpened pencils, a good pen or two, and in his pants pocket a roll of writing paper or a notebook pushed down into the back pocket. He never wore a tie, and when I met him, he didn't even have a warm coat. In the cold, wintery days, he wore an old army jacket that seemed much too big. His bony fingers stuck out, and his cowboy boots seemed to have been worn down to paper. Yet he walked with a stride – a fast walker when he had to go somewhere, a dawdly one when he was strumming and coming down the street. He talked concisely, a few short words, to the point, with a funny little laugh as he seemed to reflect on his own words. His eyebrows always seemed to be raised in question over his small beady eyes. He had what appeared to be leathery, tough sun-tanned skin, his face had smile lines, and his thin lips curled up at the ends.

I liked walking down the street holding hands. His grip was firm, and despite his "country" appearance he felt "special." We shared hours of talk and dreams. We liked dreaming and teasing about the future. We made up stories about what our life would be about, how our kids were going to grow up and be "world changers and hope-ers" – how we were going to be the "singing Guthries" – how we would travel as a family – making this world a better place with songs and dance and that "good union feeling." We were like any young couple in love – planning for the tomorrows and believing that we could do anything that we set out to do – as long as we were together.

Woody had been married before and already had three children. We shared a little room in a typical rooming house on 14th Street in New York City, one window, one bed, a small sink, a chest of drawers, one chair, one small closet.

When I went off in the morning to my rehearsals or classes, he would sit down with his typewriter on the chest of drawers or sit in the chair and fill up a ten-cent notepad and sip a container of coffee. Sometimes, when I returned, I would find funny drawings or notes telling me he was out walking or grabbing a bite to eat across the street or going to see Joy Homer, who was then editing his autobiography, "Bound for Glory." Those were busy, productive days. After long hours of work both of us would put our thoughts together, and either he or I would read what he had written that day out loud, so that the other one could type it up properly for Joy to read the next day.

One day he wrote about his mother, describing how she had become disheveled and neglected the house and even had temper tantrums and threw things around the house and was often found sitting in the little movie house of Okemah, Oklahoma, where the Guthries lived. After his older sister Clara died from a fire in the house, his "mama" was taken to the "insane asylum" in Norman, Oklahoma.

I asked Woody what kind of sickness this was. He said that the doctor told them she had Huntington Chorea. I asked him if he could get sick like his mother, and he said that only females get this chorea so he did not have to worry.

And we didn't worry. We went on building our dreams, working hard at our professions, he writing, me teaching and dancing. Sometimes, at a party with our friends, I would feel so bad when Woody would drink too much and become angry over little things — or perhaps disappear with a friend — and I would go home crying and hurt. When I protested that I didn't see why he had to drink so much, he would explain that where he came from everybody drinks this cheap wine from the time they were four years old. His body was used to it and it wouldn't hurt him one bit! And he resumed his writing, with an occasional trip to record his songs for Moe Asch at the Folkways recording office on 46th Street.

During the war, Woody and his good friend, Cisco Houston, shipped out in the Merchant Marine. Cisco was not one to knuckle down to anybody, but he always handled Woody so tenderly. He told us wonderful stories about Woody at sea, and we would all laugh together about Woody's antics on the ship. Instead of setting the tables for the thousands of men who were on their way to fight in Europe, Woody would write the day's news on a blackboard with cartoons all around. This was supposed to be the day's menu, but his humor and his songs had become part of Woody that everybody could enjoy, so there were no complaints. They made three trips together and were torpedoed twice. Woody wore his medals proudly. He believed in the fight against Hitler, and on his guitar he had a large sign: THIS MACHINE KILLS FASCISTS. He wrote many songs about the defeat of Hitler — some serious and some satire — always with the hopes for a better world — a positive picture of what that world could be like, would be like. He was not one to be defeated or to let us believe in defeat.

Meanwhile, our family had grown. Our little girl, Cathy, whom Woody called "Stackabones," had died in a fire, and now we had three little ones, all of us living in three tiny rooms in Coney Island. I liked color — the linoleum floor was bright blue — the book shelves went from the floor to the ceiling, and Woody's desk was a piece of wood, cut on an angle, nailed to the wall in the corner of our living-room. Our bedcouch opened up at night and touched the little piano that I had bought during one of Woody's trips, so that if you wanted to get out of the bed at night you had to climb out either end. Our three kids slept on little nursery cots side by side, and we used a gate between their room and ours so that they could all play together, yet we could see them. Many days when I was away teaching, Woody was left in charge of the children until my friends who helped to care for them would arrive later in the day. He would write, sing, feed, tease, and read all day, alternating whenever he felt like it from one activity to another. Sometimes he would make a sketch or two or write whatever the children said about his drawing on the paper.

In the beginning, I felt good leaving him with the children. I knew he had the patience to do things with them. I also knew that my mother or my helper would be there in time. It was a good family life with all the usual ups and downs. Sometimes his anger was tough to take. There were times when we parted for a day or two — sometimes for a week or more — when he would be away singing somewhere and not return as I had expected. But there would come in the mail another ten-cent notepad telling me how much he loved me and the kids and that he wasn't good enough for us.

He would return dirty and tired, I would set him down into a tub, wash him up, and he would dance around our little room and say how good it was to be home again. And I would sit at the piano chording the way he said his mother used to do, with him brushing my long hair down my back, as he used to do for her. I always felt that in many ways I was not only Woody's wife, but also the mother that he never had and always wanted. We had wonderful, friendly neighbors in those days. Young and old came to our apartment, listening to our records, playing chess on our tiny kitchen table. Woody enjoyed our neighbors and loved Coney Island, which was where we could live and still have "wide open spaces," something that Woody felt was missing in the city, since he identified with the wheat fields and the crops and trees and rivers where he had slept in his travels.

Signs of Huntington Disease

I recall very clearly how one day Woody was walking in front of me and his guitar was not on his back, and yet he seemed to be walking a bit lopsided. I remember thinking "that's funny, he looks like his guitar is on his shoulder pulling him over, but it's not there." (I used to carry my little bag with all of my dance clothes in my hand and I always felt so unbalanced when I did not have it. I recalled thinking "that's the way I feel when I walk without my bag.")

I know now that this walk was one of the first signs of Woody's chorea.

I thought nothing of it at the time, but little by little his uneven walking became worse. Also, in retrospect, his beautiful diction on his recordings became more and more difficult to maintain. He had a marvelous way of saying the t's or d's at the end of a word, and he made every effort to speak clearly. To do this, he seemed to gather his breath and the words seemed to explode from his lips. I began to notice that his anger seemed longer or more severe than before. Thinking that maybe it was the pressure of three kids disturbing his work, we moved into a larger apartment, where Woody could have a special room nearby with his books and typewriter, where no one would disturb his thinking. We set up a great studio, using orange crates, for his writing and drawing paraphernalia. He worked there beautifully for a while, Then little by little he would bring home a book he was reading, or a few pages for me to read, then the typewriter. Little by little he soon moved back in. He worked at home and several weeks later would try moving to another place. Once we used a store around the corner and had to set up a big curtain to cover the storefront so people would not knock on the window and want to come in.

Recognizing that none of these places was working out, we moved to a new apartment, where Woody had his own room in his own home. We thought surely that was going to help him become more stable.

I was still teaching, earning a living, and had to leave home regularly. I began to leave with more and more concern as I noticed the heavier drinking, and he seemed to tire more. He would rest on our bed for longer periods in the middle of the day. When he was resting, he seemed to be glad to be away from it all. If I wanted to ask a question, I waited until I felt he would be more responsive. I was aware of what I was doing, but one day I noticed that my daughter, who at that time was about two years old, would walk up to the bed and if he did not seem to want to talk to her, she would quietly walk away, sensing that this was not the time to talk to Daddy.

Without knowing, I think all of us were aware that there was something wrong with Woody. A young musician who loved Woody began to imitate his explosive speech as though that was his real speech pattern. There were numerous outbursts of temper, and one frustrating day Woody agreed that "there was something wrong" and consented to seek medical help.

Doctors and Hospitals

After three weeks in a local hospital for observation, we were told that Woody was an alcoholic. Later, after several weeks in Bellevue Hospital, there was still no diagnosis of his condition. Then one day Woody suddenly called. The doctor had told him to go home. They gave him a subway token and a dime to call me. He was already on his way! I panicked. I called the hospital and asked the doctor if it were true that he was told to go home. No diagnosis! Just go home! The doctor said, "Mrs. Guthrie, your husband is a very sick man, and WE DON'T KNOW WHAT TO DO WITH HIM." I replied that I didn't know what to do with him either. I was worried about my children. What could we do now?

This was the real beginning of anguish! Whom would I talk to? Whom would I consult? How should we live? Was it safe to leave him with the children?

To my surprise, Woody looked well. The food and rest in the hospital had been good for him. He seemed calm and ready to work again. He did work. He wrote songs and articles, typing away, sometimes writing with his collection of pens and pencils, sometimes drawing wonderful funny sketches. He was Woody

again. It was wonderful to see him busy, active, and smiling. Yet underneath
all this were my own fears. The words of the doctor were ringing in my ears,
and I became more and more concerned about leaving him in the house, but I
knew I had no choice. Our mother's helper was more experienced with life than
I. She handled Woody calmly and took care of the children. As the weeks went
by I managed to keep up a good front with her help.

One day, Woody said that he wanted to take a trip to California, and I rushed
at the opportunity to have him leave home. Our good friends Will and Herta Geer
welcomed him, and I felt relieved that Woody was in good hands. He wrote regularly, notebooks full of ideas for songs, telling about life with the Geers. This was
a time of respite for me. It did not last too long, and soon he was on his way back
to New York.

For the next two or three years, with more involuntary movement, with more
difficulty swallowing, and difficulty with speech, he signed himself in and out of
Brooklyn State Hospital. The first time we went to this hospital he told the doctors
that he knew something was wrong and hoped they could find out. I recounted his
background and begged that they find out, for whatever it was we could find a way
to face it, but the not-knowing was killing us! Eventually it was suggested that
Woody should have some shock treatments, and he was moved to a ward to wait
his turn for these treatments. He and I just accepted this as a possible hope that
something could be done. It was while waiting in this ward that a young physician
came up with the diagnosis of Huntington chorea.

We were stunned! Woody believed that he couldn't have his mother's illness because "men did not get chorea." We were told there was no treatment.
HOPELESS.
HELPLESS.
For days after, we talked at the hospital about what we should do. There was no
question but that he would have to stay in the hospital. We would keep our family
together. I would bring him home on weekends. We would find a way to tell the
children when it was appropriate. He would try to keep writing in the hospital. We
would stick by each other as best we could. We found OUR way.

We stumbled a lot over the following years. We listened to what others said, and
then we did what we thought was best for ourselves and our children, and it usually
was NOT what others had advised. One doctor suggested (along with most of my
friends) we should tell the children that Woody had died, so that they would not have
to see him deteriorate. This was so unreal to me at the time. What would happen
if they found out that I had lied? And how could I help to take care of him if we
wiped him out of our lives? He did not seem so ill. There were many, many good days
when he walked rather well and enjoyed our visits. He began to show more of the
involuntary movements, but he always joked that his "vitaphones" (the loads of
vitamins that he was taking) were going to make him better. When we went to
our local hot-dog stand on weekends, he ordered several, ate the hot-dogs, threw

the rolls away, and drank six or seven root beers. He enjoyed riding in the car, and particularly liked to lie down in the sun in our backyard. By now, I had bought a house in Queens, and while Woody never lived in this house, our neighbors knew who he was and shared in our pleasure as Woody became better known to the public. A newspaper article told about Woody's sickness and the Secretary of the Interior, Stewart Udall, honored him with an award for the songs that expressed his love for our country. He could not go down to Washington to receive the award, but we took his picture as he held it, seemingly happy that people were still singing his songs.

Towards the end he was confined to his wheelchair and found speech and swallowing very difficult. He almost choked several times, and on several occasions I received a telegram telling me that he was dying of pneumonia. Each time he pulled through and each time he laughed about how he was "still here".

All this time he was trying to write. His beautiful handwriting was deteriorating, but he still wanted me to bring long yellow pads to the hospital. He filled them up with his "scrabbles," and I replaced them with additional tablets. He loved the feel of his pencils and tried to keep one always on him, which wasn't easy in a ward with 40 men, mostly patients with mental disorders. All during the years when I came to visit and to read his fan mail, there were always letters from young people. I would read parts, and he would enjoy hearing the good thoughts. I had been told that he probably did not understand one word, but his response was so evident and obvious, that I would ask him questions to prove to myself that he did understand all I was reading and saying. He had many moments of extreme tiredness when his concentration would wane. He would show such exasperation when he waved two open fingers in the air (meaning that he wanted a cigarette placed there) and no one cared to accommodate him, even though I left cartons of cigarettes for him each week. His inability to express a need and the frustration of being ignored were the greatest hardships of all for him. I understood his sign language and his frustration, and I began to think of ways to try to get the hospital attendants to become more responsive to his needs. I made three cards "YES," "NO," and "?," and I spread them either on his bed or on the tray of his wheel chair. I teased him and said that he must help me prove to the attendants and the doctors that he was fully competent despite his appearance, and he must answer some questions to show that he did know what I was saying. I asked a series of questions to which I knew the answers, and despite an annoyed look on his face that he had to prove his sanity, he invariably moved his arms to the correct card. This is when I began to wonder whether the doctors really knew all about Huntington. We "tested" him in this way continually, and then, towards the end, we used one or two eye blinks to answer yes or no. I changed the number occasionally to be sure that we were still communicating. In this way I learned that there was a whole man locked up inside this shell of a person. I learned that he had no physical pain, although his nervous system was deteriorating and affected him in many ways. He could not feel or taste, which was why he wanted more seasoned foods, candy, and strong coffee.

He was tied into his wheel-chair to avoid falling, but this also hastened the wasting of his muscles. He could no longer stand and could no longer walk or come home. I suggested loosening his bonds in the chair, so that he might try some simple exercises to build up his thigh muscles so that he could walk. When I came to visit and asked if he had done the exercises, he replied by popping up and down in his chair. One day, another patient remarked that he had walked. Sure enough, when I untied him, he walked several steps away from the chair and then returned, collapsing into it with a big grin on his face.

It was then I began to believe there were things that we could do to help the patient who had Huntington. Each time I visited, I questioned and observed. For years, I came with my friend Shirley. I found that it was getting more difficult for me to converse with Woody, knowing that he could not respond without great effort. I found that if Shirley and I sat on each side of him and we talked so that he could hear all our news and hear what we were doing with the children and all the usual family gossip, he enjoyed being a part of what he was hearing and often smiled and shook his head in response.

On his dying day he heard us come into his room, opened his eyes, and made a grunting sound when I asked him if he would like some water. I fed him a spoon of water to wet his dry lips. He was still a whole person, but this person was dying and he knew it. We knew it too, and the hospital chaplain who was standing by asked if he might say a prayer. He recited the Lord's Prayer, and we all looked at each other, listening quietly. I told the chaplain that Woody had always loved to read the Bible and was more versed in the Bible than most people. He had always enjoyed studying the religions of the world, and throughout this conversation he was listening with his eyes sometimes closed and sometimes open. When I left the hospital, I stroked his forehead. I knew it was the last time.

Early the next morning, they called. Woody had died.

HELPING OTHERS TO COPE

I began to live, however, with a new vigor and determination. I had already talked to Dr. Whittier about what I might do to help him and other scientists find families with this disease, because there was a feeling that this "rare disorder," was not so rare. Several months before Woody died, I did find three other affected families, and that is when I organized The Committee to Combat Huntington Disease, in 1967. I had told Woody of my plans, and I do think that he understood. Now, relieved of the care of Woody, I could devote my energy and whatever talents I had to this task of finding Huntington families and bringing attention to this disease, and thereby maybe even helping my own children.

With each passing year, I meet and talk with mothers and fathers, children and friends of affected families as I travel across the country, and I hear in their stories remnants of my own. Today, there is better understanding of how Huntington progresses. The "team approach" has been recognized as the best method for helping a patient and family through the various stages of the disease. Neurologists, family physicians, genetic counselors, social workers, nurses, and a variety of health therapists are working together, starting at the earliest symptoms, to offer better care and treatment. Now, we recognize that every member of the family is a patient whose needs must be assessed with each passing year. Huntington is a chronic disorder which requires a great variety of care.

The Future Is Unpredictable

Each person who lives in an environment that is unpredictable develops fantasies, some unrealistic, some closer to reality. All are trying to find ways to cope with the unknown. These are common threads, but I believe the answers for coping depend on many factors that need to be explained.

When should one talk about Huntington when a parent has just begun to show symptoms and has young children? Regardless of what the spouse might wish to say, one must consider the kind of person the patient was and is, the temperament of the children, their ability to cope with their friends who might visit the home, the kind of community in which the family lives, the educational background of the family, their way of coping with any problem, and who their physician is.

Each member of a family expresses himself or herself in an individual way when a family first learns about Huntington or when a diagnosis has been confirmed. Much depends on how the doctor tells the patient, how the doctor looks when he says there is no treatment, or "there is nothing I can do, come back in a year." Sometimes a family does not go to its physician because they know what he will say, and the patient or the spouse does not want to face the facts yet. A person may have had the experience of seeing Huntington in his or her parent as a child and may wish to protect the family from this diagnosis.

In my own family, one child thought he knew something about father's disease, but did not think that I, his mother, was truly aware of the facts, and, wanting to spare his mother, suffered quietly and alone.

These are only some of the challenges people are dealing with in their personal lives.

Difficult Practical Decisions

What of practical problems? Should the patient live in an institution? Is this just an escape? Can the patient be cared for at home? Are there other places where a patient might go and still function at his or her own best level? Who can afford to pay for this kind of care? Will the family have to sell everything they own in order to qualify for medical care? What happens to the remaining family? Where will they live or find schools or work? Do you tell your employer that you seem to or might have Huntington? What should you do about your workman's compensation form, your insurance, your will, your various legal problems? After many days and nights of anguish over these kinds of thoughts . . . how does a patient learn to live with Huntington?

The Healing Effect of Time

Many people have written of the coping mechanisms which all of us eventually either do or do not develop. I have come to certain truths for me. Most important is that time is the great teacher. In time we learn many things. Our parents have told us this over and over, but it is beginning to become a reality as I think about my life. If there is time, we can hope to resolve our thoughts and our ways of accepting or finding new ways to solve problems. In talking with affected families, I find that those who begin to face their reality — not mine or yours but their own vision of what life is all about — as early as possible, make the best adjustments. If you are a child, and you know that someday you might have Huntington like your parent, perhaps the fact that in your family the adult form may not show symptoms until 35 or 40 can help you rationlize that there is no need to worry because it is still far off.

When you are deeply worried, the fears wax and wane depending on what happened that day or that night. We bring to each day an accumulation of experiences, and they melt into feelings that change from day to day. These are different when you are alone from when you are among friends. Sometimes we share our fears with our peers; sometimes we cannot find the words to use with them; or we try and are frustrated in the effort.

As time goes by, a child may find his or her Huntington problems are either increasing or becoming forgotten, sunk deep into the subconscious, or they come and go depending on who or what arouses these thoughts again. The child has become familiar with his fears. The more we feel at home with our fears, the easier it is to accept the reality of what is or what might be.

I think most adults recognize this pattern of growth in all kinds of living. Being familiar with life itself helps most of us to wake up in the morning and do what must be done. Our hospitals are filled with people who could not or did not practice coping with their reality. And it takes a lot of practice and much help and inspiration and examples from the kinds of people we see around us or read about. Heroes begin to take shape when we are young, and they help us to define ourselves as we look into the mirror. We "make believe" that we are a favorite school teacher, and we talk or walk or imitate what we like about him. Our reaction to sickness and deformity is learned early in life from those around us. What happened in a family when a grandparent dies, or becomes ill, and who does what for whom? Did the family console together, or cry at the gravesite, or was death a celebration of life? Was there something in accepting that all of us have a limited time? Who is first to talk about the "quality of life?" A parent, a teacher, or a friend? Children do talk about these thoughts and we the adults are like a mirror in which they look to learn about themselves.

HELPING MYSELF TO COPE

This is the way I thought about living with Huntington in my family. Woody was my mirror at first. In those early days, when our life was full of living, creating, and believing that we had many tomorrows, we saw in each other a partner toward common goals. Our dream was to make a better world. Woody came from a rural Midwest background, and I came from an urban big city background. Each of us had parents who set us examples, gave us the courage to work hard, imbued in us the faith to believe that we were here for a wonderful purpose, which we could achieve with hard work. Woody liked to make long lists of all the different kinds of work he had done. My list was shorter, but it was there for me to reflect on; what we did together became another list; what we did with our family was another list. We extended these lists to our neighbors and our community. We saw all these wonderful opportunities because we were looking for them.

In the long years of hospitalization, one of the questions I used to ask was "Do you want to live?" and Woody always answered that he did. I guessed his desire was to see what was going to happen next. When I asked "What do you do here all day, think about the past?" he answered with a nod of his head. "Do you worry about the future?" He would smile and say no. He had enough of his life stored in his bank of memories to keep himself going.

I do not know how much of this has rubbed off onto our children. I do not know their inner fears or what they share with their partners, but I hope that time will help them too. We have talked together as a family, and whatever they say today, I know they will say it differently tomorrow. Knowing that I am trying to do something to help may or may not be of comfort to them, if and when they ever show symptoms of Huntington. But we are learning many things about it that we did not know yesterday. My experiences with Woody have helped me to learn that our understanding of this disorder was wrong from the start.

PROFESSIONAL SUPPORT FOR FAMILIES

Today, with help from a "team" of professionally trained persons, I believe we must begin by exploring the whole background and history of a family which has concerns about Huntington. All the empty spaces should be filled in not only regarding those who had Huntington in the past, but how their family responded, and how the individuals who did or did not develop it conducted their lives.

I believe we should try to hold up a mirror for those who seek our help. We should help them see where they came from, how they feel about themselves and their way of life. With guidance from the professional "life-givers," we should try to draw out from each person a vision of the path which that person might begin to walk. Every now and then, there will be a new turning, but we should try to keep our people moving along the projected path, sometimes jumping over a hurdle, sometimes stopping to catch their breath.

I am convinced that a Huntington patient should not be hospitalized too soon. He or she needs to be able to live each day to his full potential. Many patients are capable of developing new skills commensurate with their handicap. They need to be encouraged to participate in every phase of family life. Relatives who are "at-risk" may choose to hide from reality for a while, but if they could be helped to sense, early in life, that living is one big "risk," they will begin the coping process early and accumulate enough strength to fill their days doing the things they can and want to do.

In our experience, learning about the possibility of having Huntington close to the "age of onset" (35–45) can be devastating. An "at risk" person has the least time to learn to cope and usually has the greatest difficulty in accepting the facts. Here again, we should emphasize that, despite the dreaded truth, there are still years of living to be experienced. You do not just drop off tomorrow with Huntington. When I look back, I marvel at the way Woody lived in a ward with 40 or more mentally handicapped people all those years and yet somehow managed to maintain his sanity. Today we encourage patients to live at home as long as possible. We believe that work and recreational day facilities should be available on an out-patient basis, instead of leaving these patients alone all day without any social contact. If it becomes necessary to live in a nursing home facility, there should be incentives for productive living for as long as possible. Even in later stages of Huntington proper care facilities should be provided which should include social and therapeutic resources [1]. Physical, occupational, and speech therapies are essential to preserve mobility, morale, and communication as long as possible.

We encourage patients to participate in experimental drug therapy for the control of the involuntary movements, as well as to alleviate depression and irritability with the newly developed drugs. Sometimes meeting and talking with a similarly affected patient has given new courage and purpose to one newly diagnosed. Now I know that Woody should not have been strapped to a chair, without any physical excercise, those last four years. We recommend starting a course of therapy as early as possible, to prevent muscles from wasting away. We know that with speech therapy we can maintain better communication, which is itself one of the major causes of stress and frustration, and these in turn aggravate involuntary movements. Some families have learned ways to prepare foods that are easier to swallow and to design clothes that are easier to put on and take off. Enabling patients to dress and care for themselves is essential for maintaining a sense of human dignity. When institutional care becomes unavoidable, having one's loved one close by — caring — is perhaps one of the most important strengths needed by the patient.

Recently, I have come to realize that my comments about living with Huntington are valid for anyone living with any chronic debilitating disorder. Huntington disease has become a prototype for neurogenetic conditions. As the commonality of the problems in these families becomes recognized, I believe that they should speak as one constituency, as members of society.

But we do need the help of trained professionals, who should reflect a positive feeling about his or her own life. We need to transmit hope. Without giving advice, I believe in sharing thoughts and in helping people to live with their reality, remembering that this reality is constantly changing.

We need the mirror and the sounding board to see and hear ourselves. Sensitive support and counseling is becoming more urgently needed, as more inherited disorders become identified. Counseling must not create more problems; otherwise it would be better to hide our family secrets, and suffer quietly and alone, as it was for centuries. Effective counseling should help families learn to live with their problems and make wise decisions. This could strengthen family relationships, as loved ones work together to make the most of the time they have.

To this day, I have not changed my youthful dreams of wanting to be a world "changer and hoper," but I think I have learned how to accept my reality through change and experience. Let's help others do so too.

Postscript. After this article was written, the United States Congress, in response to our appeal for help, mandated the Commission for the Control of Huntington's Disease and Its Consequences. Nine concerned persons, scientists and representatives of Huntington families, served for one year. As chairperson of the Commission, I presented the summary report to Congress on October 17, 1977, and this document is available to the public [1]. Many of the thoughts which I have expressed here have been greatly expanded and substantiated through the scientific work groups and by the testimony of over 2,000 persons who apeared before the Commission.

REFERENCES

1. Commission for the Control of Huntington's Disease and Its Consequences: Vol I: Overview; Vol II: Technical Report; Vol III Part 2: Work Group Reports – Social Management; Vol IV Part 1: Public Testimony – Summaries and Indexes; Vol IV Part 2: Public Testimony – Ann Arbor, Atlanta, Boston; Vol IV Part 3: Public Testimony – Chicago, Dallas; Vol IV Part 4: Public Testimony – Denver, Los Angles; Vol IV, Part 5: Public Testimony – New Orleans, New York, Seattle; Vol IV Part 6: Public Testimony – Washington D.C., Wichita.
   Bethesda, Maryland: 1977. National Institute of Neurological and Communicative Disorders and Stroke.

Index